STUDENT WORKBOOK FOR
Clinical Pharmacology and N

ROBERTA TODD SPENCER, R.N., M.S.
Adjunct Assistant Professor, College of Nursing
University of Florida, Gainesville, Florida
Associate Professor Emeritus
State University College, Plattsburgh, New York

LYNN WEMETT NICHOLS, B.S.N., M.S.N.
Associate Professor, Department of Nursing
State University of New York, Plattsburgh, New York

GLADYS B. LIPKIN, R.N.C., C.S., M.S., F.A.A.N.
Nurse Psychotherapist in private practice
Childbirth (Lamaze) Instructor; Lecturer
Certified by ANA as Generalist and Specialist
in Psychiatric-Mental Health Nursing and
by ANA and MAACOG in Obstetric Nursing
Bayside, New York

HELEN M. SABO, B.S.N., M.S.N.
Associate Professor, Department of Nursing
State University of New York, Plattsburgh, New York

FRANCES M. WEST, R.N., B.S.N., M.S.N
Vice-President, Nursing Service Division
Champlain Valley Physicians Hospital Medical Center
Plattsburgh, New York

Contributors

Mary X. Britten, R.N., Ed.D.
Associate Professor of Nursing and Coordinator, Graduate Program
State University of New York
Binghamton, New York

Martha Fortune, R.N., M.S.
Holistic Nurse Practitioner
Rochester, New York

Patricia Hryzak Lind, R.N., M.S.
Pediatric Manager, Anthony L. Jordan Health Center
Rochester, New York
Adjunct Faculty, School of Nursing
University of Rochester
Rochester, New York

Charlotte Torres, R.N., M.S
Assistant Professor of Clinical Nursing
School of Nursing
University of Rochester
Rochester, New York

STUDENT WORKBOOK FOR Clinical Pharmacology and Nursing Management THIRD EDITION

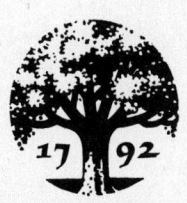

J. B. LIPPINCOTT COMPANY
Philadelphia
Cambridge New York St. Louis San Francisco
London Singapore Sydney Tokyo

Coordinating Editorial Assistant: Ellen Campbell
Manuscript Editor: Irene Glynn
Production: Till & Till, Inc.
Compositor: C. L. Hutson Company, Inc.
Printer/Binder: Malloy Lithographing, Inc.

Third Edition
Copyright © 1989, by Roberta Todd Spencer, Lynn Wemett Nichols, Gladys B. Lipkin, Helen M. Sabo, and Frances M. West

Copyright © 1986, by Roberta Todd Spencer, Lynn Wemett Nichols, Gladys B. Lipkin, Helen Pianta Waterhouse, Frances M. West, and Esther Graber Bankert. All rights reserved. No part of this book may be used or reproduced in any manner whatsoever without written permission except for brief quotations embodied in critical articles and reviews. Printed in the United States of America. For information write J. B. Lippincott Company, East Washington Square, Philadelphia, Pennsylvania 19105.

6 5 4 3 2

ISBN 0-397-54704-8

The author and publisher have exerted every effort to ensure that drug selection and dosage set forth in this text are in accord with current recommendations and practice at the time of publication. However, in view of ongoing research, changes in government regulations, and the constant flow of information relating to drug therapy and drug reactions, the reader is urged to check the package insert for each drug for any change in indications and dosage and for added warnings and precautions. This is particularly important if the recommended agent is a new or infrequently employed drug.

Preface

The purpose of this workbook is to assist students in mastering the content of *Clinical Pharmacology and Nursing Management*. The workbook contains exercises that involve students with material from the text to develop further relationships between facts and to provide repetition conducive to learning. Completion of the workbook promotes a degree of overlearning favorable to the retention of essential content. Students are stimulated to relate pharmacology to their own life experiences by analyzing personal exposure to and attitudes toward chemicals used as drugs.

A variety of approaches to learning are used in this workbook. For the most part, each chapter stands alone. In a few instances, however, mainly relating to the student's self-study, an exercise may relate to previous work. With these exceptions, each workbook chapter can be completed without reference to previous chapters. Answers are provided in the back of the book.

It is our hope that this workbook will function as both an aid to learning and a means for measuring progress in the mastery of content in pharmacology relative to nursing practice.

—*The Authors*

Contents

UNIT ONE: INTRODUCTION TO PHARMACOLOGY

1. Orientation to Pharmacology: Historical Overview   1
2. Standards and Controls   5
3. Nursing Process in the Management of Drug-Related Problems   9
4. Development of a Knowledge Base in Pharmacology   13
5. Toxicology   17

UNIT TWO: THERAPY WITH DRUGS

6. Approaches to Drug Therapy   19
7. Pharmacodynamics and Pharmacokinetics   21
8. Drug Preparations   27
9. Drug Reactions and Interactions   31
10. Interactions between Food and Medications   35
11. Psychological Aspects of Drug Therapy   41
12. Cultural Aspects of Drug Therapy   43

UNIT THREE: ADMINISTRATION OF MEDICATIONS

13. Basic Principles of Medication   47
14. Special Skills Related to Drug Administration   51

UNIT FOUR: DRUGS USED FOR INFLAMMATIONS AND INFECTIONS

15. Major Antimicrobial Drugs   61
16. Antimycobacterial Agents, Miscellaneous Antimicrobials, and Urinary Tract Antiseptics   65
17. Drugs Used to Treat Infections Caused by Viruses and Fungi   69
18. Drugs Used to Treat Rickettsiae, Protozoa, Helminths, and Ectoparasites   73
19. Antipyretics   79
20. Agents Used in Debridement of Wounds   83
21. Anti-inflammatory and Related Agents   85

UNIT FIVE: DRUGS AFFECTING THE NERVOUS SYSTEM

22. Autonomic Drugs	87
23. Central Nervous System Stimulants	95
24. Central Nervous System Depressants	101
25. Anticonvulsants	109
26. The Psychoactive Drugs	115

UNIT SIX: DRUGS AFFECTING THE CARDIOVASCULAR SYSTEM

27. Cardiac Drugs	119
28. Vascular Drugs	127
29. Drugs Affecting Coagulation	137

UNIT SEVEN: DRUGS AFFECTING THE GASTROINTESTINAL SYSTEM

30. Agents Affecting the Upper Gastrointestinal Tract	145
31. Agents Affecting the Lower Gastrointestinal Tract	157

UNIT EIGHT: DRUGS AFFECTING THE ENDOCRINE SYSTEM

32. Steroid Hormones and Their Antagonists	165
33. Protein Hormones: Insulin and Other Drugs Affecting Blood Glucose	175
34. Thyroid, Parathyroid, Pituitary, and Hypothalamic Hormones	181

UNIT NINE: DRUGS AFFECTING SPECIFIC BODY SYSTEMS

35. Drugs Affecting the Respiratory Tract	193
36. Drugs Affecting the Reproductive Systems and Sexuality	197
37. Drugs Affecting the Musculoskeletal System: Skeletal Muscle Relaxants and Antispastic Agents	199
38. Drugs Affecting the Kidneys: Diuretics	201

UNIT TEN: DRUGS USED FOR NEOPLASTIC DISEASE

39. Theoretic Base for Chemotherapy, Alkylating Agents, and Antimetabolites	207
40. Natural Products, Hormones, and Miscellaneous Agents	209

UNIT ELEVEN: DRUGS AFFECTING THE IMMUNE SYSTEM

41. Drugs Used in the Treatment of Allergy	211
42. Drugs Used for Immunity	213

UNIT TWELVE: NUTRITIONAL SUPPLEMENTS

43. Oral Supplements	215
44. Parenteral Preparations	225

UNIT THIRTEEN: MISCELLANEOUS DRUG FAMILIES

45. Diagnostic Agents	229
46. Enzymes and Drugs Affecting Enzymes	237
47. Complexes: Chelators and Ion-Exchange Compounds	241

UNIT FOURTEEN: SPECIAL CONSIDERATIONS IN DRUG THERAPY

48. Substance Abuse	243
49. Drug Therapy in Maternal Care	245
50. Drug Therapy in Pediatric Nursing	249
51. Drug Therapy in Gerontologic Nursing	251
52. Drug Therapy in Community Health Nursing	253
53. Drug Therapy for Pain Relief	255
54. Self-Medication with Over-the-Counter Drugs	261

ANSWER SECTION

1. Orientation to Pharmacology: Historical Overview	265
2. Standards and Controls	267
3. Nursing Process in the Management of Drug-Related Problems	268
4. Development of a Knowledge Base in Pharmacology	269
5. Toxicology	270
6. Approaches to Drug Therapy	271
7. Pharmacodynamics and Pharmacokinetics	272
8. Drug Preparations	277
9. Drug Reactions and Interactions	278
10. Interactions between Food and Medications	280
11. Psychological Aspects of Drug Therapy	281
12. Cultural Aspects of Drug Therapy	282
13. Basic Principles of Medication	284
14. Special Skills Related to Drug Administration	286
15. Major Antimicrobial Drugs	293
16. Antimycobacterial Agents, Miscellaneous Antimicrobials, and Urinary Tract Antiseptics	295
17. Drugs Used to Treat Infections Caused by Viruses and Fungi	297
18. Drugs Used to Treat Rickettsiae, Protozoa, Helminths, and Ectoparasites	299
19. Antipyretics	300
20. Agents Used in Debridement of Wounds	301
21. Anti-inflammatory and Related Agents	302
22. Autonomic Drugs	304
23. Central Nervous System Stimulants	306
24. Central Nervous System Depressants	308
25. Anticonvulsants	310
26. The Psychoactive Drugs	311
27. Cardiac Drugs	312
28. Vascular Drugs	314
29. Drugs Affecting Coagulation	317
30. Agents Affecting the Upper Gastrointestinal Tract	320
31. Agents Affecting the Lower Gastrointestinal Tract	323
32. Steroid Hormones and Their Antagonists	325
33. Protein Hormones: Insulin and Other Drugs Affecting Blood Glucose	327
34. Thyroid, Parathyroid, Pituitary, and Hypothalamic Hormones	328
35. Drugs Affecting the Respiratory Tract	331
36. Drugs Affecting the Reproductive Systems and Sexuality	334
37. Drugs Affecting the Musculoskeletal System	335
38. Drugs Affecting the Kidneys	336
39. Theoretic Base for Chemotherapy, Alkylating Agents, and Antimetabolites	338
40. Natural Products, Hormones, and Miscellaneous Agents	340
41. Drugs Used in the Treatment of Allergy	342
42. Drugs Used for Immunity	343
43. Oral Supplements	344

44. Parenteral Preparations	347
45. Diagnostic Agents	348
46. Enzymes and Drugs Affecting Enzymes	349
47. Complexes: Chelators and Ion-Exchange Compounds	350
48. Substance Abuse	351
49. Drug Therapy in Maternal Care	353
50. Drug Therapy in Pediatric Nursing	355
51. Drug Therapy in Gerontologic Nursing	357
52. Drug Therapy in Community Health Nursing	358
53. Drug Therapy for Pain Relief	359
54. Self-Medication with Over-the-Counter Drugs	361

STUDENT WORKBOOK FOR
Clinical Pharmacology and Nursing Management

UNIT ONE: INTRODUCTION TO PHARMACOLOGY

1
Orientation to Pharmacology: Historical Overview

Pharmacology is one of the oldest sciences known to humankind. It is the study of the effects of chemical substances on living tissue. An interdisciplinary study, pharmacology helps us to find a balance between the use of drugs in preventing or ameliorating illness and the danger of toxicity and user dependence.

Sequences
Arrange the following in chronologic order by numbering each in sequence.
- _____ Ebers Medical Papyrus (Egypt)
- _____ Use of foxglove by William Withering
- _____ Codification of mixtures for medicine (China)
- _____ Sophisticated Arabian pharmacology
- _____ Injection techniques
- _____ Drug production as a major technical industry
- _____ Roman Materia Medica

Checklist
Using a check mark, indicate the five basic problems with which pharmacology is concerned:
- _____ 1. Dose–effect relationships
- _____ 2. Nurse–patient relationships
- _____ 3. Handling of drugs by bodily processes
- _____ 4. Localization of the site of action of drugs
- _____ 5. Chemistry versus botany
- _____ 6. Mechanisms of drug action
- _____ 7. Relations between chemical structure and biologic activity of substances

Short Answer Questions
List six major characteristics of the 20th century, relative to pharmacology.

Matching
Match the substance in the left-hand column with the result in the right-hand column. Place your answer in the space provided.

Common substances have been used historically for mood alteration and as laxatives. Match the following:

_____ 1. Alcohol
_____ 2. Coca
_____ 3. Senna
_____ 4. Tobacco
_____ 5. Opium
_____ 6. Rhubarb
_____ 7. Marijuana
_____ 8. Betel

a. Mood alteration
b. Laxative

Completion Exercises

Read each question carefully and place your answer in the space provided.
1. Another substance not mentioned above but used historically as a laxative is _____.
2. Other mood-altering substances are _____
_____.
3. Pure drugs were first available for scientific study in the _____ century.
4. The types of drugs used by homeopaths are _____.
5. One value of homeopathy was that it _____.

Personal Exercise: History of Pharmacologically Active Substances

As completely as possible, list in the table the pharmacologically active substances to which your body has been exposed over the past week; describe your response(s) to them and identify whether each response was desirable or undesirable.

DRUG NAME	RESPONSE	DESIRABLE	UNDESIRABLE
		(Check one)	
Prescription Drugs			
_____	_____	_____	_____
_____	_____	_____	_____
_____	_____	_____	_____
_____	_____	_____	_____
_____	_____	_____	_____
Patent Medicines			
_____	_____	_____	_____
_____	_____	_____	_____
_____	_____	_____	_____
_____	_____	_____	_____
_____	_____	_____	_____
Folk Remedies			
_____	_____	_____	_____
_____	_____	_____	_____
Herbs			
_____	_____	_____	_____
_____	_____	_____	_____

DRUG NAME	RESPONSE	DESIRABLE	UNDESIRABLE
		(Check one)	

Foods

_____	_____	_____	_____
_____	_____	_____	_____
_____	_____	_____	_____
_____	_____	_____	_____

Social Drugs

_____	_____	_____	_____
_____	_____	_____	_____
_____	_____	_____	_____
_____	_____	_____	_____
_____	_____	_____	_____
_____	_____	_____	_____

Poisons

_____	_____	_____	_____
_____	_____	_____	_____

Pollutants

_____	_____	_____	_____
_____	_____	_____	_____

(Save this list. You will be asked to refer back to it in later exercises.)

2
Standards and Controls

Controls on drug use range from formal laws to cultural mores and family customs. Standards for drug quality are used to judge a drug's purity, potency, efficacy, bioavailability, and safety.

Matching

A. Match the drug in the left-hand column with the constraint(s) that currently exist in the United States in the right-hand column. Place your answer(s) in the space provided. (There may be more than one constraint for each drug.)

    _____ 1. Alcohol
    _____ 2. Caffeine (tea, coffee)
    _____ 3. Marijuana
    _____ 4. Heroin
    _____ 5. Aspirin
    _____ 6. Diazepam (Valium)
    _____ 7. Tobacco (cigarettes)

a. Legal control (federal, state, local)
b. Institutional policies in, for example, hospitals and nursing homes
c. Religious proscriptions
d. Cultural mores

B. Match the drug in the left-hand column with its classifications in the right-hand column according to the standards presented in the Controlled Substance Act of 1970. Place your answer in the space provided.

    _____ 1. Diazepam (Valium)
    _____ 2. Peyote
    _____ 3. Heroin
    _____ 4. Cough syrups with codeine
    _____ 5. Meprobamate (Miltown)
    _____ 6. Methadone
    _____ 7. Secobarbital ("reds")
    _____ 8. Amphetamines ("speed")
    _____ 9. LSD
    _____ 10. Nalorphine

a. Schedule I
b. Schedule II
c. Schedule III
d. Schedule IV
e. Schedule V

Correct the False Statement

Indicate in the blanks whether the following statements are true or false; if false, correct the underlined words or phrases.

    _____ 1. The federal agency charged with the task of controlling the smuggling of heroin or cocaine into the United States is the <u>Food and Drug Administration</u>.

    _____ 2. According to the text, penalties for drug infractions in many countries are <u>more lenient</u> than in the United States.

    _____ 3. In the United States, the first federal legislation that dealt with drug controls was the <u>Food, Drug, and Cosmetic Act of 1906</u>.

    _____ 4. In the United States, the first official standards designated for drugs were the <u>United States Pharmacopeia</u> and the <u>Homeopathic Pharmacopeia of the United States</u>.

    _____ 5. The Shirley Amendment of 1912 <u>was effective in requiring that efficacy of drug remedies be proven</u>.

    _____ 6. The first federal controls on habit-forming drugs were established by the <u>Controlled Substance Act of 1970</u>.

_____ 7. The Food, Drug, and Cosmetic Act of 1938 placed specific controls on the labeling of drugs.

_____ 8. In Canada, drug laws are amended regularly at frequent intervals, whereas in the United States, drug laws tend to be enacted in response to public concern over incidents or occurrences involving drugs.

_____ 9. A legend drug may be sold without a prescription.

_____ 10. Only physicians can file adverse drug reaction reports with the Food and Drug Administration.

Multiple Choice Questions

For each of the following, choose the one best answer.
1. The cheapest and most valid test for drug evaluation is usually through
   a. Chemical assay
   b. Bioassay
   c. Bioimmunoassay
   d. Animal trials
   e. Clinical trials on humans
2. An important nursing responsibility related to clinical trials of experimental drugs on humans is
   a. Recording data identifying subjects as members of either the experimental or the control group
   b. Testing blood samples to determine the drug level in the serum
   c. Assessing subjects' responses to treatment
   d. All of the above
3. The Ames test measures
   a. Carcinogenicity of chemicals in animals
   b. Bioavailability of chemicals in humans
   c. Potency of chemicals in animals
   d. Mutagenicity of chemicals in bacteria

Completion Exercises

Read each question carefully and place your answer in the space provided.
1. A drug that causes congenital absence or severe deformity of the limbs in children exposed to it *in utero* is _____.
2. Inadequate control of production in the manufacture of the drug _____ caused permanent paralysis in some recipients.
3. A drug for which there is substantial evidence of effectiveness would be rated _____ according to the rating scale adopted by the National Research Council of the National Academy of Sciences.
4. The law requiring that the effectiveness of drugs must be established by substantial evidence is the _____.
5. The factor most important in determining a person's drug use is _____.

Short Answer Questions

1. According to the provisions of the Controlled Substance Act of 1970, how does drug dependence differ from drug addiction?

2. List one or more examples of United States legal drug controls that have been more strict than the customs or mores of the population at large or of a substantial subculture. What happened as a consequence?

3. Identify the drug property described in the following:
   a. The relative strength of drug action: _____
   b. The magnitude of the difference between safe and toxic doses: _____
   c. Ability to produce desired therapeutic responses: _____
   d. Freedom from contaminating substances: _____
   e. Degree to which a drug is absorbed and transported to target tissues: _____

4. What is the Ames test used for?

5. List the attitudes and practices in your family that exert control over drug use—for example, the use of social drugs and illegal drugs, adherence to physicians' orders for prescription drugs, and preferred patent medicines. Include avoidance of drugs known to cause adverse reactions, such as those causing allergies or idiosyncratic reactions.

3
Nursing Process in the Management of Drug-Related Problems

The nursing process provides the framework for logical scientific problem solving in nursing care. The process includes the following: assessment, diagnosis, planning, intervention, and evaluation. The nurse uses the nursing process to promote optimal response to chemicals, to decrease the risk of adverse reactions, and to assist clients to achieve optimal health through the proper use of drugs.

Personal Exercise: Nursing Care Plan

Select one medicinal substance that you use regularly or sporadically. Using the nursing process, develop a nursing care plan tailored to your own personal needs. Identify interventions in the care plan of which you had not previously been aware that will enhance the effectiveness of the medication and minimize adverse reactions to the drug.

Correct the False Statement

Indicate in the blanks whether the following statements are true or false; if false, correct the underlined words or phrases.

_____ 1. Nursing responsibilities for clients receiving therapeutic drugs is limited primarily to the dependent function of administering drugs prescribed by the physician.

_____ 2. The nursing care plan should include consideration of potential as well as actual problems arising from drug use.

_____ 3. Detailed teaching regarding drug properties is particularly important for institutionalized clients receiving drugs for treatment of acute health problems.

_____ 4. Nurses should teach clients to avoid the use of drugs whenever possible.

_____ 5. Criteria for evaluation should be formulated at the time evaluation data are collected.

Short Answer Questions

1. Name three general objectives of nursing care related to the proper use of drugs.

2. Name the steps in the nursing process.

3. Identify four categories of data required for assessing drug use.

4. Identify five types of goals that are appropriate in the care of clients receiving therapeutic drugs.

5. Identify five types of reactions that should be investigated while taking a drug history.

6. Why are data about unusual drug reactions in family members important?

7. What elements are desirable in a measurable criterion for evaluating nursing care?

Multiple Choice Questions

For each of the following, choose the one best answer.

1. Information regarding the properties of drugs used by a client may be considered to be part of the
   a. Objective data base
   b. Subjective data base
   c. Analysis
   d. Plan
2. A comparison of drug data and client data to identify potential problems in the planned drug regimen is part of the
   a. Data base
   b. Analysis
   c. Diagnosis
   d. Plan
3. Consulting with a physician or pharmacist regarding the drug regimen is usually considered part of the
   a. Assessment
   b. Diagnosis
   c. Plan
   d. Intervention
   e. Evaluation
4. When treating a client for drug overdose, the most important question to ask is:
   a. What substance was taken?
   b. How much drug was taken?
   c. When was the drug taken?
   d. Is the client dependent on the drug?
5. To find out if the client is dependent on a drug, an appropriate question would be:
   a. How much of the drug do you take at one time?
   b. How often do you use the drug?
   c. How long have you used the drug?
   d. What happens when you stop taking the drug?
6. The identification of contraindications for a drug to be used is the primary responsibility
   a. Of the nurse
   b. Of the physician
   c. Of the pharmacist
   d. Equally of all of the above
7. Consultation with a pharmacist is likely to be required when clients
   a. Cannot metabolize or eliminate normal dosages of the drug
   b. Experience severe adverse reactions to drugs
   c. Receive many drugs concurrently
   d. All of the above

Selection of Options

For each of the following, select *all* appropriate responses. Circle the correct answers.

1. The part(s) of the nursing diagnosis that must be amenable to nursing interventions is (are) the
   a. Problem
   b. Cause of the problem
   c. Underlying factors that contribute to the cause of the problem
2. Clients who are most likely to need a drug dosage smaller than the usual range for their age and body size are clients with
   a. Malabsorption
   b. Impaired circulation
   c. Renal impairment
   d. Hepatic impairment

3. Inherited factors affecting response to drugs include
   a. Ability to absorb oral doses
   b. Microsomal enzymes in the liver
   c. Kidney function
   d. Allergic tendencies

4
Development of a Knowledge Base in Pharmacology

The nurse must know the facts pertaining to any and all drugs a particular client is using. This requires a basic knowledge of pharmacology. Drugs used frequently can and should be memorized, but it is not possible to memorize all drugs. Personal drug files are helpful references. No single source provides all the pertinent information for such files. A sound scholarly approach and the use of a variety of sources promote the development of a solid knowledge in the discipline.

Personal Exercise: Drug File

The following exercises will introduce you to several drugs widely used in health care and will assist you in beginning your personal drug file. Determine the system you prefer to use.

Following directions given in the text, look up the following drugs and make out cards or sheets, outlining the essential information about each preparation. Use various references to gather your data, including the following, if possible: the *Physicians' Desk Reference*; *Drug Information, Facts and Comparisons*, or the *United States' Dispensing Information*; and *The Nurse's Drug Handbook* (by Loebl) or *Drugs and Nursing Implications* (by Govoni and Hayes). After completing your entries on *each* drug, answer the questions relating to that remedy. Circle, check, or fill in blanks to answer questions.

1. ASPIRIN

1. The chemical name for aspirin is _____.
2. Which of the following classifications or drug "families" are appropriate when used to describe aspirin? (Check all correct items)
   - _____ Alkaloid
   - _____ Analgesic
   - _____ Anesthetic
   - _____ Anti-inflammatory
   - _____ Antipruritic
   - _____ Antipyretic
   - _____ Diuretic
   - _____ Placebo
   - _____ Stomachic
3. Aspirin is indicated in (used for) which of the following?
   - _____ Bone infections
   - _____ Headache
   - _____ Arthritis
   - _____ Excessive fever
   - _____ Gastric distress
4. What is the current theory about aspirin's mechanism of action?
   a. Aspirin inhibits prostaglandins.
   b. Aspirin reduces immune response.
   c. Aspirin coats and soothes the stomach lining.
   d. The mechanisms of aspirin's action are not completely understood.

   (1) a, b, c, d (2) a, b (3) c, d (4) a, c (5) b, d (6) a, d (7) b, c (8) Only d
5. A side effect of aspirin is
   1. Inhibition of platelet aggregation
   2. Drowsiness
   3. A lowering of the pain threshold
   4. Miosis
6. Adverse reactions to aspirin include
   a. Asthmatic attacks in susceptible persons
   b. Epigastric distress
   c. Increased bleeding tendency

   (1) a, b (2) b, c (3) a, c (4) Only b (5) a, b, c
7. Toxic effects usually seen in aspirin poisoning include
   a. Acid–base disturbances
   b. Hypothermia
   c. Dehydration

   (1) a, b (2) b, c (3) a, c (4) All of the above (5) None of the above

8. Is an antidote used in the treatment of aspirin poisoning? _____ If so, what is it? _____
_____

9. Contraindications to the use of aspirin include
   a. Cardiovascular disease
   b. A history of asthma, nasal polyps, and tartrazine sensitivity
   c. A history of peptic ulcer disease

   (1) a, b
   (2) b, c
   (3) a, c
   (4) All of the above
   (5) None of the above

10. The usual adult analgesic dose of aspirin is
    1. 1 g daily
    2. 10 mg q4h
    3. 50 mg q6h
    4. 600 mg q4h

11. Most aspirin is administered orally. Another route used to obtain a systemic effect is
    1. Subcutaneous
    2. Intramuscular
    3. Intravenous
    4. Topical (mucous membrane)
    5. Inhalation

12. How is aspirin metabolized and eliminated by the body?

13. When aspirin is prescribed, the nurse should observe the client for
    1. Abnormally low temperature
    2. Abnormal or excessive bleeding
    3. An increase in pain caused by the aspirin
    4. All of the above

14. Aspirin is best administered
    1. With food
    2. On an empty stomach
    3. With only small amounts of water
    4. Only for minor pain, because severe pain does not respond to it

2. REGULAR INSULIN

1. Insulin is properly categorized as which of the following? (Check all that apply.)
   _____ Hormone   _____ Protein   _____ Pyretic
   _____ Steroid   _____ Diabetogenic   _____ Analgesic
   _____ Alkaloid

2. What is the mechanism of action of insulin?

3. What is its therapeutic effect?

4. One side effect of insulin is
   1. Lipodystrophy at the sites of injection
   2. A reduction in appetite
   3. An elevation of the blood sugar level
   4. All of the above

5. In toxic doses, insulin causes
   1. Rapid cardiovascular degeneration
   2. Ketoacidotic coma
   3. Hypoglycemia
   4. Tissue breakdown at the site of injection

6. The main nontoxic adverse reaction to insulin is
   1. An allergic response (rash)
   2. A lowering of the blood sugar level
   3. Inhibition of the pancreatic secretion of insulin
   4. Visual disturbance

7. A contraindication for the use of insulin would be
   1. Chronic hyperglycemia
   2. Chronic hypoglycemia
   3. Visual loss by vascular degeneration
   4. All of the above

8. By which of the following routes are maintenance doses of insulin _usually_ administered?
   1. Oral
   2. Subcutaneous
   3. Intramuscular
   4. Intravenous

9. Which of the following statements are true of the body's metabolism of insulin? (Check all that apply.)
    _____ a. Insulin is broken down to inactive compounds by the digestive process.
    _____ b. Insulin enters the enterohepatic cycle and is excreted in the feces.
    _____ c. Insulin antibody production may delay or decrease the effects of insulin.
    _____ d. Most insulin is metabolized by the liver and by other tissues before excretion.
    _____ e. The major pathway for excretion of insulin and its metabolites is exhalation through the lungs.
10. What is (are) the antidote(s) for insulin toxicity?

11. A nurse caring for a client receiving insulin should monitor closely lab data concerning
    1. Hemoglobin level
    2. Calcium serum levels
    3. Cytology reports
    4. Blood sugar levels
12. If a double dose of insulin were given to a client by mistake, the nurse should
    1. Force fluids to increase elimination of the insulin
    2. Administer oxygen to prevent brain malfunction
    3. Obtain an order for an emetic to prevent absorption of the entire dose
    4. Feed the client carbohydrates
    5. Do nothing except notify the physician because insulin has a wide safety margin
13. How should insulin be stored between uses?

14. Insulin doses are currently measured in
    1. Milligrams
    2. Grains
    3. Units
    4. All of the above
15. The term "lipodystrophy" means
    1. Weakening of the muscles
    2. Abscesses in subcutaneous tissue
    3. Either hypertrophy or wasting of fatty tissue
    4. Abnormalities of blood lipids

3. MEPERIDINE

1. Meperidine is also known as
    1. Morphine
    2. Demerol
    3. Opium
    4. Darvocet
2. Indicate in the blanks whether the following statements are true or false; if false, correct the underlined words or phrases.

    _____ a. Meperidine is classified as a narcotic analgesic.

    _____ b. Meperidine is a central nervous system stimulant.

    _____ c. A frequent side effect of meperidine is insomnia.

    _____ d. One toxic effect of meperidine is respiratory depression.

    _____ e. Meperidine is detoxified mainly by the liver and excreted by the kidneys.

3. What is meperidine's mechanism of action?

4. The major clinical use for meperidine is
   1. As a hypnotic
   2. As an antiemetic
   3. The treatment of minor pain
   4. The treatment of severe pain
5. A frequent adverse reaction to meperidine is
   1. Hyperpnea
   2. Increased tendency to bleed
   3. Acute anaphylaxis
   4. Nausea and vomiting
6. Meperidine is contraindicated
   1. During pregnancy
   2. When respirations are fewer than 12/min
   3. For clients suffering severe trauma (e.g., broken bones)
   4. For clients who cannot take oral medication
7. A given dose of meperidine is least effective when administered
   1. Orally
   2. Subcutaneously
   3. Intravenously
   4. Intramuscularly

Matching

Match each item in the left-hand column with the most appropriate reference in the right-hand column. Place your answer in the space provided.

_____ 1. Contains extensive material on adverse reactions

_____ 2. Is the best reference for determining the generic name for a new trade name drug

_____ 3. Contains extensive material on nursing implications

_____ 4. Is written primarily for practicing physicians

_____ 5. Is written primarily for medical students

_____ 6. Is written primarily for practicing nurses

_____ 7. Contains pharmaceutical data but has few medical or nursing implications

a. The USP
b. Gilman, Goodman, and Gilman: *The Pharmacological Basis of Therapeutics*
c. The PDR
d. Loebl et al.: *The Nurse's Drug Handbook*

Short Answer Question

Whom should the nurse consult if printed information about a drug that is to be administered is unavailable?

5
Toxicology

The study of toxicology enables the student to develop an awareness about the differences between the therapeutic use of pharmacologic agents and their poisonous potential in lethal doses. The following exercises will provide a broad base of information related to poison intervention and control.

Short Answer Questions

1. Define the following terms:
   a. Antidote

   b. Toxicology

   c. FEP

   d. Chelate

2. Give the route of entry of a toxin and provide an example of each.

TOXIN ROUTE	EXAMPLE

3. Briefly describe first-aid steps to be taken when intervening in a poison emergency under the following conditions:
   a. Ingestion in a conscious victim

   b. Inhaled poison

   c. Skin contamination

   d. Eye contamination

4. List five methods used to prevent absorption of poisons.

5. List five methods used to enhance excretion of a poison.

6. Identify the four criteria needed to diagnose plumbism positively.
    a.

    b.

    c.

    d.

UNIT TWO: THERAPY WITH DRUGS

6
Approaches to Drug Therapy

Drug therapy has evolved from primitive cultures to modern times, reflecting the quest for knowledge about the world and its natural resources and the desire to influence the outcomes of natural events. Drug therapy has evolved from three major areas: (1) development and transmission of oral tribal traditions in drug folklore (magical approach); (2) experience, observation, and analysis of cultural traditions in the use of environmental elements (empiric protopharmacologic approach); and (3) development of chemical and biologic research methodologies (scientific rational approach).

Matching

Match the definition in the left-hand column with the approach in the right-hand column. Place your answer in the space provided.

_____ 1. Use of antibiotics to treat a sore throat without a throat culture
_____ 2. Development of designated methodologies to demonstrate cause and effect
_____ 3. Use of religious amulets
_____ 4. Development and communication of traditional cures
_____ 5. Experience, observation, and analysis of traditional uses.

a. Rational approach
b. Empiric approach
c. Magical approach

Completion Exercise

Read the question carefully and place your answer in the space provided.
1. Reflect on your most recent use of medicinal agents. As accurately as possible, identify the following aspects of your selection and use of these drugs.

SUBSTANCE USED	WHO PRESCRIBED	REASON FOR USE	TYPE OF APPROACH REPRESENTED

Short Answer Questions
1. Trace the evolution of pharmacology by briefly describing the contributions of each of the following in the development of modern science. Identify the time period during which they lived.
   a. Hippocrates

   b. Galen

   c. Pliny

d. Magendie

e. Thales

2. List five problems addressed by scientists using the rational approach for the evaluation of pharmacologic agents.
   a.

   b.

   c.

   d.

   e.

Multiple Choice Questions

For each of the following, choose the one best answer.

1. The magical approach to the use of medicines represents which of the following beliefs?
   a. Demonic possession was the cause of illness
   b. Dreams, divine revelation, and chance account for the use of certain medicinal substances
   c. A specific remedy was used for a particular disease
   d. A specific remedy was used because of known effects on certain body organs
      (1) a only
      (2) a, b
      (3) b only
      (4) a, b, c
      (5) a, c, d

2. Which of the following represents the empiric approach to drug use?
   a. Prescribing the use of antacids following a complaint of gastric distress after eating spicy foods
   b. Prescribing penicillin in the treatment of venereal disease
   c. Using garlic to prevent a cold
   d. None of the above

3. Localization of the site of drug action was a factor in the development of which approach to pharmacology?
   a. Magical
   b. Empiric
   c. Rational

7
Pharmacodynamics and Pharmacokinetics

Individual response to drugs is determined in large part by inherited processes affecting the absorption, distribution, storage, receptor interaction, and excretion of active chemicals. The following exercises relate to these processes of pharmacokinetics and pharmacodynamics.

Matching

A. Match the term in the left-hand column with the most appropriate item in the right-hand column. Place your answer in the space provided.

_____ 1. Urinary acidifier
_____ 2. Osmotic diuretic
_____ 3. Lubricant
_____ 4. Agonist
_____ 5. Saline cathartic
_____ 6. Antacid
_____ 7. Antagonist
_____ 8. Endorphin

a. Alteration of the physical environment of the cell
b. Alteration of the chemical environment of the cell
c. Interaction with a cell receptor

B. Match the tissue in the left-hand column with the most appropriate item in the right-hand column. Place your answer in the space provided.

_____ 1. Tissue that tends to store metallic ions
_____ 2. Tissue that tends to store acidic drugs
_____ 3. Tissue that tends to store hydrocarbons
_____ 4. Tissue that most actively breaks down drugs

a. Fat
b. Bone
c. Liver
d. Plasma proteins
e. Brain

C. Match the phrase in the left-hand column with the term in the right-hand column. Place your answer(s) in the space provided. (More than one answer may be correct.)

_____ 1. Movement across a membrane requiring dissolution in the lipid portion of the membrane
_____ 2. Transport mechanism(s) that requires energy expenditure
_____ 3. Transport mechanism that is most specific (i.e., is highly selective of the type of molecule transported)
_____ 4. Movement of water across a membrane that is impervious to some or all of the chemicals in the solution
_____ 5. Movement across a membrane by means of encapsulation in an envelope of membranous material
_____ 6. Movement across a membrane against a pressure gradient
_____ 7. Mechanism whose maximum capacity is limited only by the area of the membrane
_____ 8. Mechanism that allows free movement of polar compounds

a. Active transport
b. Diffusion
c. Pinocytosis
d. Osmosis

Computation

Compute the therapeutic index for the following:

DOSE PRODUCING A THERAPEUTIC RESPONSE IN 50% OF ANIMAL SUBJECTS	DOSE PRODUCING DEATH IN 50% OF ANIMAL SUBJECTS
1. 100 μg	2 g (2,000,000 μg)
2. 0.24 mg	0.45 mg
3. 10 mg	100 mg

Checklist

Using a check mark, indicate the administration routes involving absorption by mucous membranes.

- _____ 1. Sucutaneous
- _____ 2. Sublingual
- _____ 3. Intrathecal
- _____ 4. Intramuscular
- _____ 5. Rectal
- _____ 6. Buccal
- _____ 7. Nasal
- _____ 8. Intra-arterial
- _____ 9. Vaginal

Correct the False Statement

Indicate in the blanks whether the following statements are true or false; if false, correct the underlined words or phrases.

- _____ 1. Desensitization may involve an increase in the number of cell receptors.
- _____ 2. Refractoriness may involve a decrease in the number of cell receptors.
- _____ 3. The greater the specificity of a drug, the narrower is the margin of safety.
- _____ 4. The wider the margin of safety of a drug, the lower is its therapeutic index.
- _____ 5. A drug with a therapeutic index of 1.0 would have a wide margin of safety.
- _____ 6. Water-soluble drugs are absorbed most readily by the skin.
- _____ 7. Inflamed tissue such as the meninges and skin tend to absorb drugs more readily than normal tissue.
- _____ 8. Drugs are applied to the skin only for a local effect.
- _____ 9. Salts in solution ionize more readily than nonelectrolytes.
- _____ 10. Drugs that are basic in nature are absorbed rapidly by the gastric mucosa.
- _____ 11. The administration of large doses of antacids with oral acidic drugs facilitates the absorption of the drug.

_____ 12. The absorption of basic drugs is retarded in persons with low levels of or no hydrochloric acid in gastric secretions.

_____ 13. Enteric-coated tablets are designed to disintegrate rapidly in the stomach.

_____ 14. Oral administration of medications is desirable because it is convenient and provides for rapid absorption.

_____ 15. A given dose of drug (corrected for body weight) is likely to exert a greater effect in normal young adults than in an infant or an elderly person.

_____ 16. Starvation is likely to make a person more sensitive to drug effects.

_____ 17. Induction of liver enzymes is likely to increase a person's response to a given dose of drug.

_____ 18. Loading doses are recommended when beginning therapy with most drugs.

_____ 19. Clients in shock caused by trauma are likely to receive medication by inhalation and by intravenous injection.

_____ 20. The organ that is most active in metabolizing drugs is the brain.

_____ 21. The organ that is most active in excreting drugs is the kidney.

_____ 22. The metabolism of drugs is not affected by the sex of the recipient.

_____ 23. The results of pharmaceutical research involving animals are not always applicable to humans.

Completion Exercises

Read each question carefully and place your answer in the space provided.
1. Two routes of administration that provide higher concentrations of drug at the target tissues than in the systemic circulation are _____ and _____ .
2. A drug used to facilitate absorption of subcutaneous medication is _____ .
3. A drug used to delay absorption of local anesthetics is _____ .
4. Water-soluble compounds with a molecular weight of _____ are usually eliminated by the kidneys.
5. Large molecules are usually excreted by the _____ .
6. A steady state blood level of drug is usually best achieved by means of the _____ _____ method of administration.

Draw a Drug Map

Using standard pharmacologic references, determine the usual pharmacokinetic processes involved when each of the following drugs is administered. Complete the diagram by drawing arrows to delineate the pathways the drug takes and by identifying the specific organs and tissues involved in the process. Note any special characteristics (e.g., protein binding in the blood, active secretion in the kidneys).

1. penicillin G procaine

Sites of Absorption		Sites of Biotransformation
_____		_____
_____		_____

Vascular Compartment
_____
_____

Sites of Inactive Storage	Target Tissues	Sites of Excretion
_____	_____	_____
_____	_____	_____
	_____	_____

2. prednisone

Sites of Absorption		Sites of Biotransformation
_____		_____
_____		_____

Vascular Compartment
_____
_____

Sites of Inactive Storage	Target Tissues	Sites of Excretion
_____	_____	_____
_____	_____	_____
	_____	_____

3. insulin

Sites of Absorption		Sites of Biotransformation

Vascular Compartment

Sites of Inactive Storage	Target Tissues	Sites of Excretion

4. milk of magnesia

Sites of Absorption		Sites of Biotransformation

Vascular Compartment

Sites of Inactive Storage	Target Tissues	Sites of Excretion

5. morphine sulfate

Sites of Absorption		Sites of Biotransformation
_____		_____
_____		_____

Vascular Compartment
_____
_____

Sites of Inactive Storage	Target Tissues	Sites of Excretion
_____	_____	_____
_____	_____	_____

6. methotrexate sodium

Sites of Absorption		Sites of Biotransformation
_____		_____
_____		_____

Vascular Compartment
_____
_____

Sites of Inactive Storage	Target Tissues	Sites of Excretion
_____	_____	_____
_____	_____	_____

8
Drug Preparations

The drugs produced by pharmaceutical firms today are ready-to-use products that have been purified, modified, formulated, named, and packaged to appeal to the consumer. Some basic knowledge of these preparations is essential for safe use by both nurses and their clients.

Matching

For each name in the left-hand column, select *all* appropriate items in the right-hand column.

_____ 1. Abbreviation
_____ 2. Trade name
_____ 3. Official name
_____ 4. Chemical name
_____ 5. Generic name
_____ 6. Proprietary name
_____ 7. Brand name

a. Tends to be long and cumbersome
b. In the United States, is printed in the *United States Pharmacopeia* and *National Formulary*
c. In the United States, is chosen by the United States Adopted Name Council
d. Is protected by copyright
e. Is usually an acronym
f. Is capitalized when written
g. Denotes molecular structure of a drug
h. Often has no written standard

For each item in the left-hand column, select the most appropriate item from the right-hand column.

_____ 8. Binders
_____ 9. Disintegrators
_____ 10. Dyes
_____ 11. Fillers
_____ 12. Preservatives
_____ 13. Vehicles

a. Aid in identifying unlabeled drugs
b. Prevent microbial growth in injectable solutions
c. Decrease the risk of tablets crumbling
d. Give form and substance to a drug
e. Enable a manufacturer to adjust dosage of a preparation
f. Make drugs more palatable
g. Promote dissolution of a tablet.

Correct the False Statement

Indicate whether the following statements are true or false; if false, correct the underlined words or phrases.

_____ 1. A single drug may have multiple generic names.
_____ 2. The proprietary name identifies the manufacturer of the drug.
_____ 3. Individual drugs may be members of more than one drug family.
_____ 4. Acids and salts are among the drugs derived from mineral sources.
_____ 5. In most cases, synthetic drugs are not as effective as are natural drugs.
_____ 6. The purpose of adding lubricants to tablets is to make them easier to swallow.
_____ 7. Fixed oils evaporate easily, leaving no greasy residue.
_____ 8. A foam is a homogeneous mixture of two liquids that do not dissolve in each other.

Multiple Choice Questions

For each of the following, choose the one best answer.
1. If a drug label is difficult to read, the nurse should
   a. Ask a colleague to verify the name
   b. Contact the physician to verify the order
   c. Return drug and container to the pharmacist
   d. Rewrite the label clearly
2. If successive prescriptions for a drug use different names, the client is *most* apt to
   a. Refuse to take the second prescription
   b. Skip doses of the drug
   c. Take a double dose of the drug
3. If the name of the durg ordered is not the same as the name on the medication container, the nurse should *first*
   a. Omit the dose
   b. Look up the names in a drug reference book to verify them
   c. Call the pharmacy to verify the names
   d. Call the physician to verify the names
4. Aspirin is usually manufactured
   a. From a plant source
   b. From a mineral source
   c. From animal tissues
   d. By synthesis in a laboratory
5. Which of the following drugs is *least* likely to be prescribed for oral administration?
   a. Polypeptides
   b. Steroids
   c. Glycosides
   d. Salts
6. Which of the following drugs is *least* likely to be compatible with morphine sulfate?
   a. Atropine sulfate
   b. Sodium pentobarbital
   c. Meperidine hydrochloride
   d. Magnesium chloride
7. Which of the following drug families contains substances whose pharmacologic action is attributed to the formation of charged ions upon dissolution?
   a. Polypeptides
   b. Steroids
   c. Glycosides
   d. Salts
8. Which of the following substances is *not* a steroid?
   a. Cholesterol
   b. Estrogen
   c. Digitalis
   d. Glycerin
9. Asthmatic clients are *most* apt to experience allergic reactions to dyes that color tablets
   a. Red
   b. Blue
   c. Green
   d. Yellow
10. Tartrazine is added to drug formulations for the purpose of
    a. Making pills taste better
    b. Making tablets look more attractive
    c. Preventing tablets from crumbling
    d. Increasing the bulk of a tablet without increasing the dose

11. Which of the following types of medication should be swallowed with a glass of liquid?
    a. Enteric-coated tablets
    b. Troches
    c. Sublingual tablets
    d. Buccal tablets
12. Which of the following preparations is *most* likely to contain a soap?
    a. Liniment
    b. Suppository
    c. Paste
    d. Lotion
13. Which of the following is *most* likely to taste sweet?
    a. An extract
    b. A fluidextract
    c. An elixir
    d. An aromatic water

Selection of Options

For each of the following, select *all* appropriate responses
1. Techniques frequently employed in the laboratory production of drugs include
    a. Maintaining a natural drug in its crude form in order to preserve all active principles
    b. Modifying natural drugs to increase specificity
    c. Building complex molecules from pure chemical elements
    d. Altering genes of microorganisms to induce production of drugs in short supply
    e. Altering drug molecules to reduce toxicity
2. Data appropriate to a drug history include
    a. Chemical names of drugs used by the client
    b. Generic names of drugs used by the client
    c. Trade names of drugs used by the client
    d. Allergic reactions to drugs
    e. Allergic reactions to foods
3. Why are enteric coatings applied to tablets?
    a. To make them easier to swallow
    b. To make them taste better
    c. To delay their absorption
    d. To protect the stomach from irritation
    e. To protect the drug from stomach secretions
4. The term lozenge is synonymous with
    a. Tablet
    b. Pill
    c. Capsule
    d. Troche

Rank-Order Question

Arrange the following in rank order according to their viscosities, starting with the most viscous.
a. Magma

b. Solution

c. Suppository

d. Cream

e. Ointment

f. Paste

Short Answer Questions

Name the type of drug preparation described by the following:
1. Mixtures of oil, water, and drug ingredients

2. Compressed powders or granulated ingredients

3. Molded mixtures of drug's ingredients in a firm base with a low melting point

4. Drug ingredients mixed with alcohol, oil, soap, or water

5. Saturated solutions of water and volatile substances

6. High concentrations of alcohol solution of vegetable drugs

7. Mixtures of alcohol, volatile oils, and sweeteners

8. Generic names ending in "ine"

9
Drug Reactions and Interactions

Every physiologically active drug has the potential to cause an undesirable reaction that may induce illness in the recipient. Such conditions are termed "iatrogenic." A drug interaction occurs when an interactant chemical modifies the therapeutic results that have been anticipated with a drug. Drug interactions may be beneficial or detrimental, and may differ from person to person.

Adverse reactions are of many types and include side effects, allergic reactions, idiosyncratic reactions, chain reactions, cumulative reactions, tolerance and dependence, and detrimental drug interactions.

Short Answer Questions

1. Define the following terms:
   a. Iatrogenic:

   b. Adverse reaction:

   c. Side effect:

   d. Allergic reaction:

   e. Idiosyncratic reaction:

   f. Chain reaction:

   g. Cumulative reaction:

   h. Tolerance:

   i. Dependence:

   j. Detrimental drug interaction:

2. Look up phenylbutazone in the text.
   a. List the side effects.

   b. Identify drugs and classes of drugs that may interact with phenylbutazone.

3. Look up penicillin in the text. Describe (a) the most frequent, and (b) the most serious allergic reaction seen with this drug.
   a.

   b.

4. List six drugs whose absorption will be decreased by concurrent administration of another drug, and list the interactant drug responsible for the decreased absorption.

DRUG WITH DECREASED ABSORPTION	INTERACTANT DRUG

5. Explain how drug interactions during the absorptive phase can be avoided. Give one specific example.

6. Drugs do compete with other drugs for drug-binding sites on albumin, but often the drug–drug interaction is really a result of a second mechanism. List three examples of drugs that interact as a result of displacement and of another mechanism.
   a.
   b.
   c.

7. Define the terms "drug inhibitor" and "drug inducer." Give three examples of each type of drug.
   a. Drug inhibitor:

   b. Drug inducer:

8. Name two drugs that can be both inhibitors and inducers.

9. Look up allopurinol in the text. Describe how metabolic inhibition occurs when allopurinol is used.

10. Explain how tyramine could cause an accentuated hypertensive effect.

11. Smoking (nicotine) appears to be a drug inducer. How would you explain the effects of smoking on an interactant drug to a heavy smoker?

12. List seven routes by which drugs may be excreted.

13. How could you increase the rate of excretion of salicylates?

Matching

A. Read the section in the text about commonly abused substances. Study the description of the opiate withdrawal syndrome.
Match the signs and symptoms of the syndrome in the left-hand column with the phase of the syndrome in the right-hand column. Place your answer in the space provided.

_____ 1. Abdominal cramps
_____ 2. Diaphoresis
_____ 3. Diarrhea
_____ 4. Extreme restlessness
_____ 5. Yawning
_____ 6. Mydriasis
_____ 7. Nausea and vomiting
_____ 8. Insistent drug-demanding behavior
_____ 9. Muscle twitching
_____ 10. Hyperglycemia
_____ 11. Elevated vital signs
_____ 12. Rhinorrhea

a. First phase
b. Second phase
c. Third phase
d. Fourth phase

B. Match the mechanism of drug interaction in the left-hand column with its pharmacokinetic phase in the right-hand column. Place your answer in the space provided.

_____ 1. Competition for carrier mechanism for secretion
_____ 2. Acceleration of metabolism
_____ 3. Dissolution rate change
_____ 4. Insufficient ingestion of solvent
_____ 5. Displacement
_____ 6. Change in pH of urine
_____ 7. Inhibition of metabolism
_____ 8. Direct interaction

a. Absorption
b. Distribution
c. Biotransformation
d. Excretion

C. Drug excretion may be affected by drug–drug interaction. The secretion of digoxin, penicillin, and acetohexamide (hydroxyhexamide) will be decreased by certain other drugs. Match these drugs in the left-hand column with their interactant drug in the right-hand column. Place your answer in the space provided.

_____ 1. Digoxin
_____ 2. Penicillin
_____ 3. Acetohexamide (hydroxyhexamide)

a. Acetylsalicylic acid
b. Indomethacin
c. Phenylbutazone
d. Spironolactone
e. Lithium
f. Probenecid

Completion Exercises

Read each question carefully and place your answers in the spaces provided.
1. Study this diagram, which illustrates a chain reaction to cortisone. Fill in the blanks.

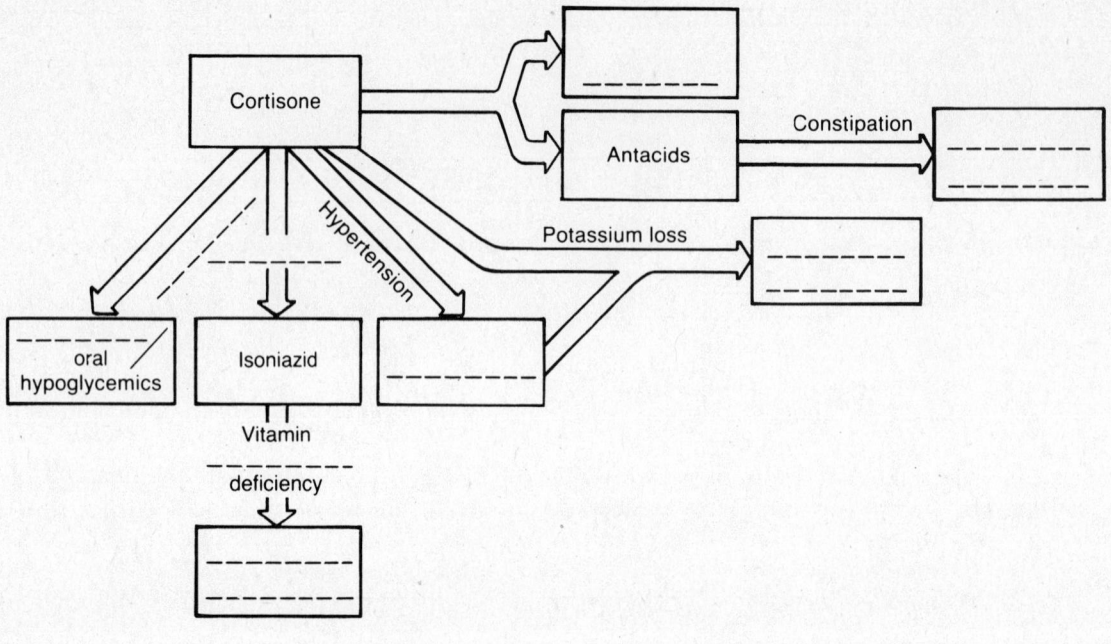

2. _____ acids are excreted _____ rapidly in _____ urine. Weak _____ are excreted more _____ in _____ urine.

Short Answer Questions

1. List some factors that might be elicited through taking a detailed client history that would indicate to the nurse that the client may well be a candidate for a drug–drug interaction.

2. List appropriate nursing approaches to ameliorate the following problems:
   a. Anorexia, nausea, and/or vomiting

   b. Postural hypotension

   c. Itching

   d. Diarrhea

   e. Constipation

10
Interactions between Food and Medications

Foods and beverages contain nutrients, natural and artificial toxins, and pharmacologic substances. All of these can produce therapeutic effects or adverse reactions when ingested in large quantities or when taken with certain drugs. The following exercises relate to this material.

Matching

A. Match each food listed in the left-hand column with the appropriate toxin from the right-hand column.

    _____ 1. Potatoes   a. Cyanide
    _____ 2. Apple seeds   b. Vitamin A
    _____ 3. Moldy rye flour   c. Oxalic acid
    _____ 4. Cabbage   d. Parasympathomimetic chemicals
    _____ 5. Cassava   e. Solanine
    _____ 6. Poisonous mushrooms   f. Ergot
    _____ 7. Polar bear liver   g. Goiterogens
    _____ 8. Turnips
    _____ 9. Spinach

B. Match the medications listed in the left-hand column with their physiologic antagonists from the list of nutrients in the right-hand column.

    _____ 10. L-dopa   a. Calcium
    _____ 11. Coumarin anticoagulants   b. Potassium
    _____ 12. Digoxin   c. Sodium
    _____ 13. Hydrochlorothiazide (a diuretic)   d. Zinc
                                                 e. Vitamin A
                                                 f. Vitamin B_6
                                                 g. Vitamin B_{12}
                                                 h. Vitamin C
                                                 i. Vitamin D
                                                 j. Vitamin K

C. Match each nutrient listed in the left-hand column with all the signs and symptoms of its deficiency syndrome.

    _____ 14. Vitamin A   a. Anemia
    _____ 15. Vitamin B_6 b. Leg pains
    _____ 16. Vitamin B_{12} c. Dermatitis
    _____ 17. Niacin   d. Abnormal gastrointestinal bleeding
    _____ 18. Riboflavin   e. Loss of night vision
    _____ 19. Vitamin C   f. Hypotension
    _____ 20. Vitamin K   g. Petechiae
    _____ 21. Sodium   h. Sore tongue

Correct the False Statement

Indicate in the blanks whether the following statements are true or false; if false, correct the underlined words or phrases.

    _____ 1. Plants containing toxins <u>are not used as foods</u>.
    _____ 2. Adverse reactions to the many toxins present in white potatoes are rare because <u>the potato contains an adsorbent chemical that prevents absorption of these toxins</u>.

_____ 3. Daily ingestion of a gram of vitamin C <u>helps prevent respiratory infection caused by common cold viruses</u>.

_____ 4. Daily ingestion of capsules containing garlic extracts <u>helps prevent cardiovascular disease by altering blood lipids</u>.

_____ 5. Baked beans can cause excessive flatus because they contain <u>indigestible sugars</u>.

_____ 6. A client known to have food allergies should avoid eating <u>foods known to act frequently as allergens</u>.

_____ 7. Ginger acts as <u>an antinauseant</u>.

_____ 8. A food additive that is listed on the FDA's GRAS list <u>can be considered safe to use</u>.

_____ 9. A side effect of beta-carotene is <u>vitamin A toxicity</u>.

_____ 10. According to the Feingold theory, food additives <u>contribute to hyperkinesis in children</u>.

_____ 11. Most labels on processed foods <u>must list specific ingredients and additives</u>.

_____ 12. According to the Feingold theory, hyperkinesis in children may be reduced by <u>substituting for processed food, foods prepared from fresh natural ingredients</u>.

_____ 13. Charcoal broiled foods are known to <u>facilitate absorption of tetracycline</u>.

_____ 14. Dissolution of most drugs is promoted by the ingestion of <u>warm liquids</u>.

_____ 15. Enteric-coated tablets should be administered with <u>milk to facilitate absorption</u>.

_____ 16. Treatment of epilepsy often causes deficiency of <u>B complex vitamins</u>.

Multiple Choice Questions

For each of the following, choose the one best answer.

1. According to Katona-Apte and Anderson (1978), how many toxic substances are present in white potatoes?
   a. None
   b. Fewer than 10
   c. About 100
   d. More than 150

2. An excellent dietary source of vitamin A is
   a. Cranberries
   b. Polar bear liver
   c. Calves liver
   d. Orange juice

3. Cyanide is a component of
   a. Tea
   b. Raw beet greens
   c. Unprocessed cassava
   d. Applesauce

4. Which of the following foods are likely to be goiterogenic?
   a. Red meats
   b. Milk
   c. Cereals
   d. Vegetables

5. Foods containing live lactobacilli should be
   a. Avoided because they can cause enteritis and diarrhea
   b. Avoided because the microorganisms deprive the body of nutrients
   c. Added to the diet to reduce vitamin D deficiency
   d. Added to the diet to inhibit superinfection caused by broad-spectrum antibiotics

6. According to recent research, garlic
   a. Has no medicinal value
   b. Contains essential nutrients
   c. Will prevent a common cold
   d. Tends to lower harmful blood lipids

7. A food rich in avidin is
   a. Orange peel
   b. Raw eggs
   c. Seafood
   d. Legumes

8. Substances in foods that inhibit thyroid function are called
   a. Cyanides
   b. Goiterogens
   c. Phytates
   d. Thiaminases

9. Cardiac patients who take both digitalis and diuretic medications should be sure to include in their diets foods rich in
   a. Potassium
   b. Sodium

c. Iron
   d. Calcium
10. What juice would you offer to a client who is recovering from barbiturate poisoning?
   a. Cranberry juice
   b. Tomato juice
   c. Ginger ale
   d. Milk
11. If a child eats too much candy on Easter Sunday, he or she is likely to experience
   a. Restlessness and insomnia
   b. Diarrhea, frequent urination, and thirst
   c. Water retention and bloating
   d. Hypertension and headache
12. A food substance that destroys biotin is
   a. Avidin
   b. Citral
   c. Lathyrogen
   d. Phytate
13. Urinary calculi can be caused by excessive intake of
   a. Citric acid
   b. Lactic acid
   c. Magnesium
   d. Oxalic acid
14. Absorption of dietary minerals such as zinc and calcium is inhibited by concurrent ingestion of
   a. Cereals
   b. Fruits
   c. Potatoes
   d. Green leafy vegetables
15. If mineral oil is taken with meals, it is likely to cause a deficiency of
   a. Univalent cations
   b. Fat-soluble vitamins
   c. Trace minerals
   d. Water-soluble minerals
16. A food or foods used to reduce the risk of calcium stones in the urinary tract is
   a. Citrus fruits
   b. Cranberries
   c. Green leafy vegetables
   d. Milk
17. High potassium intake is dangerous to individuals with
   a. Hepatic impairment
   b. Malabsorption
   c. Hypertension
   d. Renal impairment
18. A food additive that is banned in the United States but is available in Canada is
   a. Aspartame
   b. Cyclamate
   c. Fructose
   d. Saccharin
   e. Sorbitol
19. Sorbitol and mannitol should not be consumed in large quantities because they increase the risk of
   a. Bladder cancer
   b. Cataracts
   c. Constipation
   d. Water intoxication
20. A food additive known to act as a teratogen is
   a. Ascorbic acid
   b. Corn syrup
   c. Tartrazine
   d. Vitamin A
21. A high intake of licorice flavoring is most likely to cause
   a. Excessive flatus
   b. Goiter
   c. Hypertension
   d. Restlessness
22. Preliminary reports on aspartame toxicity indicate that the substance may cause
   a. Cancer in laboratory animals
   b. Acute allergic reactions
   c. Cataract formation
   d. Nervous system damage
23. The absorption of tetracycline is inhibited by
   a. Citrus juices
   b. Egg whites
   c. Ginger ale
   d. Milk
24. A food component that antagonizes the action of L-dopa is
   a. Vitamin A
   b. Vitamin B_6
   c. Vitamin K
   d. Potassium
25. Metoclopramide (Reglan) acts as
   a. An antidiarrheal
   b. An astringent
   c. A histamine$_2$ receptor antagonist
   d. A stimulator of peristalsis
26. Long-term therapy with cimetidine is most likely to cause a deficiency of
   a. Vitamin A
   b. Vitamin B_6
   c. Vitamin B_{12}
   d. Potassium
   e. Zinc

27. Malabsorption during antibiotic therapy is most likely to be caused by
    a. Complexation of nutrients
    b. An enteric yeast infection
    c. Inhibition of active transport systems
    d. Chemical damage to the gastrointestinal mucosa
28. Antineoplastic drugs are likely to cause malnutrition by
    a. Combining with nutrients to form indigestible compounds
    b. Preventing absorption by adsorbing nutrients
    c. Inhibiting active transport systems in the gut
    d. Damaging the gastrointestinal mucosa
29. A drug used to reduce nausea during cancer chemotherapy is
    a. Alcohol
    b. Dramamine
    c. Heroin
    d. Marijuana
30. The most frequent single vitamin deficiency is inadequate supply of
    a. Vitamin A
    b. Vitamin B_6
    c. Vitamin B_{12}
    d. Folic acid
    e. Niacin
    f. Riboflavin
    g. Thiamin
31. Moldy rye flour is most apt to cause
    a. Cyanide poisoning
    b. Ergotism
    c. Altered sensory perception
    d. Diarrhea
    e. Constipation

Selection of Options

For each of the following, select *all* appropriate responses. Circle correct answers.

1. The pharmacologic actions of tea include
    a. Central nervous system sedation
    b. Increased alertness and restlessness
    c. Inhibited secretion of intestinal mucus
    d. Enhanced absorption of medications
    e. Irritation of the bowel
2. A client complaining of "loose bowels" should probably avoid ingesting
    a. Rhubarb pie
    b. Blueberry pie
    c. Yogurt
    d. Eggs
    e. Fresh apples
    f. Fresh pears
    g. Cranberry jelly
    h. Raisins
    i. Prunes
3. Foods rich in potassium include
    a. Apples
    b. Apricots
    c. Bananas
    d. Cranberries
    e. Orange juice
    f. Soup
4. Which of the following should *not* be used as foods because they contain high levels of toxins?
    a. Fresh rye bread
    b. Turnip peelings
    c. Potato sprouts
    d. Beet tops
    e. Rhubarb leaves
    f. Apple seeds
5. Foods containing lactobacilli include
    a. Butter
    b. Buttermilk
    c. Cream
    d. Eggs
    e. Yogurt
6. People who tend to become constipated should be careful *not* to consume large amounts of
    a. Berries
    b. Coffee
    c. Pears
    d. Prunes
    e. Tea
7. Minerals that exert a direct effect on cardiac function include
    a. Aluminum
    b. Copper
    c. Calcium
    d. Iron
    e. Potassium
    f. Phosphorus
    g. Zinc
8. A person wishing to determine whether a field mushroom is edible should consult
    a. A dietician
    b. A pharmocognosist
    c. A nurse
    d. A physician
    e. A pharmacist
9. Use of tea helps to ameliorate
    a. Calcium deficiency
    b. Constipation
    c. Dehydration

     d. Diarrhea
     e. Potassium deficiency
     f. Sodium deficiency
10. Sulfites are used as preservatives in
     a. Baked goods
     b. Fresh salads
     c. Meats
     d. Wines
11. Foods or food components that may contribute to hyperkinesis in children include
     a. Accent
     b. Coffee
     c. Cola drinks
     d. Coloring agents
     e. Preservatives
12. Additives likely to cause allergic reactions in asthmatic individuals include
     a. Accent
     b. BHT
     c. Caffeine
     d. Sulfites
     e. Tartrazine
     f. Vinegar
13. Medications likely to impair intestinal absorption include
     a. Broad-spectrum antibiotics
     b. Digestants
     c. Diuretics
     d. Laxatives
     e. Tetrahydrocannabinol
14. Diuretics that conserve body potassium include
     a. Ethacrynic acid
     b. Furosemide
     c. Hydrochlorothiazide
     d. Spironolactone
     e. Triamterene

Short Answer Questions

1. List at least four factors that can contribute to the development of constipation.

2. List at least six types of food additives.

3. Name at least ten food additives considered by Jacobson to be safe.

4. List at least four foods that should not be ingested by individuals receiving monoamine oxidase inhibitors.

5. List at least ten factors predisposing to drug-induced nutritional deficiency.

11
Psychological Aspects of Drug Therapy

A person's physiologic response to a particular drug is affected by the psychological response to drugs, as is the reverse. Each person's response is unique. An understanding of these factors helps the nurse to obtain a more effective response from the client when administering drug therapy.

Short Answer Questions

1. Drug effectiveness is influenced by psychological response and pharmacodynamic actions. Identify the three resulting degrees of effectiveness and define each term.
   a.

   b.

   c.

2. List various emotional responses a person may have to drug therapy.

3. Give several instances in which placebos are used.

4. Ways in which the angry client might respond to drug therapy include the following:

5. Ways in which the "good" client might respond to drug therapy include the following:

Matching

Match the behavioral response in the right-hand column with the supporting statement in the left-hand column. Place your answer in the space provided.

_____ 1. Hidden beliefs unconsciously affecting the emotional state and responsiveness to drug therapy

_____ 2. A positive or negative attitude affecting the therapeutic value of a drug

_____ 3. State of mind, or opinions, that influence behavior

_____ 4. Behavior arising from attitudes held toward people, drugs, drug therapy, health care, and self

_____ 5. Acuteness or chronicity of illness, leading to positive or negative responses

_____ 6. Causative factors activating behavior for need satisfaction

a. Attitude
b. Motivation
c. Meaning attached to drugs
d. Power of suggestion
e. Type of illness
f. Nurses' behavioral response

Multiple Choice Questions

For each of the following, choose the one best answer.

1. Placebos are thought to be effective because of the
   a. Production of endorphins in the brain
   b. Pharmacologic action of the active drug in the placebo
   c. Nurturing attitude of health-care providers

2. Mrs. Brown has continued to take her digitoxin regularly, as prescribed by her physician, although she has experienced extreme nausea and vomiting, headaches, and drowsiness for the last 5 days. Mrs. Brown could be
   a. Exhibiting anger and resentment about her condition
   b. Gaining a feeling of security from taking the digitoxin
   c. Manifesting fear over her drug dependency
   d. Exhibiting physical symptoms of psychological origin

3. In this instance, an appropriate nursing diagnosis for Mrs. Brown would be
   a. Ineffective coping (displaced anger) related to feelings of helplessness
   b. Overcompliance related to knowledge deficit and the need for security
   c. Fear related to knowledge deficit
   d. Anxiety related to chronic physical illness

4. An important nursing intervention for Mrs. Brown would be
   a. Encourage verbalization of anger
   b. Provide information on digitoxin toxicity and her responsibilities
   c. Explore with Mrs. Brown her fears about drug dependency
   d. Discuss with Mrs. Brown the relationship between her physical symptoms and her anxiety

5. When assessing a client for drug therapy, one of the first areas to be assessed is
   a. Length of time of therapy
   b. Family support of drug therapy
   c. Types of drugs available
   d. Client attitude toward drugs and drug taking

6. Successful drug therapy is most apt to be accomplished when
   a. Both client and health-care providers strive toward the same goal
   b. The nurse is knowledgeable about the drugs administered
   c. The right drug in the right dosage is given at the right time
   d. The client substitutes drugs for the sick role

12
Cultural Aspects of Drug Therapy

The study of ethnopharmacology has developed an awareness of the influences brought to bear on the choices made by peoples of different backgrounds when confronting illness or seeking health care in the United States today. Sensitivity to and knowledge about health and illness beliefs, and methods of remediation practiced, are essential for the development of effective interventions in health-care delivery.

Short Answer Questions

1. Define the following terms:
   a. Ethnomedicine:

   b. Medicinal plant:

   c. Ethnopharmacology:

   d. Doctrine of signatures:

   e. Decoction:

   f. Tisane:

   g. Maceration:

   h. Infusion:

2. Identify the most characteristic aspects of the health and illness beliefs of the following ethnic groups:
   a. Black Americans:

   b. Hispanic Americans:

   c. Native Americans:

   d. Asian Americans:

3. List five factors that generally determine the health and illness beliefs and practices of different ethnic groups.

4. List four factors that may affect the potency and usefulness of an herbal plant.

Completion Exercises

Read each question carefully and place your answers in the spaces provided.
1. For each cultural group listed, identify folk remedies used in the treatment of common illnesses.

GROUP	COMMON ILLNESS	REMEDY
Black Americans	Cold	
	Fever	
	Boil	
Hispanic Americans	Stomachache	
	Pneumonia	
Native Americans	Cough	
	Stomachache	
European Americans	Sore throat	
	Burns	

2. Complete the table, giving potential body effects caused by the following common chemical components of plants.

CHEMICAL COMPONENT	EFFECT ON THE BODY
Vitamins	
Alkaloids	
Antibiotics	
Heterosides (sugars)	
Acids	
Minerals	

44

3. Listed below are several known medicinal plants. Identify the active ingredients and their therapeutic uses.

MEDICINAL PLANT　　　　　　　ACTIVE INGREDIENT(S)　　　　　MEDICINAL USE

Purple foxglove
　(*Digitalis purpurea*)
Rauwolfia (*Rauwolfia serpentina*)

American mandrake
　(*Podophyllum peltatum*)
Periwinkle
　(*Catharanthus roseus*)
Cocaine (*Erythroxylon coca*)
Opium poppy
　(*Papaver somniferum*)

Checklist

Using a check mark, indicate the category of the body fluids listed according to traditional Hispanic practices.

1. Blood
   _____ a. Hot, wet
   _____ b. Hot, dry
   _____ c. Cold, wet
   _____ d. Cold, dry
2. Yellow bile
   _____ a. Hot, wet
   _____ b. Hot, dry
   _____ c. Cold, wet
   _____ d. Cold, dry
3. Black bile
   _____ a. Hot, wet
   _____ b. Hot, dry
   _____ c. Cold, wet
   _____ d. Cold, dry
4. Phlegm
   _____ a. Hot, wet
   _____ b. Hot, dry
   _____ c. Cold, wet
   _____ d. Cold, dry

UNIT THREE: ADMINISTRATION OF MEDICATIONS

13
Basic Principles of Medication

Many people are involved in the various processes required for the manufacture, distribution, prescription, administration, and monitoring of drugs used to treat human diseases, but it is vital that the nurse be aware of all drugs taken by the client, that the client be evaluated regularly and comprehensively for therapeutic response and adverse reactions, and that intervention be initiated when necessary to ensure optimal effects of drug therapy.

Matching

A. Match the medication procedure (as described in the text) in the left-hand column with the strengths listed in the right-hand column. Place your answer in the space provided. (More than one answer may be given.)

_____ 1. Procedures using medication cards
_____ 2. Procedures using medication carts

a. Provides continuous written identification of drugs
b. Is most efficient (requires least time to complete the procedure)
c. Provides continuous written identification of the client to be medicated
d. Keeps drugs most secure against accidental spillage
e. Keeps drug supplies most secure against diversion to unauthorized recipients
f. Provides privacy for preparation of drugs
g. Allows immediate charting of medications
h. Provides best protection against omission of drug dosages

B. Match the health-care personnel in the left-hand column with their legal rights in the right-hand column. Place your answer in the space provided.

_____ 1. Physicians
_____ 2. Physician's assistants
_____ 3. Pharmacists
_____ 4. Nurses
_____ 5. Dentists

a. May compound drugs
b. May dispense drugs
c. May administer drugs to clients

Correct the False Statement

Indicate whether the following statements are true or false; if false, correct the underlined words or phrases.

_____ 1. When the route is not specified in a medication order, <u>the drug is administered orally</u>.

_____ 2. In hospital situations, <u>only physicians and nurses</u> commonly administer drugs to clients.

_____ 3. In administering drugs, the nurse must <u>adhere to the order as written by the physician</u>.

_____ 4. For most drugs, the time required for elimination of residues from the body in a normally healthy adult is <u>2 weeks</u>.

Multiple Choice Questions

For each of the following, choose the one best answer.

1. Your client is to receive digoxin 0.375 mg PO. In the drug supply you find that all the digoxin tablets are scored and that each contains 0.25 mg. There are three whole tablets and one half-tablet. You would
   a. Give the half-tablet and one whole tablet to the client
   b. Break another tablet; give the half-tablet and a whole one to your client and leave the original half-tablet for the nurse who broke it to administer
   c. Call the pharmacy for a tablet containing 0.125 mg digoxin to administer with one 0.25-mg tablet
   d. Call the physician to request an order consistent with the drug preparations available.

2. The most critical nursing responsibility related to medication is
   a. Preparing and administering the dose with 100% accuracy
   b. Explaining the purposes of therapy to the client
   c. Warning the client of the risk of drug use
   d. Assessing client response to drugs

3. In which of the following settings is the nurse likely to have the greatest latitude in the administration of medications and the greatest influence on drug regimens?
   a. Care of clients in the home (community nursing)
   b. Skilled nursing care (nursing home)
   c. Acute care facility (hospital)
   d. Primary practice (private office for independent nursing)

4. In hospital settings, professional nurses are responsible for the accuracy of medications administered to clients by them and also for those administered by
   a. Vocational–technical nurses
   b. Respiratory therapists
   c. Physicians
   d. a and b above
   e. All of the above

5. If the required dose of a drug is half of a tablet, the drug can be administered provided that
   a. The tablets furnished are scored
   b. The tablets furnished are enteric-coated
   c. The tablets furnished are water-soluble
   d. None of the above; fractional parts of a tablet should not be given

Selection of Options

For each of the following, select *all* appropriate responses. Circle correct answers.

1. A nurse working in a physician's office could appropriately advise a client to
   a. Inform the physician if improvement does not occur as expected
   b. Discontinue drug therapy when symptoms subside
   c. Adjust the dosage in accordance with severity of the symptoms
   d. Report adverse reactions associated with taking the medication

2. To measure accurately an 18-ml dose of liquid medication, you could use a
   a. Medicine glass
   b. Measuring teaspoon
   c. Fluted paper cup
   d. 6-ml syringe

3. What should the nurse do when a medication order specifies a dose that is more than the usual dosage range?
   a. Give the dose as ordered; physicians are responsible for their actions
   b. Consult with the physician to clarify the accuracy of the order
   c. Refuse to give the drug if the dose is likely to harm the client

4. To assess client response to drug therapy, the nurse must have knowledge of
   a. Therapeutic effects expected of the drug
   b. Side effects of the drug
   c. Signs and symptoms of drug toxicity
   d. The specific dose administered to the client

Sequences

A nurse caring for a hospital client notes that the signs and symptoms of infection remain unabated 3 days after an oral antibiotic has been ordered. (Acute signs and symptoms of infection usually subside about 24 hours after effective antibiotic treatment is begun.) Arrange the following steps in the order in which the actions should be taken.

_____ Notify the physician of the client's failure to improve.

_____ Check the chart to see how many doses of antibiotic the client has received.

_____ Interview the client to determine whether the oral antibiotic has been retained.

Short Answer Questions

1. Identify the five "rights" of medications.

2. How many serum half-lives ($t_{\frac{1}{2}}$) elapse before drug residues in the blood are reduced to less than 1%?

3. If a drug has a half-life of 24 hours, how long would it take for 99% of a given dose to be eliminated from the body of a normally healthy adult? (Ignore the factor of storage in tissue depots.)

Completion Exercises

1. Distribution of a drug supply is termed _____ .
2. When a physician or dentist recommends a medicinal substance and specifies the way it is to be used, this is known as _____ .
3. Preparation of medicinal substances from raw ingredients is termed _____ .

Situational Exercises

What would you do in the following situations? Write your answers on a separate sheet of paper.

1. To prevent the development of a stress ulcer in a client suffering from renal failure who is beginning hemodialysis treatment, the physician orders the following medication: cimetidine, 150 mg PO q6h. Assume that the cimetidine is marketed in only one dose form: a glazed, unscored tablet containing 300 mg.
2. A physician with a heavy German accent gives you a telephone order to give one of his patients "one Eva Coogan." You know he means to order a medication, but you do not recognize this drug name.
3. When you offer your client his daily dose of allopurinol at 10 AM, he asks you to leave it, saying that he doesn't want to take it until his dinner tray arrives because he experiences stomach distress when taking it on an empty stomach.

Personal Exercise: Drug History

Pretend that you are acutely ill with abdominal pain and are admitted to the hospital. What information should you give the nurse who is taking your drug history? Write your answer on a separate sheet of paper, using the form in the textbook appendix as a guide.

14
Special Skills Related to Drug Administration

Effective drug therapy depends on the delivery of accurate doses of active chemicals to the body tissues at the proper site of action for the drug involved. To complete this process successfully, the practitioner must master certain technical skills: proper storage and handling of drugs; command of the language used in drug therapy; accurate computation of drug doses; and techniques used in delivering drugs by specific routes to specific sites. The following exercises will help you to develop knowledge and skills in storage and handling, language, and computation.

Matching

Match each measure of weight in the left-hand column with the letter designating the equivalent volume(s) (of water) in the right-hand column. Place your answer(s) in the space provided.

_____ 1. Dram
_____ 2. Ounce
_____ 3. Gram
_____ 4. Grain
_____ 5. Pound
_____ 6. Kilogram

a. Milliliter
b. Pint
c. Fluidounce
d. Cubic centimeter
e. Tablespoon
f. Minim
g. Fluidram
h. Liter

Correct the False Statement

Indicate whether the following statements are true or false; if false, change the underlined words or phrases.

_____ 1. Insulin should be stored in the refrigerator at all times.

_____ 2. The best way to warm a medication to body temperature is to place the container in warm water.

_____ 3. The best place to store most drugs in the home is in the bathroom medicine cabinet.

_____ 4. In health-care institutions, narcotics are usually stored in areas secured by at least two locks.

_____ 5. A bottle of elixir of phenobarbital used to pour medication for all clients receiving the drug is an example of unit dosage.

_____ 6. When a medication order does not specify the route to be used, the drug is administered by mouth.

_____ 7. Once a physician has verified a drug order that the nurse has feared may harm the client, the nurse may administer the dose.

_____ 8. After a telephone order is written by the nurse on the physician's order sheet, it must be countersigned as soon as possible by the physician.

_____ 9. The nurse who administers a drug in accordance with a verbal order can be charged with <u>practicing medicine without a license</u> if the physician later repudiates the order.

_____ 10. The substance used as a standard for equating measures of weight and volume in both the apothecary and metric systems is <u>wine</u>.

Multiple Choice Questions

For each of the following, choose the one best answer.

1. The label on a container of liquid medication has become soiled from spilled medication. The nurse should
   a. Relabel the container clearly, verifying the accuracy of the new label by checking three times
   b. Return the container to the pharmacy for relabeling
   c. Discard the container and medication and secure a new supply
   d. Ask the nursing supervisor to assist in relabeling the container to ensure against error

2. Child-protective packaging should be used for all medications
   a. Without exception
   b. Except topical ointments, eye drops, and nose drops
   c. Except for drugs used by clients with impaired manual dexterity
   d. Except for drugs given by injection

3. The best organization for storage of stock drug supplies is
   a. Separation of injectable preparations from topical and oral drugs
   b. Separation of ingestible drugs from preparations for external use
   c. Arrangement in alphabetical order
   d. Separation of light-sensitive from light-stable drugs

4. When the medication nurse leaves a unit for lunch, what should be done with the key to the medication cart (closet)? The key is
   a. Kept in the possession of the medication nurse
   b. Left with the charge nurse
   c. Left with the ward secretary or manager
   d. Hidden in a place known only to members of the nursing staff

Selection of Options

For each of the following, select all appropriate responses. Circle correct answers.

1. Most drugs maintain their safety, potency, and stability longest when stored in environments that are
   a. Light
   b. Airy
   c. Cool
   d. Moist
   e. Dark
   f. Dry
   g. Warm
   h. Clean

2. Drugs likely to require refrigeration include
   a. Elixirs
   b. Suppositories
   c. Vaccines
   d. Parenteral fluids
   e. Liquid antibiotics
   f. Oral liquids with a bitter taste
   g. Eye and ear drops

Short Answer Questions

Define the following abbreviations:
1. IV
2. OD
3. od
4. ac
5. hs
6. gtt i
7. ℨ i
8. mg
9. g
10. ml
11. SOS
12. PRN

13. pc
14. qd
15. qh
16. stat
17. IM
18. H
19. v
20. ss
21. SSKI
22. SSE
23. ms
24. MOM
25. MO
26. TWE
27. gm
28. μg
29. kg
30. cc
31. l
32. ASA

Completion Exercises

Read each question carefully and place your answer in the space provided.

1. Protocols are defined as _____

2. The three essential parts of a prescription are _____

3. Name the three systems used to measure drugs: _____

4. Which system is preferred for medication? _____

Computation: Review of Mathematics

Compute the following:
1. Convert to arabic numbers:
   a. xx
   b. xi
   c. iv
   d. ii
   e. xxiv
   f. xv
   g. viiss
   h. xxxii
   i. lx
   j. iss
   k. ix
   l. xlii
   m. cliv
   n. lxv
   o. mm
   p. vc
2. Write in Roman numerals:
   a. 2
   b. 10
   c. 6
   d. 14
   e. 29
   f. 96
   g. 144
   h. 63
   i. 39
   j. 86
   k. 17
   l. 1984
   m. $7\frac{1}{2}$
3. Change these improper fractions to mixed numbers:
   a. $\frac{5}{2}$
   b. $\frac{16}{3}$
   c. $\frac{25}{4}$
   d. $\frac{15}{12}$
   e. $\frac{16}{7}$
   f. $\frac{43}{10}$
   g. $\frac{56}{9}$
   h. $5\frac{90}{11}$
4. Change these decimals to fractions:
   a. 0.5
   b. 0.03
   c. 0.305
   d. 0.011
   e. 0.13
   f. 0.0025
   g. 0.125
   h. 0.0875
   i. 0.326
   j. 0.4004
   k. 0.00007
5. Change to decimals:
   a. $\frac{3}{4}$
   b. $\frac{2}{3}$
   c. $\frac{1}{8}$
   d. $\frac{3}{10}$

- e. $\frac{7}{8}$
- f. $\frac{1}{6}$
- g. $1\frac{1}{2}$
- h. $3\frac{3}{8}$
- i. $10\frac{7}{9}$
- j. $3\frac{5}{16}$

6. Give the metric equivalent for these:
   - a. 1 teaspoon
   - b. 1 tablespoon
   - c. 1 ounce
   - d. ʒ i
   - e. gr i
   - f. min i
   - g. fluidram i
   - h. 1 pint
   - i. 1 quart

7. Reduce these fractions to their lowest terms:
   - a. $\frac{24}{60}$
   - b. $\frac{12}{16}$
   - c. $\frac{10}{15}$
   - d. $\frac{300}{60}$
   - e. $\frac{21}{42}$
   - f. $\frac{48}{78}$
   - g. $\frac{24}{32}$
   - h. $\frac{32}{78}$
   - i. $\frac{26}{65}$
   - j. $\frac{225}{300}$
   - k. $\frac{144}{256}$
   - l. $\frac{51}{119}$
   - m. $\frac{39}{53}$
   - n. $\frac{0.125}{0.25}$

8. Convert these improper fractions to mixed numbers:
   - a. $\frac{3}{2}$
   - b. $\frac{5}{4}$
   - c. $\frac{10}{4}$
   - d. $\frac{20}{12}$
   - e. $\frac{650}{325}$
   - f. $\frac{40}{15}$
   - g. $\frac{22}{5}$
   - h. $\frac{57}{6}$
   - i. $\frac{0.6}{0.4}$
   - j. $\frac{40}{25}$
   - k. $\frac{300}{250}$
   - l. $\frac{0.25}{0.125}$
   - m. $\frac{\frac{1}{2}}{\frac{1}{3}}$
   - n. $\frac{\frac{2}{3}}{\frac{1}{4}}$

9. Express these ratios as fractions:
   - a. 1:3
   - b. 2:7
   - c. 2:3
   - d. 2:300
   - e. 5:1000
   - f. 125:2000
   - g. 6:100
   - h. 3:500
   - i. 1:1000
   - j. 4:300
   - k. 1:150

10. Convert these to decimals:
    - a. $\frac{2}{5}$
    - b. $\frac{7}{15}$
    - c. $\frac{5}{8}$
    - d. $1\frac{3}{4}$
    - e. $2\frac{3}{5}$
    - f. $\frac{100}{60}$
    - g. $\frac{0.125}{0.25}$
    - h. $\frac{0.625}{0.3}$
    - i. $\frac{1}{0.5}$
    - j. $\frac{0.6}{0.4}$
    - k. $\frac{50}{40}$
    - l. $\frac{30}{18}$
    - m. $\frac{7}{9}$
    - n. $\frac{0.45}{0.9}$

11. Convert these decimals to fractions and reduce to the lowest terms:
    - a. 0.7
    - b. 1.35
    - c. 0.875
    - d. 0.4
    - e. 0.89
    - f. 0.75
    - g. 0.375
    - h. 1.67
    - i. 7.3
    - j. 3.1625
    - k. 5.66
    - l. 8.125
    - m. 0.11
    - n. $6.33\frac{1}{3}$

12. Add these fractions and mixed numbers:
    - a. $\frac{1}{7} + \frac{3}{7}$
    - b. $\frac{7}{30} + \frac{9}{30} + \frac{1}{30}$
    - c. $\frac{1}{2} + \frac{1}{3}$
    - d. $\frac{1}{6} + \frac{3}{4}$
    - e. $\frac{1}{14} + \frac{1}{7} + \frac{1}{2}$
    - f. $\frac{1}{18} + \frac{1}{9} + \frac{1}{12} + \frac{1}{4}$
    - g. $2\frac{1}{2} + 1\frac{1}{3}$
    - h. $3\frac{1}{6} + \frac{2}{9} + 1\frac{1}{2}$
    - i. $3\frac{1}{3} + \frac{1}{9} + \frac{3}{4} + 8\frac{1}{12}$

13. Subtract these fractions and mixed numbers:
    - a. $\frac{3}{4} - \frac{1}{4}$
    - b. $\frac{7}{12} - \frac{5}{12}$
    - c. $\frac{5}{18} - \frac{2}{9}$
    - d. $\frac{1}{2} - \frac{5}{12}$
    - e. $\frac{3}{4} - \frac{7}{12}$
    - f. $\frac{7}{12} - \frac{2}{9}$
    - g. $\frac{11}{15} - \frac{1}{4}$

h. $10\frac{7}{9} - 6\frac{1}{6}$
i. $30\frac{11}{13} - 2\frac{1}{3}$
j. $1\frac{1}{2} - \frac{7}{11}$

14. Multiply these fractions:
    a. $\frac{1}{2} \times \frac{1}{3}$
    b. $\frac{3}{4} \times \frac{1}{5}$
    c. $\frac{3}{8} \times \frac{2}{3}$
    d. $\frac{1}{3} \times \frac{9}{10}$
    e. $\frac{5}{12} \times \frac{3}{4}$
    f. $\frac{50}{60} \times 60$
    g. $\frac{100}{60} \times 12$
    h. $\frac{300}{125} \times 5$
    i. $\frac{75}{20} \times 5$
    j. $\frac{25}{50} \times 2$
    k. $1\frac{1}{2} \times 325$

15. Divide these:
    a. $\frac{1}{4} \div \frac{1}{6}$
    b. $\frac{3}{32} \div \frac{1}{8}$
    c. $\frac{7}{10} \div \frac{3}{5}$
    d. $\frac{1}{150} \div 2$
    e. $\dfrac{\frac{1}{10}}{\frac{1}{2}}$
    f. $\dfrac{\frac{1}{200}}{\frac{1}{150}}$
    g. $\dfrac{\frac{1}{2}}{\frac{1}{2}}$
    h. $\dfrac{\frac{3}{4}}{3}$

16. Change these mixed numbers to improper fractions:
    a. $4\frac{1}{2}$
    b. $16\frac{9}{10}$
    c. $10\frac{3}{4}$
    d. $13\frac{3}{8}$
    e. $26\frac{1}{11}$
    f. $13\frac{5}{12}$

17. Add these decimals:
    a. $0.5 + 0.05$
    b. $0.33 + 0.66$
    c. $1.5 + 0.75$
    d. $0.125 + 0.25$
    e. $0.75 + 0.5$
    f. $4.302 + 1.88 + 0.009$

18. Subtract these decimals:
    a. $19.83 - 4.51$
    b. $3.75 - 1.5$
    c. $4 - 0.8$
    d. $3.7 - 1.9$
    e. $10.05 - 3.88$

19. Multiply these:
    a. 0.125×10
    b. 0.5×100
    c. $10{,}000 \times 0.75$
    d. 0.1×1000
    e. 2.1×3.4
    f. 1.5×8.04
    g. 0.125×5
    h. $0.25 \times \frac{1}{2}$
    i. $0.6 \times \frac{3}{4}$

20. Divide these:
    a. $0.60 \div 2$
    b. $0.125 \div 5$
    c. $10{,}000 \div 2$
    d. $0.25 \div 0.125$
    e. $0.5 \div 4$
    f. $5.5 \div 10$
    g. $0.100 \div 1000$
    h. $8.75 \div 100$
    i. $0.3 \div 1000$

21. Express these as percentages:
    a. $\frac{1}{4}$
    b. $\frac{3}{5}$
    c. $\frac{3}{8}$
    d. $\frac{1}{6}$
    e. 3:5
    f. 7:100
    g. 1:1000
    h. 9:1000
    i. 0.06
    j. 3.5
    k. 0.10
    l. 0.0002
    m. 0.005

22. Express these as decimals:
    a. 0.09%
    b. 50%
    c. 3%
    d. 75%

23. Express these as fractions:
    a. 10%
    b. $37\frac{1}{2}\%$
    c. $66\frac{2}{3}\%$
    d. $9\frac{1}{11}\%$
    e. 25%
    f. 60%
    g. $87\frac{1}{2}\%$
    h. $16\frac{2}{3}\%$

24. Compute these:
    a. 50% of 250
    b. 25% of 36
    c. 10% of 45
    d. 12% of 1000
    e. 0.1% of 25
    f. 20% of 0.01
    g. What percent of 18 is 9?
    h. What percent of 50 is 10?
    i. What percent of 100 is 9?
    j. What percent of 2 is 0.1?
    k. What percent of 0.1 is 2?
    l. What percent of 150 is 50?

25. Write these as ratios:
    a. $\frac{3}{4}$
    b. $\frac{1}{2}$
    c. $\frac{7}{8}$
    d. $\frac{13}{20}$
    e. $\frac{65}{83}$
    f. 10 ÷ 30
    g. 22 ÷ 30
    h. 3 ÷ 100
    i. 10
    j. 8
    k. 75%
    l. $33\frac{1}{3}$%
    m. $\frac{\frac{1}{4}}{10}$
    n. $\frac{\frac{1}{10}}{100}$
26. Solve these:
    a. 10:5::x:1
    b. 1:0.5::x:1
    c. 1 g:500 mg::x tab:1 tab
    d. 0.4 mg:0.6 mg::x ml:1 ml
    e. x mg:50 mg::1 ml:2 ml
    f. $\frac{2}{3}$:x::$\frac{3}{4}$:1
    g. 2:x::5:7
    h. 0.5:x::0.25:1
    i. $\frac{x}{9} = \frac{2}{63}$
    j. $\frac{3}{x} = \frac{9}{15}$
    k. $\frac{50}{2} = \frac{25}{x}$
    l. $\frac{325}{1} = \frac{650}{x}$
    m. $\frac{400\ \mu g}{1\ mg} = \frac{x}{1\ ml}$
    n. $\frac{0.4}{x} = \frac{0.6}{1}$
27. Complete these equivalents:
    a. 1 cc = _____ ml
    b. 1 liter = _____ ml
    c. 1000 cc = _____ liter
    d. 3.0 liters = _____ ml
    e. 5.3 liters = _____ cc
    f. 500 ml = _____ liter
    g. 1.9 liters = _____ ml
    h. 350 cc = _____ liter
    i. 4.03 liters = _____ cc
28. Add these:
    a. 1 liter + 50 ml + 30 cc + 0.4 liter
    b. 180 ml + 3 liters + 30 cc + 60 cc
29. Convert these:
    a. 2 g to mg
    b. 0.5 g to mg
    c. 0.25 mg to g
    d. 600 mg to g
    e. 100 µg to mg
    f. 30 µg to mg
    g. 0.4 mg to µg
    h. 1000 µg to g
    i. 3000 µg to mg
    j. 5 µg to g
30. What are the ratio and percentage strength of each of the following solutions?
    a. 1000 ml of solution containing 50 g glucose in water
    b. 500 ml of solution containing 350 ml alcohol in water
    c. 200 ml of solution containing gr xxx of boric acid in water
31. How much penicillin solution will be needed to give the following doses?
    a. 200,000 U from a solution containing 500,000 U/ml
    b. 300,000 U from a solution containing 200,000 U/ml
    c. 70,000 U from a solution containing 100,000 U/ml
    d. 150,000 U from a solution containing 200,000 U/ml
    e. 15,000 U from a solution containing 40,000 U/ml
    f. Zephiran chloride solution 1:5000 is ordered for irrigation. How much 1:2000 stock solution is needed to prepare 1000 ml?
32. Solve these conversion problems:
    a. Change gr x to milligrams (mg).
    b. Change 150 mg to grains (gr).
    c. Change 400 µg to mg.
    d. Change 0.5 g to gr.
    e. Change gr $1\frac{1}{2}$ to mg.
    f. Change gr $\frac{1}{300}$ to mg. How many micrograms is this?
    g. Change 200 mg to gr.
    h. How many milliliters (ml) are in 3 ounces (oz)? 8 oz?
    i. How many minims are in $\frac{3}{4}$ ml? $\frac{1}{3}$ ml?
33. For the following, determine the number of tablets to give:

PHYSICIAN'S ORDER	DOSE PER TABLET
a. gr x	0.3 g
b. gr $\frac{1}{12}$	2.5 mg
c. 2 g	gr viiss
d. gr $\frac{3}{4}$	gr $1\frac{1}{2}$
e. gr $\frac{1}{150}$	0.2 mg
f. 500 mg	0.25 g
g. 0.125 mg	0.25 mg
h. 60 mg	gr ss
i. 0.4 g	gr iss

34. Determine the amount of solution to give:

	PHYSICIAN'S ORDER	LABEL ON DRUG BOTTLE
a.	100 mg	125 mg/5 ml
b.	gr v	200 mg/4 ml
c.	gr $\frac{1}{2}$	125 mg/5 ml
d.	15 mg	gr i/fl oz
e.	gr i	gr iii/ml
f.	75,000 U	50,000 U/ml
g.	90 mg	gr $\frac{1}{2}$/fl oz
h.	gr $\frac{1}{100}$	60 mg%
i.	500 mg	0.25 g/fl oz
j.	gr i	50 mg/ml

35. How much pure drug is contained in each of the following solutions?
    a. gtt iv of Neo-Synephrine $\frac{1}{2}$% nose drops. (Assume the drops are equivalent to 1 min.)
    b. 15 ml of 2% cocaine solution applied topically
    c. 100 ml of 5% boric acid solution

Sequences

Arrange the following in descending order, from largest to smallest.
1. $\frac{2}{3}, \frac{1}{2}, \frac{1}{4}, \frac{3}{4}, \frac{5}{12}$
2. $\frac{3}{8}, \frac{5}{6}, \frac{3}{4}, \frac{1}{12}, \frac{1}{2}$
3. $\frac{1}{3}, \frac{2}{7}, \frac{1}{6}, \frac{3}{13}, \frac{5}{6}$
4. 4.48, 0.219, 60.001, 3.00125, 125.1
5. 0.32158, 10.038, 0.000976, 4.0680, 0.902
6. 134.6, 3.209, 0.832, 29.10, 1.999

Completion Exercise

Complete the following table:

DRUG	RATIO	%	FRACTION	DECIMAL
Normal saline solution		0.9		
Epinephrine	1:1000			
Disinfectant alcohol			$\frac{7}{10}$	
Rubbing alcohol				0.5
Neo-Synephrine nose drops		$\frac{1}{4}$		
D_5W				

Situational Exercises

A. What would you do in the following situations?
1. A stock vial of heparin solution for injection is labeled 10,000 U/ml. How much solution would you give to administer the following doses?
   a. 6000 U
   b. 5000 U
   c. 2500 U
2. Prednisone is available as scored tablets containing 5 mg, 20 mg, and 40 mg. Which tablets and how many would you give for the following dosages?
   a. 50 mg
   b. 35 mg
   c. $32\frac{1}{2}$ mg
   d. 25 mg
   e. $17\frac{1}{2}$ mg
3. On hand are morphine solutions containing 6 mg (gr $\frac{1}{10}$)/ml and 15 mg (gr $\frac{1}{4}$)/ml. How much of each strength solution would you need to administer the following doses?
   a. 4 mg (gr $\frac{1}{15}$)

   b. 10 mg (gr $\frac{1}{6}$)

c. 8 mg (gr 1/8)

d. 30 mg (gr 1/2)

e. 6 mg (gr 1/10)

f. 12 mg (gr 1/5)

4. On hand are 1-ml vials of atropine sulfate for injection containing 1.0 mg/ml, 0.6 mg/ml, or 0.4 mg/ml each. How many milliliters of each would you need to administer the following doses?
   a. Atropine 0.6 mg

   b. Atropine 0.3 mg

   c. Atropine 400 µg

   d. Atropine 200 µg

   e. Atropine gr 1/100

   f. Atropine gr 1/150

5. If Phenergan HCl tablets are available in 0.0125-g and 0.025-g sizes, which tablets and how many of them would you use to administer the following doses?
   a. 50 mg

   b. 40 mg

   c. The physician orders ascorbic acid 0.5 g bid for 3 days. Ascorbic acid is stored in bottles containing scored tablets of 50 mg, 100 mg, and 1000 mg each. Which tablets would you use to administer a single dose? How many tablets would you need to administer *all* the drug ordered?

B. For each of the following, describe what you would do. If the medication cannot be given, give your reason and explain whom you would contact to remedy the situation. If the medication can be given, describe how you would prepare it. Write your answers on a separate sheet of paper.
   1. Order: saline enema. On hand: tap water and salt.
   2. You wish to prepare a saline mouthwash for your patient. On hand: tap water and salt.
   3. Order: 5% soda bicarbonate douche.
   4. Order: Azulfidine 1.0 g tid PO. On hand: Azulfidine 500-mg scored tablet.
   5. Order: $FeSO_4$ gr iv tid PO. On hand: $FeSO_4$, 324-mg enteric-coated tablets.
   6. Order: Thorazine 30 mg q4h PRN for agitation. On hand: IM ampules of Thorazine containing 50 mg/ml.
   7. Order: Lanoxin 1.25 mg PO stat. On hand: digoxin 0.125-mg scored tablets and digoxin 0.25-mg scored tablets.
   8. Order: 1% hydrogen peroxide mouthwash pc. On hand: 3% hydrogen peroxide stock bottle.
   9. Order: Soak foot in 1:1000 potassium permanganate solution bid. The patient's foot has been wounded and the skin is still open. On hand: tablets of potassium permanganate containing 20 mg each.
   10. Order: 0.4 mg atropine IM preop. On hand: atropine solution in a vial marked 0.6 mg/ml.
   11. Order: 50 mg Demerol, 0.4 mg atropine, and 25 mg Vistaril preop (all IM). On hand: meperidine 75 mg in 1-ml Tubex, atropine in a vial containing 1 mg/ml, and Vistaril in a vial containing 50 mg/2 ml. (Prepare so as to give as few injections to the client as possible, and so as not to contaminate vials that could be used for subsequent doses.)

12. Order: K-Lyte 15 mEq bid PO. On hand: K-Lyte powder, 25 mEq per packet with directions to dissolve in 3 to 4 oz water just before administering.
13. Order for a kidney failure patient: 175 mg cimetidine tid PO. On hand: Tagamet 350-mg tablets (hard-coated, unscored).
14. Order: elixir of phenobarbital, 70 mg bid by nasogastric tube. On hand: elixir of phenobarbital, 30 mg/5 ml.
15. Order: phenytoin 300 mg by nasogastric tube. On hand: phenytoin suspension containing 125 mg/5 ml of solution.
16. You wish to prepare a small amount of rubbing alcohol from alcohol disinfectant (rubbing alcohol = 50% alcohol in water, disinfectant alcohol = 70% alcohol in water).

UNIT FOUR: DRUGS USED FOR INFLAMMATIONS AND INFECTIONS

15
Major Antimicrobial Drugs

Antimicrobials are a major class of curative drugs frequently used in clinical medicine. Treatment protocols are fairly well developed for many agents, but certain aspects of therapy such as client education have not always been fully addressed. The nurse's role is vital to the success of chemotherapy involving these drugs.

Personal Exercise: Antimicrobials

Review the list of drugs developed for Exercise 1 in the workbook material for Chapter 1. Were any antimicrobials on the list? In relation to this or to some other antimicrobial treatment given to you, evaluate the prescribed regimen. Did the health-care provider inform you fully about the effects of the medicine(s)? Was the drug regimen clearly explained? Did you experience any adverse reactions to the drug(s)? What type were they? How severe? Do you now wear a medical identification device warning of adverse reaction to antimicrobials? Should you?

Short Answer Questions

1. List the six properties of an ideal antimicrobial.
    a.
    b.
    c.
    d.
    e.
    f.
2. Identify five bacterial cell structures or processes that are damaged or disrupted by antimicrobial drugs.

3. Name four processes by which resistance to anti-infectives develops and spreads among microbial populations.

4. Define "spectrum of activity."

5. List four hygienic measures that reduce the risk of recurrent cystitis in women.

6. The drug of choice for initiating treatment of anaphylaxis is _____ .

7. List the characteristics that distinguish cephalosporins of the three "generations."
   First-generation cephalosporins: _____

   Second-generation cephalosporins: _____

   Third-generation cephalosporins: _____

Crossword Puzzle

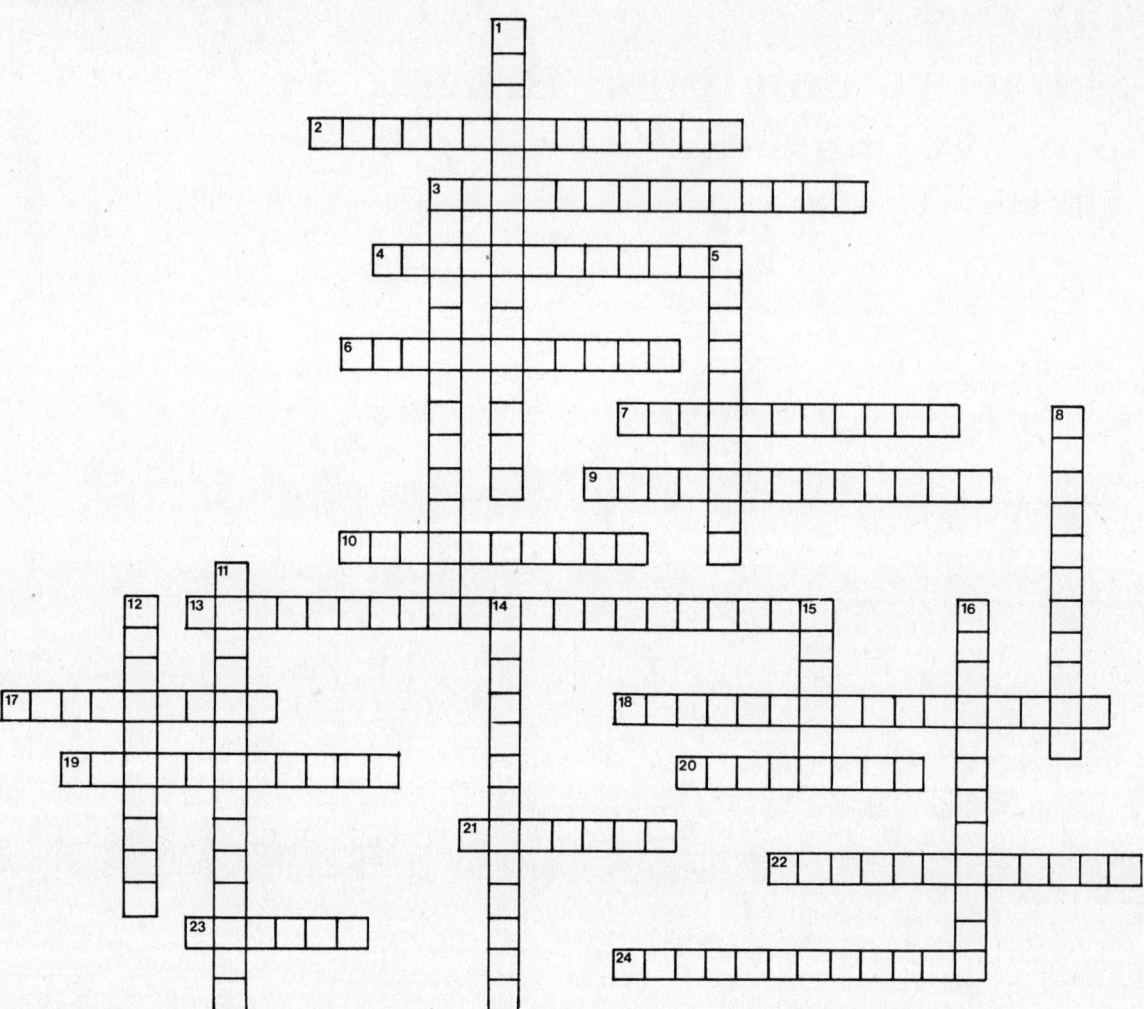

ACROSS

2. Drugs that exhibit cross sensitivity with penicillins.
3. Incorporation by a microbe of genes from the environment that were previously released by another microbe.
4. Staining property characteristic of microbes affected by penicillin.
6. An early antimicrobial currently used most often to treat and prevent urinary tract infections.
7. A serious side effect of prolonged aminoglycoside therapy.
9. An enzyme produced by penicillin-resistant organisms.
10. The property that enables microbes to thrive in the presence of an antimicrobial drug.
13. Laboratory test used as a guide to choice of anti-infective medication.
17. A juice administered to produce an acid urine.
18. A basic requirement for infection control in health-care institutions.
19. Exchange of genetic material by two microbes connected by a corridor from cytoplasm to cytoplasm.
20. The number and types of organisms affected by an antimicrobial.

21. Route of drug administration most likely to induce allergic sensitivity in the recipient.
22. An antibiotic that should not be given to young children.
23. Body organ most likely to be damaged by sulfonamide therapy.
24. Transfer of genetic material from one organism to another by a virus.

DOWN

1. A drug that may cause gray syndrome in babies.
3. One method by which resistance is spread from one organism to another without direct contact.
5. A macrolide anti-infective used to treat the eyes of newborns.
8. The drug of choice for treatment of anaphylaxis.
11. Overgrowth of organisms in the body that are not affected by anti-infective therapy.
12. An inhibitor of renal tubule excretion of several antibiotics.
14. Organisms frequently responsible for resistant nosocomial infections.
15. A substance given orally to reduce the risk of superinfection.
16. An antibiotic effective against gram-negative organisms.

Multiple Choice Questions

For each of the following, choose the one best answer.

1. The original source of sulfonamide drugs was
   a. Vegetable dyes
   b. Coal tar
   c. Bacterial cultures
   d. Fungal cultures
2. By what route are the sulfonamides most frequently administered?
   a. PO
   b. PR
   c. IM
   d. IV
3. Sulfonamide therapy can cause bleeding in persons who are on long-term warfarin therapy by
   a. Reducing metabolism of warfarin by the liver
   b. Reducing excretion of warfarin by the kidney
   c. Exerting an antiplatelet effect
   d. Decreasing vitamin K absorption
4. Sulfonamides are not used to treat newborns because
   a. The newborn's immature liver cannot metabolize them
   b. The newborn's immature kidneys cannot excrete them
   c. The drugs can stimulate the newborn's thyroid gland
   d. The drugs tend to increase kernicterus and jaundice
5. The action of sulfonamides is
   a. Bacteriostatic
   b. Bactericidal
   c. Both bacteriostatic and bactericidal
   d. Neither bacteriostatic nor bactericidal
6. Sulfonamides are most easily excreted in
   a. Acidic urine
   b. Alkaline urine
   c. Neutral urine
   d. None of the above; the only consideration is that the urine be dilute
7. Penicillin is most effective in combating
   a. Gram-positive organisms
   b. Gram-negative organisms
   c. Acid-fast organisms
   d. Fungi
8. Penicillin is
   a. Bacteriostatic
   b. Bactericidal
   c. Both bacteriostatic and bactericidal
   d. Neither bacteriostatic nor bactericidal
9. Severe adverse reactions to penicillin usually take the form of
   a. Acute hepatitis
   b. Anaphylaxis
   c. Aplastic anemia
   d. Loss of hearing
10. Drugs that are most effective in the treatment of infections caused by gram-negative organisms are the
    a. Penicillins
    b. Aminoglycosides
    c. Cephalosporins
    d. Erythromycins
11. An antimicrobial drug that is contraindicated in pregnancy is
    a. Penicillin
    b. Sodium sulfasuxidine
    c. Streptomycin
    d. Tetracycline

12. Immunmosuppressed clients who experience infections require treatment with
    a. Narrow-spectrum bactericides
    b. Narrow-spectrum bacteriostatics
    c. Broad-spectrum bactericides
    d. Broad-spectrum bacteriostatics
13. Your neighbor's child has been receiving penicillin for a strep sore throat. Her mother tells you she has recovered now and asks what should be done with the rest of the prescription. You would advise her to
    a. Save the medication and resume treatment if the symptoms return
    b. Discard the medication and destroy by burning
    c. Continue to administer the drug until the original prescription is used up
    d. Contact the physician for specific instructions about the medicine
14. A life-threatening adverse reaction likely to occur in clients receiving chloramphenicol is
    a. Anaphylaxis
    b. Bone marrow depression
    c. Kidney impairment
    d. Liver degeneration
15. When antimicrobials are prescribed for the treatment of infection
    a. The intial dose of antimicrobial must be given without delay
    b. Cultures should be taken before the initial dose of antimicrobial is administered
    c. Cultures are never taken after antimicrobial treatment is in progress
    d. It is irrelevant when cultures are taken in relation to antimicrobial therapy
16. Is antibiotic therapy with a combination of a bactericidal drug and a bacteriostatic drug an example of synergism?
    a. Yes, the effect will be greater than the sum of the effects of each drug used alone
    b. No, the effect is additive
    c. No, the effect is less than the effect of either drug alone
    d. No, the effect of one drug decreases the effectiveness of the other drug

Selection of Options

For each of the following, select *all* appropriate responses. Circle correct answers.

1. Drugs derived from sulfonamides include
    a. Antimycobacterials
    b. Antifungals
    c. A diuretic
    d. Hypoglycemics
    e. Antithyroid compounds
    f. Antihistamines
2. Probenecid inhibits the excretion of
    a. Penicillin
    b. Streptomycin
    c. Tetracycline
3. Drugs that are toxic to the eighth cranial (acoustic) nerve include
    a. Streptomycin
    b. Tetracycline
    c. Kanamycin
4. How does penicillin become an environmental contaminant?
    a. It is used in animal husbandry and is found in meat and milk
    b. It is found in the urine of persons taking the drug
    c. It is spilled into the environment during preparation of doses for administration
5. Which of the following statements are valid recommendations for the use of antimicrobials?
    a. Antimicrobial therapy should be discontinued when symptoms disappear so as to decrease the development of resistant strains of organisms
    b. Antimicrobial drugs should not be used prophylactically
    c. The use of chloramphenicol should be avoided except for the treatment of serious infections caused by resistant organisms
6. Assessment of clients receiving aminoglycosides for adverse drug reactions should include monitoring of
    a. CBCs
    b. Urinary output, BUN and creatinine levels, and urinalysis
    c. Eighth cranial nerve function
    d. Respiratory function

16
Antimycobacterial Agents, Miscellaneous Antimicrobials, and Urinary Tract Antiseptics

The following exercises relate to the material from chapter 16. A few items review related material from previous chapters on anti-infectives.

Crossword Puzzle

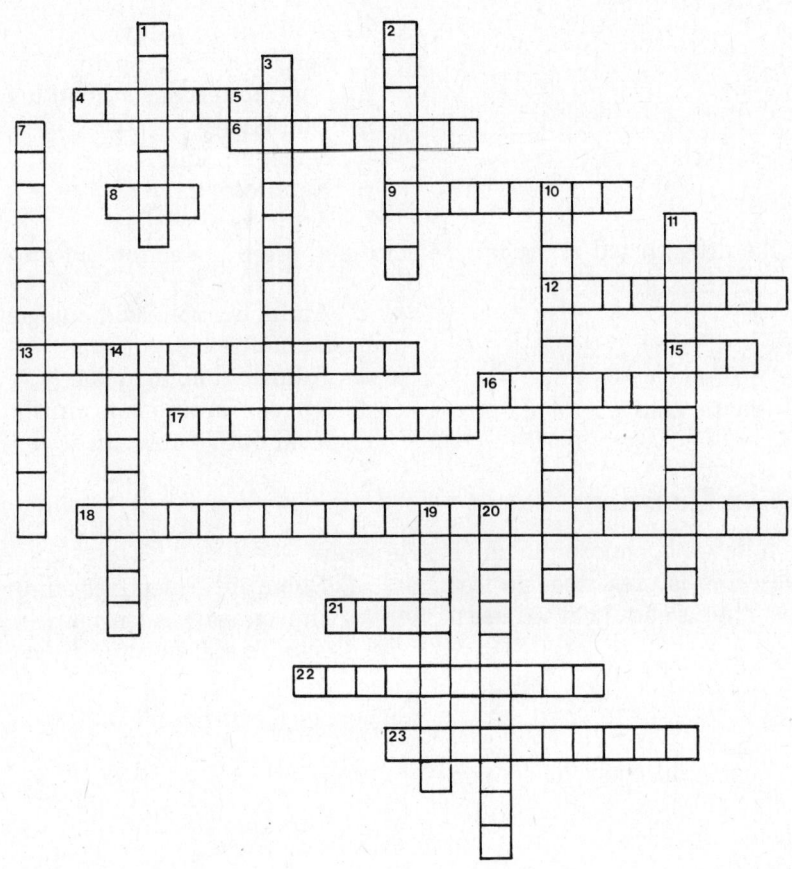

ACROSS

4. Disease caused by a mycobacterium
6. Staining property characteristic of mycobacteria
8. Abbreviated name for drug used alone to prevent active tuberculosis
9. Weak urinary antiseptic used mainly for its analgesic action
12. Color of urine during pyridium therapy
13. Serious adverse reaction to ethambutol
15. Abbreviation for para-aminosalicylic acid
16. Most frequent adverse reaction to ethionamide
17. Antibiotic that affects only mycobacteria
18. Antituberculosis drug that inhibits folic acid synthesis by the tubercle bacillus

65

21. Metabolic imbalance that may develop during pyrazinamide therapy
22. The powder form of this antibiotic must be stored in a refrigerator
23. Trade name for colistin

DOWN

1. Sulfone used to treat leprosy
2. Antimycobacterial drug excreted mainly via the liver in bile
3. Organisms susceptible to rifampin
5. One abbreviation indicating time release
7. Antituberculosis drug that is also effective against gram-negative organisms
10. Route used to administer capreomycin
11. Antituberculosis drug that must be injected parenterally
14. Generic name for INH
19. Contraindication for dapsone therapy
20. Antimicrobial that should not be used with neuromuscular agents

Matching

A. For each drug listed at the left, indicate *all* of the appropriate adverse reactions from the list at the right.

1. Capreomycin
2. Cycloserine
3. Ethambutol
4. Ethionamide
5. Isoniazid
6. Pyrazinamide
7. Rifampin

a. Anaphylaxis
b. Optic neuropathy
c. Peripheral neuropathy
d. Central nervous system toxicity
e. Ototoxicity
f. Hepatotoxicity
g. Nephrotoxicity
h. Arthritis

B. For each of the drugs listed at the left, select the appropriate action(s) from the list at the right.

1. Cycloserine
2. Dapsone
3. Isoniazid
4. Para-aminosalicylic acid

a. Aminobenzoic-acid antagonism
b. D-alanine antagonism
c. Folic-acid antagonism
d. Pyribenzamine antagonism
e. Vitamin D antagonism

Multiple Choice Questions

For each of the following, choose the one best answer.

1. When cycloserine is prescribed to treat tuberculosis, clients should avoid use of
   a. Alcohol
   b. Caffeine
   c. Nicotine
   d. All of the above

2. An antimycobacterial drug that is contraindicated for clients who must restrict sodium intake is
   a. Streptomycin
   b. Ethambutol
   c. Isoniazid
   d. p-aminosalicylic acid

3. A drug that exhibits some cross sensitivity to penicillins and cephalosporins is
   a. Streptomycin
   b. Azthreonam
   c. Bacitracin
   d. Clindamycin

4. Some anti-infectives administered intramuscularly cause pain in the injection site. To alleviate this discomfort, the nurse would
   a. Spray the site with a topical anesthetic before injection
   b. Add a small amount of procaine to the antibiotic solution
   c. Apply heat to the site after injection
   d. Apply cold to the site before and after the injection

5. The risk of serious allergic reaction to antibiotic injections is greatest in the client who
   a. Has never been exposed to the drug
   b. Has previously received the drug by injection
   c. Has previously used the drug topically with no allergic reaction
   d. Has previously taken the drug orally with no allergic reaction

6. A common household substance that has been used successfully to treat infected wounds is
   a. Salt
   b. Sugar
   c. Vinegar
   d. Soda
7. The mechanism of action by which the above substance combats infection is probably
   a. Improved nutrition of body cells in the infected tissue
   b. Mechanical removal of organic matter from the wound
   c. Reduction of *p*H in the wound environment
   d. Elevation of *p*H in the wound environment
   e. Dehydration of body cells in the infected tissues
   f. Dehydration of pathogenic microorganisms in the wound
8. To enhance the action of methenamine, the nurse may offer the client
   a. Citrus juices
   b. Cranberry juice
   c. Tomato juice
   d. Apple juice
9. Methenamine is converted in the body to a substance that acts as an
   a. Acid
   b. Alkalizer
   c. Aldehyde
   d. Oxidizer
10. The most pronounced effect of phenazopyridine (Pyridium) in the urinary tract is
    a. Antiseptic
    b. Analgesic
    c. Bacteriostatic
    d. Acidification
11. Phenazopyridine changes the color of urine to
    a. Blue
    b. Green
    c. Brown
    d. Orange
12. Superinfection caused by nitrofurantoin therapy is likely to be caused by
    a. Candida
    b. Gram-negative rods
    c. Gram-positive cocci
    d. Pseudomonas

Selection of Options

For each of the following, select *all* appropriate responses. Circle correct answers.
1. Properties of mycobacteria used for identification when viewed on slide preparations (smears) include
   a. Acid fast
   b. Gram positive
   c. Gram negative
   d. Visible on a dark field
2. Antimycobacterial drugs that change the color of body fluids include
   a. Ethambutol
   b. Isoniazid
   c. Rifampin
   d. Streptomycin
3. Factors contributing to failure of drug treatment for tuberculosis and leprosy include
   a. Compliance problems because two or more drugs are used at a time
   b. Compliance problems because drugs must be taken several times a day
   c. Compliance problems because drugs must be taken for long periods of time
   d. Development of resistance to the drugs used by the pathogens
   e. A therapeutic index that is less than 1
   f. A reduction in the recipient's resistance to infection (immunosuppressant drugs, stress, malnutrition, etc.)
4. Antimicrobial drugs that may be given parenterally include
   a. Streptomycin
   b. Ethambutol
   c. Isoniazid
   d. Rifampin
   e. Cycloserine
   f. PAS
   g. Capreomycin
   h. Ethionamide
   i. Pyrazinamide
   j. Dapsone
   k. Sulfoxone

5. Principles of antimycobacterial medication include
   a. The use of one drug at a time to prevent serious adverse reactions
   b. The use of two or more agents at a time to prevent the development of resistance
   c. The use of oral drugs over long periods of time
   d. The use of parenteral drugs for long periods of time
   e. Prophylactic regimens for exposed individuals
   f. Prophylactic regimens for individuals with arrested disease when natural resistance to active infection is reduced
6. When isoniazid is prescribed, clients will have an increased need for
   a. Vitamin A
   b. Vitamin B_{12}
   c. Niacin
   d. Pyridoxine
   e. Vitamin C
   f. Vitamin D
   g. Vitamin K
7. Antimicrobial drugs that are not absorbed well from the gastrointestinal tract include
   a. Bacitracin
   b. Ethambutol
   c. Clindamycin
   d. Colistin
   e. Novabiocin
   f. Spectinomycin
   g. Troleandomycin
8. Nursing measures that support and enhance natural resistance to infection include
   a. Encouraging fluid intake
   b. Discouraging sugar intake
   c. Providing foods rich in vitamin C
   d. Promoting rest
   e. Reducing stress
9. The proprietary drug Bactrim (Septra) is a combination of
   a. An aminoglycoside
   b. A cephalosporin
   c. A penicillin
   d. A sulfonamide
   e. Trimethoprim
   f. Vancomycin

Short Answer Questions

1. Name two diseases caused by mycobacteria.

2. An aminoglycoside used in the treatment of tuberculosis is _____.

3. Name at least two primary treatment agents for tuberculosis.

4. a. Name an antimycobacterial agent that causes body fluids to change color. _____
   b. What is the color change? _____

5. List at least four measures the nurse may use to reduce the risks of recurrent urinary tract infections.

6. Why are oral preparations of methenamine enteric-coated?

17
Drugs Used to Treat Infections Caused by Viruses and Fungi

The following exercises relate to material on antiviral and antifungal medications.

Personal Experience: Antiviral and Antifungal Drugs

Review the table of drugs developed in the workbook for Chapter 1. Does this list contain any drugs discussed in Chapter 17? Should any drugs listed in Chapter 17 be added to the list? Can you now identify measures that could have prevented or reduced the severity of the condition for which these drugs were taken? Did you experience any adverse reactions to the drugs you used?

Matching

A. Match the anti-infective drug in the left-hand column with its correct mode of action in the right-hand column. Place your answer in the space provided.

    _____ 1. Germicide
    _____ 2. Bactericidal antibiotic
    _____ 3. Bacteriostatic antibiotic
    _____ 4. Human immune globulin
    _____ 5. Interferon
    _____ 6. Vaccine
    _____ 7. Animal serum containing antitoxins

a. Confers temporary passive immunity
b. Stimulates the development of active immunity
c. Inhibits reproduction of microbial cells
d. Kills microorganisms
e. Inhibits reproduction of viruses

B. For each drug in the left-hand column, select the appropriate classification(s) from the right-hand column.

    _____ 1. Acyclovir
    _____ 2. Nystatin
    _____ 3. Gamma globulin
    _____ 4. Corticosteroids
    _____ 5. Alcohol
    _____ 6. Salicylic acid
    _____ 7. Amantadine
    _____ 8. Amphotericin B

a. Antifungal
b. Antiviral
c. Keratolytic
d. Astringent
e. Serum
f. Vaccine
g. Anti-inflammatory

Short Answer Questions

1. Give the medical name for each of the following:
    a. Measles _____
    b. Mumps _____
    c. German measles _____
    d. Chickenpox _____
    e. Polio _____
    f. Smallpox _____
    g. Whooping cough _____

2. Identify a characteristic of living organisms shared by viruses.

3. Identify a property of chemical substances shared by viruses.

4. Identify one adverse reaction to viral vaccine.

5. Name at least three common skin conditions caused by fungi.

6. Identify at least four astringents found in over-the-counter preparations.

7. List at least three measures that can reduce the risk of repeated fungal infection.

Completion Exercises

From the choices listed below each table, select the appropriate entries for each section of the table. (More than one entry may be needed for each section.) Place your answer(s) in the space provided.

1. ANTIVIRAL COMPOUND	a. TRADE NAME(S)	b. THERAPEUTIC USE(S)	c. ADVERSE REACTION(S)
Vidarabine			
Idoxuridine			
Azidothymidine			
Acyclovir			
Ribavirin			

a. Trade names: Herplex; Marboran; Stoxil; Vira-A; Virazole; Zovirax; AZT
b. Therapeutic uses: herpes simplex encephalitis; viral infections in immunosuppressed persons; lower respiratory viral infections; complications of cowpox vaccination; herpes simplex keratitis; herpes simplex keratoconjunctivitis; palliative treatment of acquired immune deficiency syndrome (AIDS); genital herpes; prevention of smallpox
c. Adverse reactions: bone marrow suppression; vomiting; renal impairment; impaired cardiac and respiratory function; local inflammation; severe tissue irritation (when combined with boric acid)

2. ANTIFUNGAL	a. ROUTE(S)	b. MODE(S) OF ACTION	c. ADVERSE REACTION(S)
Amphotericin B			
Clotrimazole			
Griseofulvin			
Ketoconazole			
Micanazole			

a. Routes: oral; topical; intramuscular; intravenous
b. Action: local; systemic
c. Adverse reactions: abnormal white blood cell counts; elevated porphyrins; gastrointestinal upset; hepatotoxicity; local tissue inflammation; nephrotoxicity; photosensitivity; skin rash; chills and fever

Correct the False Statement

Indicate whether the following statements are true or false; if false, correct the underlined words or phrases.

_____ 1. The most effective approaches to control virus infections are <u>use of high doses of vitamin C and administration of antiviral anti-infectives</u>.

_____ 2. Viral infections for which we have no effective vaccines include <u>acquired immune deficiency syndrome (AIDS) and herpes simplex</u>.

_____ 3. Acyclovir is administered <u>by intramuscular injection</u>.

_____ 4. Ribavirin is usually administered <u>by inhalation</u>.

_____ 5. Aluminum compounds used as antiperspirants act as <u>astringents</u>.

_____ 6. For reasons of economy, parenteral therapy for systemic fungal infections is likely to be conducted in <u>outpatient clinics</u>.

Multiple Choice Questions

For each of the following, choose the one best answer.

1. The treatment of infectious illness with drugs has been <u>least</u> effective for diseases caused by
   a. Lice and mites
   b. Bacteria and protozoa
   c. Fungi and viruses

2. The most effective approach to the control of viral infections to date has been the administration of
   a. Sera and vaccines
   b. Antibacterial antibiotics
   c. Viricidal drugs
   d. Interferon

3. The antiviral drug with the widest spectrum of activity is
   a. Acyclovir
   b. Azidothymidine
   c. Indoxuridine
   d. Ribavirin

4. The effect of azidothymidine on a person with AIDS infection is
   a. Rapid improvement and recovery
   b. Slow improvement and eventual recovery
   c. Delay in the progression of the disease
   d. Improvement in the symptoms of AIDS but no effect on the recipient's length of life

5. Ribavirin is usually administered by
   a. Mouth
   b. Inhalation
   c. Intravenous infusion
   d. Intramuscular injection

6. Amantadine's antiviral action results from
   a. Its ability to kill viruses
   b. Neutralization of viral toxins
   c. Inhibition of viral penetration of host cells
   d. Stimulation of interferon production

7. The antifungal drug griseofulvin is usually administered
   a. Topically to suppress fungal infections
   b. Topically to eliminate fungal infections
   c. Systemically to suppress fungal infections
   d. Systemically to eliminate fungal infections

8. Clients with diabetes mellitus should be warned against using over-the-counter preparations containing
   a. Astringents
   b. Emollients
   c. Keratolytics
   d. Insecticides

9. A medication ordered to be given as a "swish" should be
   a. Used to rinse the mouth and then swallowed
   b. Applied repeatedly to the affected skin as a rinse
   c. Sprinkled over the affected area

10. The action of nystatin is
    a. Local when administered topically and systemic when administered orally
    b. Systemic whether administered orally or parenterally
    c. Local whether administered topically or orally
    d. Local when administered topically and systemic when administered orally or parenterally

11. The drug used most often for the treatment of infections caused by *Candida albicans* is
    a. Alcohol
    b. Griseofulvin
    c. Potassium permanganate
    d. Nystatin

Selection of Options

For each of the following, select *all* appropriate responses. Circle correct answers.

1. Adverse reactions to interferon include
   a. Fever
   b. Nausea
   c. Leukocytosis
   d. Hair loss
   e. Kidney stones
2. The effects of glucocorticoids used to treat infections includes
   a. Stimulation of immune response
   b. Reduction in fever
   c. Reduction in tissue swelling
   d. Reduction in an elevated intracranial pressure
3. The antifungal drug nystatin may be administered
   a. Topically
   b. Orally
   c. Parenterally
4. Drugs classified as astringents include
   a. Alcohol
   b. Vaseline
   c. Glycerin
   d. Zinc salts
   e. Tannic acid
   f. Mineral oil
   g. Aluminum salts
5. Which of the following act as keratolytics?
   a. Alcohol
   b. Benzoic acid
   c. Aspirin
   d. Zinc salts
   e. Salicylic acid
6. Which of the following discolor skin and fabrics?
   a. Alcohol
   b. Fuchsin
   c. Gentian violet
   d. Potassium permanganate
   e. Iodine
   f. Aluminum salts
7. Substances that should be avoided by those receiving griseofulvin include
   a. Alcohol (taken orally)
   b. Phenobarbital
   c. Warfarin
8. Fungal infections include those caused by
   a. *Tinea*
   b. *Candida*
   c. Ameba

18
Drugs Used to Treat Rickettsiae, Protozoa, Helminths, and Ectoparasites

Chapter 18 discusses drugs used in the treatment of contagious illness caused by a variety of organisms. Many are transmitted by animal or insect vectors. A wide variety of chemical substances are used to prevent and treat contagious diseases caused by these life forms.

Matching

For each drug in the left-hand column, select the appropriate classification(s) from the right-hand column.

_____ 1. Elemental phosphorus	a. Anthelmintic
_____ 2. Emetine	b. Antirickettsial
_____ 3. Chlorophenothane	c. Antimalarial
_____ 4. Lindane	d. Amebicide
_____ 5. Metronidazole	e. Rodenticide
_____ 6. Piperizine	f. Insecticide
_____ 7. Pyrimethamine	g. Pediculocide
_____ 8. Quinacrine	
_____ 9. Quinine	
_____ 10. Warfarin	

Short Answer Questions

1. Give at least three principles for the safe use of insecticides.
   a.

   b.

   c.

2. Give at least two principles for the safe use of rodenticides.
   a.

   b.

3. Name the ectoparasites responsible for (a) pediculosis and (b) scabies.

Correct the False Statement

Indicate whether the following statements are true or false; if false, correct the underlined words or phrases.

_____ 1. The use of <u>rodenticides such as warfarin</u> is strictly limited to licensed personnel.

_____ 2. Clinical signs and symptoms of malaria include <u>chills, fever, and anemia</u>.

_____ 3. A public health measure used to control malaria in developing countries in which the disease is endemic is <u>the free distribution of quinine tablets</u>.

_____ 4. Populations likely to experience hemolytic reactions from primaquine include <u>northern Europeans and American Indians</u>.

_____ 5. When used to treat amebiasis, emetine and dehydroemetine are effective against <u>vegetative forms of the organism, amebic cysts, and abscesses caused by the protozoa</u>.

_____ 6. An important goal of nursing care of those under treatment for amebiasis is the maintenance of nutrition.

_____ 7. The goal of treatment of worm infestations is usually <u>thorough elimination of the parasites</u>.

_____ 8. Ascarids (roundworms) are often transmitted by ingestion of the <u>live parasites</u> eliminated by infected hosts.

_____ 9. Lindane is absorbed systemically by <u>diffusion through</u> the skin.

_____ 10. Licenses <u>are required</u> for handling certain toxic insecticides.

_____ 11. When caring for clients suffering from ectoparasitic infestations, the nurse should assign a high degree of priority to <u>emotional support and warm acceptance of the client</u>.

_____ 12. Insecticides <u>should be used regularly</u> in areas of food storage and preparation <u>to minimize contamination by infectious agents</u>.

_____ 13. Travelers to foreign countries may often avoid infectious illness by <u>eating only hot, thoroughly cooked foods</u>.

_____ 14. A household substance that acts as an antifungal is <u>sodium bicarbonate</u>.

Multiple Choice Questions

For each of the following, choose the one best answer.

1. The first effective drug for the treatment of malaria was
   a. Asafetida
   b. Quinacrine
   c. Primaquine
   d. Quinine
   e. Chloroquine

2. An herbal remedy effective in the treatment of malaria is
   a. Cinchona bark infusion
   b. Willow bark infusion
   c. Chamomile tea
   d. Comfrey tea

3. The insect vector most often responsible for the transmission of malaria is
   a. A louse that infests rodents
   b. The common housefly
   c. A wood tick
   d. The *Anopheles* mosquito

4. The drug most effective against the gametocytes of *Plasmodium falciparum* is
   a. Primaquine

b. Chloroquine
c. Quinacrine
d. Quinine

5. The mechanism of action of the rodenticide warfarin is
   a. Massive tissue damage by its corrosive action
   b. Central nervous system disturbance caused by inhibition of anticholesterase
   c. Disseminated intravascular coagulation caused by enhancement of clotting
   d. Internal hemorrhages caused by inhibition of coagulation

6. Chemotherapy for achieving a radical cure of malaria is most likely to be recommended when
   a. Active, serious malarial disease is present
   b. The disease is in remission but reinfection is likely
   c. The disease is in remission and reinfection is unlikely
   d. A person is moving to an area in which malaria is endemic

7. The antibiotics most useful for treating rickettsial disease are
   a. Penicillins
   b. Aminoglycosides
   c. Tetracyclines
   d. Erythromycins

8. The antidote for warfarin poisoning is
   a. Ipecac, administered to induce prompt emesis
   b. Parenteral injections of vitamin K
   c. Parenteral injections of heparin
   d. Parenteral injections of protamine sulfate

9. When antimalarial chemotherapy is administered, the chances of emergence of a resistant strain may be reduced by administering
   a. High doses of a single drug
   b. High doses of at least two drugs
   c. Low doses of a single drug
   d. Low doses of at least two drugs

10. The mode of transmission of amebiasis is through
    a. Lice that serve as natural reservoirs of infection
    b. Mosquitoes that serve as hosts to the protozoan during the sexual phase of development
    c. Ingestion of protozoan cysts in food or water contaminated by feces
    d. Penetration of the protozoan through the skin during contact with contaminated water

11. During the treatment of amebiasis, emetine and dehydroemetine are administered
    a. Topically
    b. Orally
    c. Intramuscularly
    d. Intravenously

12. During treatment of amebiasis with emetine or dehydroemetine, an important nursing measure is
    a. Promoting normal activity during the period of drug therapy
    b. Promoting and maintaining rest in bed
    c. Reassuring the client that the reddish brown discoloration of the urine is innocuous
    d. Monitoring the recipient for arsenical toxicity

13. Useful measures for the prevention of helminthic infestations include
    1. Maintenance of pure supplies of drinking water and food
    2. Avoidance of bathing in contaminated waters
    3. Frequent careful hand washing, especially before meals
    4. Consistent use of shoes in areas with contaminated soils
    5. Periodic prophylactic courses of treatment by anthelminthics
       a. 1, 3
       b. 2, 4, 5
       c. 1, 2, 3, 4
       d. 1, 3, 4
       e. All of the above

14. An anthelminthic drug that is contraindicated for people with roundworm infestations is
    a. Piperazine
    b. Pyrantel pamoate
    c. Pyrvinium pamoate
    d. Thiabendazole
    e. Tetrachlorethylene

15. When two or more worm infestations are present concurrently, the first drug ordered is likely to be a drug effective against
    a. Pinworms
    b. Tapeworms
    c. Hookworms
    d. Roundworms

16. Medication is likely to be ordered for everyone in a family when infestations are caused by
    a. Pinworms
    b. Tapeworms
    c. Hookworms
    d. Roundworms
17. When tetrachlorethylene is administered, the diet must be
    a. Low in carbohydrates
    b. Low in fat
    c. Low in salt
    d. High in potassium
18. Clients receiving thiabendazole for the treatment of helminthic infestations should be cautioned to
    a. Report to the physician promptly if an asparagus odor in the urine is detected
    b. Avoid use of power machinery, because the drug may produce drowsiness
    c. Disinfect stools before disposing of them in septic tanks or sewage systems
    d. All of the above
19. Another name for Kwell is
    a. Chlorophenothane
    b. Lindane
    c. DDT
    d. EDB
20. Medications used for the treatment of ectoparasitic infestations are administered
    a. Topically
    b. Orally
    c. Parenterally
    d. Intravenously
21. When chlorophenothane (DDT) is absorbed systemically, it is most likely to be stored in
    a. Bones
    b. Ovaries or testes
    c. Fat
    d. Bone marrow
22. In humans, chlorophenothane (DDT) toxicity is most likely to cause
    a. Lethargy and coma
    b. Muscle spasm and convulsions
    c. Suppression of lactation
    d. Impaired vision
23. The treatment of infectious illness with drugs has been *least* effective for diseases caused by
    a. Lice and mites
    b. Bacteria and protozoa
    c. Fungi and viruses
24. The most effective approach to the control of rickettsial diseases is
    a. Vaccination of large numbers of the population to promote active immunity to infection
    b. Suppression of animals and insects that serve as reservoirs of infection
    c. Aggressive treatment of clinical disease by the use of antibacterial antibiotics
    d. Administration of sera to confer passive immunity

Selection of Options

For each of the following, select *all* appropriate responses. Circle correct answers.

1. Alternatives to the use of pesticides in the control of vector-borne infectious disease include
    a. Screens and ratproof construction
    b. Composting of wastes in a closed system
    c. Encouragement of natural predators
2. Acute toxicity from chlorophenothane (DDT) is most likely to develop following
    a. Contamination of large areas of skin by the chemical
    b. Ingestion of contaminated food
    c. Rapid loss of weight
3. When applying ectoparasiticides, the nurse should avoid
    a. The use of protective gear so that the client will not feel rejected
    b. Inhaling the vapors of the chemicals
    c. Personal contact with the drug
4. Contraindications to the use of quinine include
    a. Active malarial infection
    b. Cinchonism
    c. Myasthenia gravis

5. Measures to prevent illness from malaria include
   a. Treating stagnant water to destroy mosquito larvae
   b. Tight screening of buildings to exclude insects
   c. Administering preventive doses of antimalarial drugs
6. Adverse reactions to antimalarial drugs include
   a. Ototoxicity
   b. Hemolysis
   c. Respiratory depression
   d. Nephrotoxicity
7. Clients who are candidates for piperazine therapy should be screened for
   a. Malnutrition and anemia
   b. Neurologic disturbance, including seizures
   c. Renal impairment

19
Antipyretics

Antipyretics are drugs that can reduce abnormally high body temperatures by suppressing inflammation or by resetting the hypothalamic thermostat toward normal levels. These drugs are used to prevent serious damage characteristic of extremely high temperatures, and to ameliorate the discomfort and debilitating effects of prolonged or pronounced fevers.

Find the Hidden Words

Hidden within the following letter grid are words and phrases from Chapter 19. They may be vertical, horizontal, or diagonal and may run from top to bottom, bottom to top, left to right, or right to left. Circle the letters as you find the hidden words.

LIST OF WORDS AND PHRASES

acetaminophen
aspirin
antipyretic
chill
crisis
dantrolene
fever
glucocorticoids
hypothalamic thermostat

hypothermia blanket
indomethacin
lysis
phenacetin
phenylbutazone
pyrogen
salicylates
thermometer
willow bark

```
l a n t k r a b w o l l i w c h d t o r a b d e l e
y s c l y s i n n a s a l i c y l a t e s a c l y n
s p h e n a c e t i n l l n p p c p n h p r o w s o
i i n d t l g l u i y g l u c o c o r t i c o i d s
r r i n d a e e m m p m p r d t h e r m r h n l a a
c i s e r d m r u y o y i n d h t l y s e o y l i c
a n l y e e c i i d h s r e f e v y s a o e l o h r
n d p h e r r n n d e l e e c r i s i s f d e e y i
t o y a i e d i e o y a v h t m c i n e a t u b n n
i m r s l t h e r h p e c r i i a s d e h e c a y e
f e v e r e t h e r p h h e c a c h i l l h r r e o
e t d e l m u u h y p o e a l b y y n y p z o k t m
t h e r m o b d d h p h e n y l b u t a z o n e h r
t a t s o m r e h t c i m a l a h t o p y h a t p e
a c e t o r l p y r r c c e s n h y p e r e s y w h
w i h h y e y h y p i h l a n k e t h y p y r o p t
a n t i y h n i p s p y r o g e n h y y n n s h y n
p h e n l t h e i n d o l l i t w o l l i s a l i c
```

Matching

Match the antipyretic drug in the left-hand column with the adverse reactions(s) caused by it from the right-hand column.

_____ 1. Aspirin
_____ 2. Acetaminophen
_____ 3. Dantrolene
_____ 4. Quinine
_____ 5. Hydrocortisone

a. Suppression of the immune system
b. Ototoxicity
c. Allergic asthma
d. Mucosal erosions
e. Liver impairment

Multiple Choice Questions

For each of the following, choose the one best answer.

1. Recordings of body temperature are apt to be highest when temperature is measured
   a. In the mouth
   b. In the rectum
   c. On the skin
   d. None of the above; temperature is consistent in various parts of the body
2. At the time a chill begins, body temperature is most likely to be
   a. Below normal
   b. Normal, or slightly above normal
   c. Markedly elevated
   d. Rapidly fluctuating
3. Dantrolene is used as an antipyretic mainly for
   a. Control of malignant hyperthermia associated with surgery
   b. Rapid reduction of potentially lethal hyperthermia regardless of cause
   c. Control of hyperthermia associated with central nervous system trauma
   d. Control of fever in clients who cannot tolerate aspirin or acetaminophen
4. Analgesic–antipyretic drugs prescribed for clients experiencing nausea and vomiting are usually administered by the
   a. Oral route
   b. Sublingual route
   c. Rectal route
   d. Intramuscular route
   e. Intravenous route
5. The glucocorticoids lower body temperature in fever by
   a. Resetting the hypothalamic thermostat
   b. Inhibiting the inflammatory response
   c. Inhibiting the growth and reproduction of pathogens
   d. Sedating the central nervous system
6. Aspirin and acetaminophen reduce body temperature by
   a. Directly stimulating perspiration
   b. Inhibiting skeletal muscle contractility
   c. Inhibiting contractility of smooth muscle in peripheral blood vessels
   d. Resetting the hypothalamic thermostat to a lower setting
7. The goal of antipyretic therapy should be to reduce body temperature to
   a. Normal (i.e., within 1° of 98.6° F PO)
   b. The client's normal temperature
   c. The maximum temperature established by the physician
   d. The lowest level possible
8. Arrange the following series of events during a chill in chronologic order:
   1. A rise in body temperature
   2. Vascular constriction and shivering
   3. An elevation of the "set" of the hypothalamic thermostat
      a. 1, 2, 3   d. 2, 3, 1
      b. 1, 3, 2   e. 3, 1, 2
      c. 2, 1, 3   f. 3, 2, 1

Selection of Options

For each of the following, select *all* appropriate responses. Circle correct answers.

1. The use of antipyretics during a febrile illness may be delayed or restricted because
   a. Fever is a valuable diagnostic sign, and early reduction of body temperature may obscure the diagnosis
   b. Fever often is harmful to pathogenic organisms causing such illnesses
   c. Fever mobilizes the body's defense systems

2. Good reasons for avoiding the use of glucocorticoids in infectious febrile disease include the following:
   a. These drugs reduce the body's defenses against infection and tend to make the underlying illness more severe
   b. Clients rapidly develop full-blown Cushing's syndrome
   c. These drugs inhibit inflammation and therefore abolish signs and symptoms that could help to diagnose the underlying illness

Short Answer Questions

1. List in chronologic order the events occurring during resolution of a febrile illness by crisis.

2. Identify at least four harmful effects of very high fevers.

3. List at least three factors associated with higher than normal body temperatures.

4. How would you establish an average basal temperature for a client?

5. Name two effective methods for reducing body temperature in clients who do not respond to antipyretic drugs.
   a.
   b.

20
Agents Used in Debridement of Wounds

In the presence of tissue debris or purulent exudate, wounds do not heal readily. Such material promotes growth of infectious organisms and stimulates inflammation in adjacent tissues. Mechanical methods may be used to remove necrotic material from wounds, but chemical agents can supplement or supplant mechanical methods.

Matching

Match the definition in the left-hand column with the appropriate term in the right-hand column. Place your answer in the space provided.

_____ 1. The tissue enzyme that catalyzes the breakdown of hydrogen peroxide to water and oxygen

_____ 2. A class of enzymes used to debride wounds

a. Lipase
b. Protease
c. Catalase
d. Monoamine oxidase

Correct the False Statement

Indicate whether the following statements are true or false; if false, change the underlined words or phrases.

_____ 1. Hydrogen peroxide causes no pain when it is first applied to wounds containing tissue debris.

_____ 2. The proper strength for hydrogen peroxide solutions used to clean infected wounds is 5%.

_____ 3. When used as a mouthwash, hydrogen peroxide solutions should be no stronger than 1%.

Multiple Choice Items

For each of the following, choose the one best answer.

1. The mechanism of action of hydrogen peroxide in the cleansing of wounds is dependent on the presence in the tissue of the enzyme
   a. Protease
   b. Catalase
   c. Monoamine oxidase
   d. Lipase

2. Hydrogen peroxide should be stored in a
   a. Warm place
   b. Refrigerator
   c. Vented container
   d. Closed brown bottle

3. An adverse reaction likely to occur when proteolytic enzymes are used for wound debridement is
   a. Suppression of the immune response
   b. Suppression of the inflammatory response
   c. A decrease in the rate of cell division
   d. Hemorrhage

4. Citrate and heparin inhibit the action of
   a. Hydrogen peroxide
   b. Dextranomer
   c. Streptodornase
   d. Fibrinolysin

5. Pharmacologic debridement of wounds accelerates healing because it
   a. Removes organic material that can be used as nutrients by the pathogenic microorganisms
   b. Increases blood supply to the affected part
   c. Reduces irritation of the affected tissues by chemical products of necrosis
   d. a and c
   e. All of the above
6. When hydrogen peroxide solutions are used for treating a wound, the nurse should be sure that
   a. Only full-strength (100%) solutions are used
   b. Only freshly prepared solutions are used
   c. Sterile aseptic technique is employed for the procedure
   d. Linens are protected from discoloration by the solution
   e. b, c
   f. a, d

Crossword Puzzle

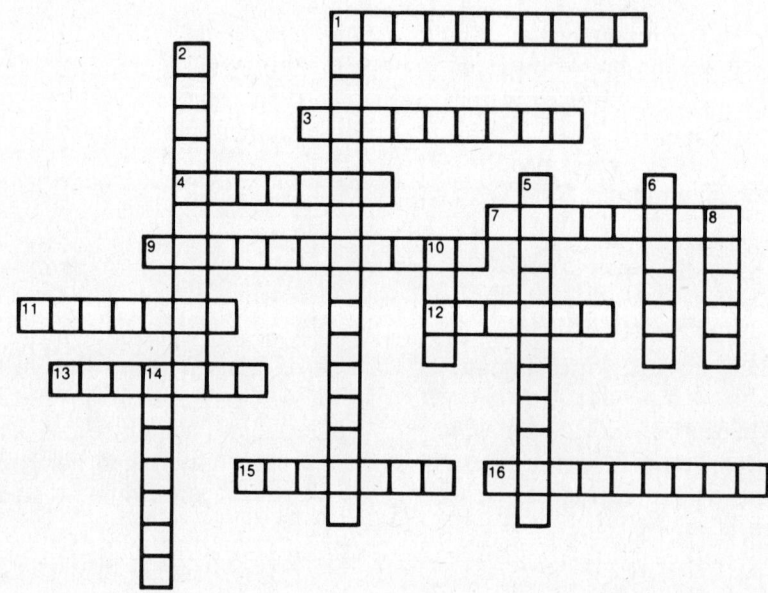

ACROSS

1. A complication caused by proteolytic enzymes used as debriding agents
3. Enzymes that break down protein
4. An adverse reaction to proteinases of animal origin
7. A tissue enzyme required for activation of hydrogen peroxide
9. The generic name for Debrisan
11. The route used for administration of debriding agents
12. The chemical classification of proteases
13. The chemical nature of most enzymes
15. Necrotic material that collects in a wound
16. The generic name for Travase

DOWN

1. A debriding agent that effervesces
2. The generic name for Santyl
5. An adverse reaction caused by prolonged use of H_2O_2 mouthwash
6. A solution used to clean wounds in preparation for application of debriding agents
8. The trade name for a preparation containing fibrinolysin and desoxyribonuclease
10. Organs to which proteases are harmful
14. A proteolytic enzyme that is a digestant secreted by the pancreas

21
Anti-inflammatory and Related Agents

The inflammatory process is composed of multiple physiologic responses to a stimulus and is primarily a protective mechanism essential for survival. Fever and pain are cardinal signs and symptoms of inflammation that may require intervention, including the use of certain medications. The drugs reviewed in this chapter include the following: the salicylates; pyrazolon, indoleacetic acid, indeneacetic acid, pyrrole acetic acid, propionic acid, fenamic acid, and para-aminophenol derivatives; gold compounds; drugs used in the management of gout; and uricosurics.

Matching
Match the following preparations listed by their generic name in the left-hand column with their trade names listed in the right-hand column. Place your answer in the space provided.

_____ 1. Phenylbutazone
_____ 2. Indomethacin
_____ 3. Ibuprofen
_____ 4. Naproxen
_____ 5. Meclofenamate
_____ 6. Mefenamic acid

a. Tolectin
b. Butazolidin
c. Ponstel
d. Tandearil
e. Meclomen
f. Dolobid
g. Indocin
h. Nalfon
i. Clinoril
j. Naprosyn
k. Motrin

Short Answer Questions
1. Explain the role of prostaglandins in the inflammatory process.

2. At what point in the process of prostaglandin synthesis do many drugs discussed in this chapter appear to interfere? How does this action help the patient?

3. Identify the four therapeutic properties of acetylsalicylic acid, and explain each.
   a.

   b.

   c.

   d.

4. List at least four specific uses for acetylsalicylic acid.
   a.
   b.
   c.
   d.

85

5. Define salicylism. What would you observe about the client experiencing this syndrome?

6. Explain how acetylsalicylic acid can have a negative effect on the process of coagulation.

7. To lessen gastric irritation, how can many anti-inflammatory medications be taken?
   a.
   b.
   c.
8. Name three drugs that would cause a drug–drug interaction complication if taken with phenylbutazone.

9. What is the most frequent side effect seen with indomethacin?

10. How do the therapeutic properties of the para-aminophenol derivatives differ from those of acetylsalicylic acid?

11. Explain what is meant by analgesic abuse nephropathy. Who is at risk? What agent(s) is (are) responsible?

12. Review the process of acute poisoning with acetaminophen. What agent is being used as an antidote?

13. How long would the typical patient have to continue with gold therapy before improvement would be noted?

14. Describe the cutaneous and mucous membrane lesions seen with gold therapy.

15. What would be considered to be the most serious complication of chrysotherapy?

16. What is the difference between primary and secondary gout?

17. Explain the mechanism of action of colchicine.

18. List two specific uses for allopurinol.
    a.
    b.
19. Describe the mechanism of action of allopurinol.

20. Describe the use of probenecid as adjunct therapy with penicillin.

21. Why is alkalinization of urine recommended with gout, and how is it accomplished?

UNIT FIVE: DRUGS AFFECTING THE NERVOUS SYSTEM

22 Autonomic Drugs

The autonomic nervous system controls vital functions of the body and the physiologic balance of the total organism. Autonomic drugs are those chemicals that change this balance, either by altering the function of the autonomic system or by augmenting or counteracting its effects. Nurses must understand autonomic functions, therefore, to understand the actions and effects of autonomic drugs.

Matching

A. Match the drug or condition in the left-hand column with the appropriate antidote from the right-hand column. Place your answer in the space provided.

_____ 1. Parathion
_____ 2. Norepinephrine
_____ 3. Mushroom poisoning
_____ 4. Nerve gas
_____ 5. Phentolamine
_____ 6. Malathion
_____ 7. Insect sting allergy

a. Norepinephrine
b. Atropine
c. Epinephrine
d. Phentolamine

B. Match the physiologic response in the left-hand column with its mode of autonomic activity in the right-hand column.

_____ 1. Miosis
_____ 2. Bradycardia
_____ 3. Bronchodilation
_____ 4. Increased respiratory secretion
_____ 5. Constriction of gastrointestinal sphincters
_____ 6. Increased contractility of the urinary bladder
_____ 7. Secretion of epinephrine and norepinephrine
_____ 8. Increased blood glucose concentration

a. Sympathetic
b. Parasympathetic

C. Match the drug in the left-hand column with its class(es) or use(s) in the right-hand column.

_____ 1. Epinephrine
_____ 2. Atropine
_____ 3. Neostigmine
_____ 4. Propranolol
_____ 5. Norepinephrine
_____ 6. Isoproterenol
_____ 7. Phenylephrine

a. Cholinergic
b. Adrenergic
c. Anticholinergic
d. Sympathetic blocking agent
e. Hyperglycemic
f. Used to control life-threatening vasogenic shock
g. Used to treat angina pectoris
h. Nasal decongestant
i. First choice for the treatment of anaphylaxis
j. Administered preoperatively to inhibit respiratory secretions
k. Used to alleviate bronchospasm
l. Used in the treatment of myasthenia gravis

Find the Hidden Words

Hidden within the following letter grid are words and phrases from Chapter 22. They may be vertical, horizontal, or diagonal. Circle the letters as you find the hidden words.

LIST OF WORDS AND PHRASES

adrenalin
adrenergic
amnesia
anticholinergic
atropine
belladonna
cholinergic
epinephrine
ergot
ganglia
levophed
midriasis
miosis
muscarine
neostigmine
nerve gas
nicotine
norepinephrine
parasympathomimetic
phentolamine
reserpine
sarin
scopolamine
soman
sympathetic
tabun

```
d a r d r s c o p b u t a n t i a a d m p h e t n
t d a d a e i o a n t i p a r a i c g r a n t i i
a h a m u s c a r i n e h y p s s y m p a m i n c
c r a t r o p n a a d r e n e p i a s i s m b a t
d x c o p o r e s e r p i n e f n a g r e n e n a
c i g a r a p p y s o i m i o s i a d e n o m p b
n e p h r i r a m m e a n i t n n a r e v o l a p
d a i t l e v o p h e d d n l g i d n e a r d a h
n e d e d o n i a n t i a r l e a i e d e p e n i
s a r i n u b a t a c i g r e n i l o h c i t n a
i i a a b o s a h i s n p n i n e r s s t i t d u
i m m a d s u m o y d e i i i p e o t n c i g r t
p n s n i i d i m n e r p p i n b r i c a i c a o
n e i t m s a p i c h e c e o p e c g d c i b c a
s y m c h a a t m p p h e n t o l a m i n e s i u
e l h c o t e p e c o t i i t o l i i e c y c b t
i n e p h t o n t l v i n p t i a n n h m c m e o
a l i e p i i n i e e e h o g a d r e n a l i n n
p e t p e p h n c r l a g r n r o g i c a t d i o
n i a h e p e d e p h r n t e c n u s a n t r i m
c r n r a r p h r i e p i a i c n t i i t a i s i
t a o e g a n g l i a d e n a m a a i o s i a h c
t n a i s c o p o l a m i n e p n b n a m o s o m
n t c w p h e d r i a s i s i t a t d r e n i m a
a i i h a p p r i o d l n i i p i r i a s i s m n
n c t p o p h i a s r d e s p a e p i n e p i n e
i c i g r e n i l o h c i t n a p h e d r e i s t
```

Correct the False Statement

Indicate whether the following statements are true or false; if false, correct the underlined words or phrases.

_____ 1. Ephedrine has a <u>shorter</u> duration of action than does epinephrine.

_____ 2. A serious adverse effect of adrenergic hormones and drugs is an <u>increased risk of cardiac arrhythmias</u>.

_____ 3. The action of dobutamide <u>is dependent</u> on release of endogenous norepinephrine.

_____ 4. It is important that the use of adrenergic vasoconstrictors to treat hypotensive shock be preceded by <u>fluid volume replacement</u>.

_____ 5. When surgery is contemplated for persons who have been receiving adrenergic blocking agents, it is important that the dosage of the medication be <u>increased on the day of the surgery</u>.

_____ 6. The active ingredients in many insecticides and nerve gas are <u>antiadrenergics</u>.

_____ 7. <u>Cholinergic or anticholinesterase</u> eye drops are often used in the treatment of chronic glaucoma.

_____ 8. The principal toxins in mushrooms are <u>nicotinic</u> compounds.

_____ 9. Nicotine <u>is absorbed through the skin</u> by workers handling tobacco.

_____ 10. The milk of lactating mothers contains nicotine concentrations <u>proportional to</u> the amount absorbed by the mother.

_____ 11. When administering eye drops, the nurse should <u>position the client so the excess medication will drain from the eye into the tear duct</u>.

Completion Exercises

On the drawing at right, identify and label the following:
1. The nerve terminal of the presynaptic nerve cell
2. The postsynaptic receptor cell
3. The synaptic contact zone
4. The postsynaptic receptor area
5. Organelles and enzymes that synthesize, store, release, and actively reuptake transmitter chemicals
6. Organelles that respond to receptor triggers

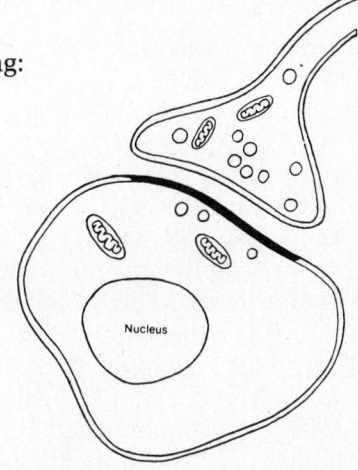

Multiple Choice Questions

For each of the following, choose the one best answer.

1. Which of the following drugs cannot safely be injected subcutaneously?
   a. Epinephrine
   b. Norepinephrine
   c. Terbutaline
   d. Bethanechol

2. Which of the following drugs is effective when administered orally?
   a. Epinephrine
   b. Norepinephrine
   c. Dopamine
   d. Ephedrine

3. Adrenergic drugs are substances that produce a physiologic response resembling that of
   a. Parasympathetic stimulation
   b. Parasympathetic inhibition
   c. Sympathetic stimulation
   d. Sympathetic inhibition

4. A cathecholamine is defined as a drug that
   a. Mimics parasympathetic nervous system activity
   b. Mimics sympathetic nervous system activity
   c. Contains a steroid nucleus in its structure
   d. Contains dihydroxybenzene in its structure

5. Isoproterenol is a(n)
   a. Acid drug
   b. Basic drug
   c. Neutral drug

6. Contraindications for the use of isoproterenol include
   a. Vasogenic shock
   b. Tachycardia
   c. Bronchoconstriction
   d. Heart block

7. Epinephrine is usually administered
   a. Orally
   b. By inhalation
   c. By injection
   d. Transdermally

8. Dopamine is usually administered
   a. PO
   b. SC
   c. IV

9. An enzyme active in the degradation and deactivation of sympathomimetic drugs is
   a. Catalase
   b. Succinyl dehydrogenase
   c. Anticholinesterase
   d. Monoamine oxidase

10. Over-the-counter preparations recommended as "decongestants" are likely to contain the following as active ingredients:
    a. Cholinergic drugs
    b. Anticholinergic drugs
    c. Adrenergic drugs
    d. Sympathetic blocking agents
11. Prolonged use or high doses of dopamine may result in gangrene secondary to
    a. Arterial thromboembolism
    b. Vascular degeneration
    c. Peripheral vasoconstriction
    d. All of the above
12. Propranolol exerts its pharmacologic actions by
    a. Stimulating β-adrenergic receptors
    b. Blocking β-adrenergic receptors
    c. Stimulating cholinergic receptors
    d. Blocking cholinergic receptors
13. A food that can cause peripheral vascular insufficiency or abortion is
    a. Hard cheese containing tyramine
    b. Moldy flour containing ergot
    c. Moldy food containing aflatoxins
    d. "Sunburned" potatoes containing solanine
14. Vascular effects of ergot alkaloids include
    a. Dilation of hypertonic vessels
    b. Constriction of hypotonic vessels
    c. Both of the above
    d. Neither of the above
15. A hallucinogen chemically related to ergot is
    a. Lysergic acid diethylamide (LSD)
    b. Dichlorodiphenyltrichloroethane (DDT)
    c. Tetrahydrocannabinol
    d. Phencyclidine hydrochloride (PCP)
16. To be effective in treating migraine headache, ergot alkaloids should be administered
    a. At least once a day as a preventative
    b. At the first signs or symptom of the attack
    c. After the initial stage of the attack, when the headache is well established
    d. Only when the severity of the headache becomes intense
17. The body tends to store phenoxybenzamine in
    a. Fat
    b. Bone
    c. The thyroid gland
    d. The cerebrospinal fluid
18. A side effect of β-adrenergic blockers is a(n)
    a. Increased heart rate
    b. Impairment of response to stress
    c. Decrease in respiratory secretions
    d. Increased concentration of glucose in the blood
19. Clients receiving drug treatment for myasthenia gravis sometimes develop impaired respirations similar to those of the untreated disease. When this problem is caused by the medication, it is called
    a. Anaphylaxis
    b. Tachyphylaxis
    c. Myasthenia crisis
    d. Addisonian crisis
    e. Cholinergic crisis
20. The above condition is usually treated by
    1. Administration of atropine
    2. Increasing the dose of cholinergics
    3. Discontinuation of the cholinergics
    4. Mechanically assisted respirations
        (a) 1, 2
        (b) 1, 3
        (c) 1, 4
        (d) 2, 4
        (e) 3, 4
21. Side effects of cholinergic drugs include
    a. Bronchodilation
    b. Relaxation of smooth muscle
    c. Urinary retention
    d. Increased peristalsis
22. A drug that is contraindicated in glaucoma is
    a. Atropine
    b. Pilocarpine
    c. Morphine
    d. Reserpine
23. Clients receiving atropine as a preoperative medication should be informed that they are likely to experience
    a. A temporary urge to defecate
    b. A temporary urge to urinate
    c. A dry mouth
    d. Heartburn
24. The usual adult dose of atropine is
    a. 300 μg to 400 μg
    b. 300 mg to 400 mg
    c. 3 g to 4 g
    d. 10 g to 12 g

25. Nurses who handle atropine carelessly are likely to develop
    a. Impairment of sexual function
    b. Urinary retention
    c. Contact dermatitis
    d. Blurred vision
26. The first drug used in the treatment of anaphylaxis is usually
    a. Atropine
    b. Neostigmine
    c. Propanolol
    d. Epinephrine
27. Nicotine acts as
    a. A nervous system stimulant
    b. A nervous system depressant
    c. Both of the above
    d. Neither of the above
28. The sites of action of nicotine are the brain and
    a. Presynaptic fibers in the autonomic system
    b. Autonomic ganglia
    c. Adrenergic cell receptors
    d. Cholinergic cell receptors
29. The action of nicotine is
    a. Antagonistic
    b. Competitive
    c. Biphasic
    d. All of the above
30. Ganglionic blocking agents are usually administered for the purpose of
    a. Blocking the effects of nicotine
    b. Reducing vasoconstriction
    c. Enhancing the effects of anesthetics
    d. Increasing blood pressure
31. An antidote for cholinergic drugs is
    a. Atropine
    b. Neostigmine
    c. Propranolol
    d. Epinephrine
32. Your client, 25-year-old Mr. Butz, tells you that he cut down from two packs of cigarettes a day to one pack per day 3 years ago. He began smoking at the age of 15. His cumulative exposure to smoking is approximately
    a. 6 pack years
    b. 10 pack years
    c. 15 pack years
    d. 17 pack years
33. According to the textbook, nicotine
    a. Causes only psychologic dependence
    b. Causes only physical dependence
    c. Causes both psychologic and physical dependence
    d. Does not produce withdrawal symptoms
34. Exposure to cigarette smoke increases the toxicity of the pollutant
    a. Acid rain
    b. Asbestos
    c. DDT
    d. Chlorine
35. People with severe allergy are often advised to carry emergency kits for self-administration of
    a. Atropine
    b. Epinephrine
    c. Norepinephrine
    d. Phentolamine

Selection of Options

For each of the following, select *all* appropriate responses. Circle correct answers.

1. Adrenergic drugs tend to cause the following side effects:
    a. Vasodilation
    b. Central nervous system stimulation
    c. Muscle tremor
2. In the autonomic nervous system the neurotransmitter acetylcholine is responsible for the transmission of impulses
    a. Across most preganglionic synapses of the parasympathetic system
    b. Across most postganglionic synapses of the parasympathetic system
    c. Across most preganglionic synapses of the sympathetic system
    d. Across most postganglionic synapses of the sympathetic system
    e. In most ganglionic synapses
3. Following transmission of an impulse, neurotransmitters in the synaptic gap are dissipated by
    a. Rapid transport away from the area by lymphatic and venous drainage
    b. Rapid breakdown by tissue enzymes
    c. Active reuptake by the axon terminal
    d. Absorption by the postsynaptic receptor area
4. Physiologic effects of epinephrine include
    a. Stimulation of α-adrenergic receptors
    b. Stimulation of β-adrenergic receptors
    c. Miosis
    d. Tachycardia
    e. Bronchodilation
    f. Release of histamine in allergic reactions

5. Routes used for administration of epinephrine include
   a. PO
   b. SC
   c. Inhalation
6. Catecholamine drugs include
   a. Ephedrine
   b. Epinephrine
   c. Norepinephrine
   d. Amphetamines
7. Contraindications for the use of epinephrine include
   a. Hypotension
   b. Angina pectoris
   c. Allergic reaction
   d. Hyperthyroidism
   e. Pheochromocytoma
8. Appropriate routes for administering norepinephrine include
   a. PO
   b. SC
   c. IM
   d. IV
   e. Inhalation
9. Isoproterenol acts by stimulating
   a. α-adrenergic receptors
   b. $β_1$-adrenergic receptors
   c. $β_2$-adrenergic receptors
10. Sympathetic drugs that are effective when administered orally include
    a. Amphetamine
    b. Ephedrine
    c. Epinephrine
    d. Terbutaline
11. Adrenergic blocking agents are likely to produce the following cardiovascular effects:
    a. Decreased blood pressure
    b. Postural hypotension
    c. Bradycardia
12. Side effects of sympathomimetic drugs include
    a. Anorexia
    b. Fatigability
    c. Drowsiness
    d. Dry skin
13. Ergot alkaloids should not be given to people suffering from
    a. Arteritis
    b. Hypotension
    c. Phlebitis
    d. Severe arteriosclerosis
14. Clients who are treated for migraine with ergot alkaloids should be monitored for
    a. Warm sweaty extremities
    b. Cold painful extremities
    c. Peripheral numbness and tingling
15. Therapeutic uses of phentolamine include
    a. Diagnosis of pheochromocytoma
    b. Prevention of tissue necrosis caused by norepinephrine infiltration
    c. Control of paroxysmal hypertension during surgical removal of pheochromocytoma
16. Therapeutic uses for β-adrenergic blocking agents include the
    a. Treatment of asthma
    b. Treatment of tachycardia
    c. Control of angina pectoris
    d. Prevention of repeated myocardial infarctions
17. Contraindications for β-adrenergic blockers include
    a. Obstructive airway disease characterized by bronchospasm
    b. Angina pectoris
    c. Bradycardia
    d. Hypertension
    e. Congestive heart failure
18. Clients receiving adrenergic blocking agents should be taught
    a. To change position slowly to prevent postural hypotension
    b. To increase salt intake to prevent hypovolemia
    c. Skills in stress management
    d. To avoid the use of over-the-counter decongestants
19. Adverse reactions to cholinergics include
    a. Bronchospasm
    b. Urinary retention
    c. Increased gastric acidity
    d. Blurred vision secondary to midriasis
20. Side effects of anticholinesterases include
    a. Dry skin
    b. Salivation
    c. Bradycardia
    d. Bronchodilation
21. Those likely to experience adverse reactions to atropine include people with a history of
    a. Bladder outlet obstruction
    b. Glaucoma
    c. Hypermotility of the bowel
    d. Hyperthyroidism
    e. Gastric hypersecretion
22. Autonomic drugs that act as miotics include
    a. Cholinergic drugs
    b. Anticholinesterases
    c. Anticholinergics
    d. Adrenergics

Short Answer Questions

1. Name the two main divisions of the central nervous system.

2. Identify the two main divisions of the brain.

3. Give at least two physiologic "centers" in the brain stem that control visceral functions.

4. Name four subdivisions of the sympathetic nervous system.

5. Identify two subdivisions of the parasympathetic nervous system.

6. Give the four main classifications of autonomic drugs.

7. Identify four uses for cholinergic drugs.

8. What is the anatomic relationship between the cranial nerves and the autonomic nervous system?

9. Name three factors to consider when scheduling doses of cholinergic drugs prescribed to treat myasthenia gravis.

10. Identify at least six signs and symptoms of acute nicotine poisoning.

11. Name at least five known health hazards associated with smoking cigarettes.

12. Define tachyphylaxis.

23
Central Nervous System Stimulants

A mechanism known as the blood–brain barrier controls the distribution of drugs within the central nervous system. Response to central nervous system drugs depends largely on the status of the person: underlying personality, physiologic function, and mental "set." Response is also influenced by the client's history and environment.

Matching

A. Match the description in the left-hand column with the appropriate drug in the right-hand column. Place your answer in the space provided.

    _____ 1. Ingredient of smelling salts   a. Strychnine
    _____ 2. Analeptic sometimes used to diagnose epilepsy   b. Picrotoxin
                                      c. Pentylenetetrazole (Metrazol)
    _____ 3. Ingredient of rat poison   d. Spirits of ammonia

Short Answer Questions

1. A xanthine used to treat apnea in premature infants is _____ .
2. List at least three nursing measures helpful to clients receiving therapeutic doses of theophylline.

3. Name at least four signs and symptoms of xanthine toxicity.

4. What is the proper procedure for administering smelling salts?

5. List at least three adverse effects of long-term use of cocaine.

6. By what route is medicinal cocaine administered?

7. What is a flashback?

8. Name two nursing measures helpful in the treatment of someone experiencing a "bad trip" following use of a hallucinogen.

9. List at least four beneficial effects of central nervous system stimulants.

10. Name at least four adverse reactions or toxic symptoms caused by central nervous system stimulants.

11. Give at least four therapeutic uses for amphetamines.

Find the Hidden Words

Hidden within the following letter grid are words and phrases from Chapter 23. They may be vertical, horizontal, or diagonal. Circle the letters as you find the hidden words.

```
b a e c c t r i s o m e t a l c h e m p n i p a n d t u c k o c o l d s
a l a b a c i t r e m e n a r c h o r o l a c o l l e b e n t o v i g l
c m e t r a l c o h y p e r a g t r i r i h o k c a b h s a l f r y r i
k u v b e s r l l s s n e s s i i t h e o p h y l l i n e v r r s a r c
t s e n s e i o e a a a n g i n a r e y e a n i x o t o r c i p e n i k
o c t e t i p n e l a t i o n t g e o m t r i c u m i b e t e l i v r e
b a n a l n p a l p i t a t i o n s e c o e s n e c t o a l e e h c o r
a n e b o n d i h e x a l g h a l a b f i n i a x h a b o s i v a a c a
c n u c t e c h y p e r a c t i v e r e f l e x e s i c o n t o i n y d
k a p t a b r a p p r e h e n s i o n t a o v a n l r p h o s d o n w i
h a h s o m t r e m o r a n g i n e j t a o c n i a s i n i f o l a e r
a b o t p e p i r n n o b b a d t r i p c o c t n r i s d s l p v b e c
n c r v q t i h t e a b i e f i a r e s t l y h h e n n i l y a l i t a
e n i m o r b o e h t c n x o i t i e n i m a i c p t o b u a m i s w r
c i a n s a n t n t a i n t n a i p a v l u m n y p a i t v g p o s i m
t a y n a z i t s i a e m o r d n y s s e t t e r u o t a n a h i a b o
o m a h v o t r i c o m m r e x n a o e i f i n t s i a n o r e c t i c
p p t a m l r d o p a m i n e c t i l b g n o i s u f n o c i n c i l c
a h a a d o r c n a a f n n f d d r o e v e s o i p f i h o c i l v i a
n a t i n a t v a i b i f a e l a t m m p a l o c h o c o l a t e a n b
t i r e r e s t l e s s n e s s u t a w i t o o m a i u c o c o l a t e
r r f a c s e t r e o n p i i a u n u t w r i h c n s l v s o d o w b n
y b a l r s h n v r r s i s e n i k r e p y h c a e i l s u d l v m e t
x t e l b e j q u t h y p o a c e b r s h i s p n b c a c o h c a i n y
a l b e l l a d o w d y m n t e s o o t y p a h t r c h i n o i l t n l
```

LIST OF WORDS AND PHRASES

agitation
ammonia
analeptic
amphetamines
angina
anorectic
anorexia
anxiety
apprehension
bad trip
bennies
betel
caffeine
cannabis sativa
chocolate
cocaine
coffee

cola
confusion
convulsions
dopamine
elation
fever
flashback
fly agaric
hallucinations
hyperactive reflexes
hyperkinesis
hypertension
insomnia
irritability
khat
LSD
levodopa

metrazol
narcolepsy
nutmeg
palpitation
panic
restlessness
ritalin
speed
strychnine
tea
theophylline
theobromine
Tourette's syndrome
tremor
wt loss
xanthine

Correct the False Statement

Indicate whether the following statements are true or false; if false, correct the underlined words or phrases.

_____ 1. Amphetamine exerts its pharmacologic action primarily by <u>directly stimulating norepinephrine receptors in the nervous system</u>.

_____ 2. Amphetamines are most likely to produce tolerance <u>when high doses are used over long periods of time</u>.

_____ 3.. Among the physiologic effects of xanthine compounds are an increased <u>basal metabolic rate and diuresis</u>.

_____ 4. Xanthines can <u>enhance</u> the performance of <u>motor skills</u> that have been incompletely mastered.

_____ 5. The metabolism of levodopa by body tissues converts it <u>to an inactive substance that is highly water-soluble</u>.

_____ 6. Dopamine is not useful in the treatment of Parkinson's syndrome because <u>it is metabolized rapidly by the peripheral tissues</u>.

_____ 7. Clients receiving phenytoin for control of seizures who develop Parkinson's syndrome may require <u>a relatively low dose of levodopa to prevent adverse reactions</u>.

_____ 8. Optimal response to levodopa therapy usually occurs <u>1 week to 10 days</u> after treatment is initiated.

_____ 9. Smelling salts are used <u>to prevent fainting</u>.

_____ 10. The abuse of central nervous system <u>depressants</u> is more likely to be associated with homicidal and suicidal tendencies than is the use of central nervous system <u>stimulants</u>.

_____ 11. Hallucinogenic drugs appear to act as <u>antagonists</u> on nerve cell receptors that normally respond to endogenous neurotransmitters.

_____ 12. Anesthetics are <u>ascending</u> central nervous system depressants.

_____ 13. Many general anesthetics pose a hazard because <u>they are flammable and explosive</u>.

_____ 14. Analgesics are <u>not</u> required during anesthesia because general anesthetics <u>completely abolish</u> pain sensations.

_____ 15. Solutions of local anesthetics containing epinephrine must not be employed if the area to be anesthetized <u>involves a large mass of tissue</u>.

_____ 16. Spinal anesthesia produces <u>temporary paralysis of the lower extremities</u>.

Multiple Choice Questions

For each of the following, choose the one best answer.

1. What is the blood–brain barrier?
   a. A lipid membrane that allows passage by diffusion of lipid-soluble chemicals only
   b. A semipermeable membrane that allows passage of ionized radicals only
   c. An active physiologic mechanism with functions similar to those of an active transport system
   d. All of the above

2. Stimulants should be used in small doses, if at all, for clients with
   a. Asthma
   b. Addison's disease
   c. Hypothyroidism
   d. Hyperthyroidism
3. Amphetamines act as stimulants to
   a. The central nervous system
   b. α-adrenergic receptors
   c. β-adrenergic receptors
   d. All of the above
4. A client known to have taken a large dose of amphetamines should be monitored for
   a. Hypotensive shock
   b. Bradycardia
   c. Hyperthermia
   d. All of the above
5. Elimination of amphetamines is enhanced by
   a. Stimulation of bile secretion
   b. Lowering the pH of the urine
   c. Raising the pH of the urine
   d. None of the above; elimination is influenced only by changes in the glomerular filtration rate
6. How do the amphetamines affect sleep?
   a. They delay or inhibit onset of sleep by increasing mental alertness
   b. They suppress REM sleep
   c. Neither of the above
   d. Both a and b above
7. One drug that can promote elimination of amphetamines, in cases of acute toxicity, is
   a. Sodium bicarbonate
   b. Ammonium chloride
   c. 5% dextrose in water
   d. Phentolamine
8. In chronic or heavy users, withdrawal of amphetamines is followed by physical and emotional symptoms. Are amphetamines considered to cause dependence?
   a. Yes, they are believed to cause psychologic dependence but not physical dependence
   b. Yes, they are believed to cause physical dependence but not psychologic dependence
   c. Yes, they are known to cause both psychologic and physical dependence
   d. The extent to which the withdrawal syndrome is caused by psychologic or physical dependence is unknown
9. Are amphetamines acceptable for use in treating obesity?
   a. No, their use is forbidden by FDA regulation
   b. Yes, provided the client is under close medical supervision
   c. Sometimes, for the first 2 weeks of a weight reduction regimen
   d. Yes, provided the client has been screened for factors that increase the risk of toxic effects
10. According to the text, the most promising approach to the problem of drug abuse is
    a. Teaching the facts about drugs to children, beginning in elementary school
    b. Promoting the growth of self-esteem and self-confidence in children
    c. Strict enforcement of drug control legislation and regulations
    d. Legalizing the use of drugs such as marijuana
11. What type of chemicals are the xanthines?
    a. Inorganic salts
    b. Catecholamines
    c. Aldehydes
    d. Alkaloids
12. At what blood concentration does theophylline usually produce toxic symptoms?
    a. 2 μg/ml or more
    b. 5 μg/ml or more
    c. 10 μg/ml or more
    d. 20 μg/ml or more
13. The *primary* medical use of the administration of the xanthine theophylline is to promote
    a. Diuresis
    b. Bronchodilation
    c. Stimulation of the respiratory center
    d. Stimulation of intestinal secretion
14. A drug used to treat convulsions caused by theophylline is
    a. Diazepam (Valium)
    b. Flurazepam (Dalmane)
    c. Phenytoin (Dilantin)
    d. Phenobarbital (Luminal)
15. A xanthine administered intravenously in the treatment of obstructive airway disease is
    a. Caffeine sodium benzoate
    b. Ethylenediamine (aminophylline)
    c. Theobromine (Theo-Dur)
    d. Xantheline

16. To reduce the severity of side effects from levodopa, the drug is usually administered in conjunction with
    a. Carbidopa
    b. Phenobarbital
    c. Diazepam (Valium)
    d. Monoamine oxidase inhibitors
17. Caffeine withdrawal is likely to be accompanied by
    a. Lethargy
    b. Headache
    c. Convulsions
    d. Hallucinations
18. When levodopa treatment is begun, the first doses are usually
    a. Larger than subsequent maintenance doses to saturate storage depots
    b. Smaller than maintenance doses to avoid toxic reactions
    c. Carefully calculated to establish the required maintenance dose
    d. Given parenterally until a therapeutic response has been achieved
19. Individuals receiving levodopa for the treatment of Parkinson's syndrome should be advised to
    a. Maintain a stable level of vitamin K in the diet
    b. Maintain a stable level of pyridoxine in the diet
    c. Avoid foods containing xanthines
    d. Eat plenty of green leafy vegetables
20. If tremors increase after initiation of levodopa therapy, the nurse should
    a. Contact the physician for an order to increase the dosage
    b. Withhold the drug and notify the physician
    c. Suggest that the physician order a muscle relaxant
    d. Inform the client that this sometimes occurs when medication is begun, but that it usually is temporary
21. Risus sardonicus is a sign of toxicity from
    a. Amphetamines
    b. Strychnine
    c. Diazepam
    d. Heroin
22. Clients receiving analeptics such as Metrazol should
    a. Receive concomitant tranquilizer medications
    b. Be placed on seizure precautions
    c. Be monitored for hypertension
    d. Be monitored for signs and symptoms of psychosis
23. Cocaine is a derivative of
    a. The opium poppy
    b. The cocoa bean
    c. The coca leaves
    d. Catecholamines
24. Medicinally, cocaine is used as a(n)
    a. Local anesthetic
    b. Central nervous system stimulant
    c. Analeptic
    d. Tranquilizer
25. Persons who "snort" cocaine regularly are likely to develop
    a. Hepatitis B
    b. Lethargy and stupor
    c. Needle "tracks" on the extremities
    d. Perforation of the nasal septum
26. The serum half-life of cocaine is approximately
    a. 2 to 5 minutes
    b. 20 to 30 minutes
    c. 1 hour
    d. 4 to 6 hours
27. What is a "speedball"?
    a. Hashish (ingestible preparation of marijuana)
    b. An ingestible preparation of amphetamine and cocaine
    c. An injection containing both amphetamine and morphine
    d. An injection containing both cocaine and heroin
28. Injecting cocaine increases the risk of
    a. Hypotensive shock
    b. Cardiac arrest
    c. Paradoxic sedation
    d. Erosion of the nasal septum
29. An hallucinogen approved for medicinal use is
    a. Lysergic acid diethylamide
    b. Psilocybin
    c. Mescaline
    d. Scopolamine

Selection of Options

For each of the following, select *all* appropriate responses. Circle correct answers.

1. Clients recovering from amphetamine overdose are likely to experience
   a. Prolongation of REM sleep
   b. Fatigue and lethargy
   c. Episodic hyperactivity
   d. Emotional depression
2. Which of the following foods contain xanthine stimulants?
   a. Coffee
   b. Ginger ale
   c. Chocolate candy
   d. Licorice candy
   e. Tea
   f. Cola beverages
   g. Wine
3. Adverse reactions to levodopa include
   a. Epigastric distress
   b. Change in bowel function
   c. Excess salivation
   d. Restlessness
   e. Inappropriate sexuality
4. Levodopa should not be given to people who
   a. Are receiving allopurinol
   b. Have narrow-angle glaucoma
   c. Have had malignant melanoma
   d. Have heart disease
5. When levodopa therapy is initiated, the client should be monitored carefully for
   a. Abnormal cardiac rhythms
   b. Change in respiratory function
   c. Signs of renal and liver impairment
   d. Gastrointestinal upset
6. When cocaine anesthesia is used for bronchoscopy, the client requires intensive nursing care during the recovery period to prevent or detect
   a. Persistent unconsciousness
   b. Cardiovascular irregularities
   c. Aspiration of secretions
   d. Respiratory problems
7. Examples of hallucinogens are
   a. Heroin
   b. Barbiturates
   c. LSD
   d. Peyote
8. How do hallucinogenic drugs affect reproduction? They
   a. Appear to be mutagenic
   b. May be teratogenic
   c. Appear to cause chromosome breakage
   d. Reduce fertility
   e. Induce abortion

24
Central Nervous System Depressants

Among the central nervous depressants discussed in Chapter 24 are many agents used to control pain and promote rest and sleep, as well as drugs of abuse. The following exercises deal with this material.

Matching

A. Match the drug or condition in the left-hand column with the pupil response in the right-hand column.

    _____ 1. Morphine   a. Midriasis (dilation)
    _____ 2. Cocaine   b. Miosis (constriction)
    _____ 3. Amphetamine
    _____ 4. Heroin
    _____ 5. Scopolamine
    _____ 6. Meperidine
    _____ 7. Withdrawal from opioids

B. Match the pathologic process in the left-hand column with the type of hallucination in the right-hand column.

    _____ 1. Opioid withdrawal   a. Visual
    _____ 2. Schizophrenia   b. Auditory
    _____ 3. Alcohol withdrawal   c. Tactile
    _____ 4. A blow on the back of the head   d. Olfactory
    _____ 5. Tumors at the base of the brain
    _____ 6. Use of ototoxic drugs

Short Answer Questions

1. Identify at least three characteristics common to toxic reactions to most central nervous system depressants.

2. List at least six types of drugs likely to be used when general anesthesia is required for surgery (include preoperative and anesthetic agents).

3. Identify at least two approaches helpful in the treatment of psychologic dependence on central nervous system depressants.

4. Under what schedule of the Controlled Substance Act of 1970 does pentazocine (Talwin) fall?

5. Does propoxyphene (Darvon) cause physical dependence?

6. Name at least four nursing measures to promote sleep.

Find the Hidden Word

Hidden within the following grid are words and phrases from Chapter 24. They may be vertical, horizontal, or diagonal. Circle the letters as you find the words.

LIST OF WORDS AND PHRASES

alcohol	halothane	nitrous oxide
analgesic	heroin	opioid
anesthetic	hypnotic	propoxyphene
apnea	meperidine	REM sleep
barbiturate	miosis	reticular activating system
coma	morphine	sedative
dissociative	naloxone	twilight sleep
ether	neurolept	

```
m o r p r o p o x e h e r o e t h e r e r h t e i r b
m e p e n e h p q a n a n i t v s l e e a n a l i g a
a n e s t h e t i c m o r t i n i l c l x j u p s e r
p i n t w i l m o r p h x a n o p t o p i u s e d a b
e d i i x w r a n g e r o u t i t a s h e r o d s i
r i t r l o c n o c t r a i l e h e r i e a n a v a s
i r i p i d a i l i w t h e m a r c o v c r e h p r o
d e m a h l s e d a p y t o n o n s i c r o s p o r p
e p s r g a j e n e p a r e r p a t i i a h s e d a e
p e r e t i c u l a r a c t i v a t i n g s y s t e m
r m s i s i c o m u l e n a i d o n e a l c i p i n e
e i v r l n r i t c i n m o e n i t r o u s o x i d e
c c g u e u a i o r a i l s p o m a s p o t o n p y h
o i l e e a b h n p y h a y l p n t a i p e l o r a l
d t a n p r o p o x y p h e n e h i m o e h t e l o h
e e n m a l e p t w i r e h t h e r o i n u h o c l a
i r a b a r b i t w i o p i a n a p c d i t t r o m l
t e r e t i c u a c t m e p e r i d i n e h s e d a f
```

Correct the False Statement

Indicate whether the following statements are true or false; if false, correct the underlined words or phrases.

_____ 1. Codeine exerts its effect on the central nervous system <u>only after it has been transformed by the tissues to morphine</u>.

_____ 2. <u>Most</u> of a given dose of morphine crosses the blood–brain barrier.

_____ 3. Heroin <u>cannot</u> legally be prescribed for medicinal use in the United States.

_____ 4. People with <u>hypothyroidism</u> are relatively insensitive to opioids.

_____ 5. Opioids are generally contraindicated in <u>severe head injury and obstructive airway disease</u>.

_____ 6. In most states, narcotic control regulations require that opioid analgesics be stored in <u>locked cabinets</u>.

_____ 7. The hypnotic drugs currently preferred for reasons of safety are the <u>barbiturates</u>.

_____ 8. Prolonged residual effects of hypnotics ("hangover") are probably caused by persistence of <u>the unchanged drug</u> in body fluids.

_____ 9. Engaging in <u>vigorous exercise</u> before bedtime will promote rest and sleep.

_____ 10. Clients who use hypnotic drugs in the home should be advised to store the medicines <u>in a bedside table</u>.

_____ 11. The class of drugs most often prescribed worldwide for medicinal use is <u>central nervous system stimulants</u>.

_____ 12. The class of drugs most often abused worldwide for psychotropic effect is <u>central nervous system depressants</u>.

_____ 13. The amounts of absolute (pure) alcohol contained in <u>a glass of wine, a mixed drink, a "shot" of whiskey, and a glass of beer</u> are usually approximately equal.

_____ 14. Dependence on distilled liquors (e.g., whiskey, brandy) <u>is more dangerous and more difficult</u> to treat than is dependence on beer or wine.

_____ 15. Alcohol is a <u>central nervous system stimulant</u>.

_____ 16. Drinkers will show few overt signs of toxicity if blood concentrations of alcohol remain <u>below 0.10%</u>.

_____ 17. A habitual drinker of alcoholic beverages <u>may show no overt signs of toxicity</u> when blood concentrations of alcohol exceed the levels that produce intoxication in naive drinkers.

_____ 18. When applied to the skin, alcohol tends to act as a <u>moisturizer</u>.

_____ 19. The medical term for alcohol withdrawal is <u>delirium tremens</u>.

_____ 20. Certain drugs produce an unpleasant reaction when combined with alcohol in the body. This reaction is called a <u>toxiholic</u> reaction.

Multiple Choice Questions

For each of the following, choose the one best answer.

1. To protect the operating room and recovery room staff from adverse reactions to drugs, it is most important to equip these suites with
   a. Ventilating systems that remove volatile drugs from the air
   b. Cleansing systems that will wash drug residues from the walls and floors
   c. Laminar air flow that will prevent contamination by antibiotic-resistant microorganisms
   d. Incinerators to destroy drug residues in vials and ampules
2. A nursing intervention that helps to reduce the risk of cardiac arrest when a general anesthetic is given is
   a. Preoperative teaching and emotional support to reduce the client's apprehension
   b. Ensuring that the preoperative anticholinergic medication is given on time
   c. Checking the ECG tracing for evidence of cardiac irritability
3. When general anesthesia is administered, which sense remains functional the longest?
   a. Touch
   b. Taste
   c. Smell
   d. Hearing
   e. Vision

4. General anesthetics are most likely to be administered by
   a. Topical application
   b. Inhalation
   c. Injection
   d. Retention enema
5. Dosages of potent analgesics used postoperatively must be reduced if anesthesia involved the use of
   a. Succinylcholine
   b. Innovar
   c. Diazepam (Valium)
   d. Nitrous oxide
6. Because they can block synaptic and neuromuscular transmission, some local anesthetics are employed medicinally as
   a. Sedatives
   b. Tranquilizers
   c. Antihypertensives
   d. Antiarrhythmics
7. A serious adverse reaction to some local anesthetics is
   a. Coma
   b. Hyperventilation
   c. Anaphylaxis
   d. Gastrointestinal atony
8. A drug often combined with local anesthetics for injection into soft tissues is
   a. Cocaine
   b. Epinephrine (Adrenalin)
   c. Phentolamine (Regitine)
   d. Diazepam (Valium)
9. Local anesthetics are eliminated primarily through
   a. The lungs
   b. The kidneys
   c. The liver
   d. Tissue metabolism to water and carbon dioxide
10. The order in which sensory function in a peripheral nerve is interrupted by local anesthetics is
    1. Warmth
    2. Cold
    3. Pain
    4. Deep pressure
    5. Touch
    a. 5, 3, 1, 2, 4
    b. 1, 2, 5, 3, 4
    c. 3, 4, 1, 2, 5
    d. 3, 2, 1, 5, 4
11. An overdose of a central nervous system depressant is characterized by
    a. Paradoxic excitation and overactivity
    b. Coma, apnea, and cardiovascular collapse
    c. Hypnosis with little or no REM sleep
    d. Respiratory paralysis without loss of consciousness
12. Withdrawal of opiates from dependent persons is often accompanied by hallucinations that are
    a. Visual
    b. Auditory
    c. Olfactory
    d. Tactile
13. Withdrawal of barbituates from a dependent client poses a significant risk of
    a. Convulsions
    b. Coma
    c. Severe fluid and electrolyte imbalance
    d. Respiratory arrest
14. Nightmares and hallucinations sometimes occur on emergence from anesthesia induced by
    a. Ether
    b. Diazepam (Valium)
    c. Innovar
    d. Ketamine
15. When administering nursing care during the night shift, care should be exercised to avoid awakening clients during
    a. The early hours of sleep
    b. The late hours of sleep
    c. The basic rest–activity cycles
    d. REM sleep
16. Which of the following beverages is most likely to promote sleep?
    a. Hot coffee
    b. A carbonated cola drink
    c. Warm cocoa
    d. Warm milk
17. An absolute contraindication for the use of barbiturates and chloral hydrate is
    a. A history of allergy to hypnotics
    b. A history of cocaine use
    c. Xanthine toxicity
    d. Acute intermittent porphyria
18. Elimination of barbiturates from the body may be enhanced by
    a. Increasing the pH of the urine
    b. Decreasing the pH of the urine
    c. Administering bile salts
    d. Administering caffeine
19. "Daymares" (waking, daytime "nightmares") have occurred following administration of
    a. Barbiturates
    b. Benzodiazepines
    c. Chloral hydrate
    d. Paraldehyde
20. Dreaming is most likely to occur during
    a. Basic rest–activity cycles (BRAC)
    b. REM sleep

c. Deep sleep
d. The first hour or two of sleep
21. Diazepam is stored in the body
    a. In fatty tissue
    b. In the central nervous system
    c. By plasma protein binding
    d. None of the above: it is not stored in the body to a significant degree
22. What is the most likely effect when naloxone is administered to a person who is feeling "high" after an active exercise session?
    a. Few, if any, effects will be discernible
    b. The "high" is likely to be decreased or abolished
    c. The "high" is likely to be enhanced
    d. Signs and symptoms of opioid withdrawal will develop
23. A frequent side effect of opioid analgesics is
    a. Hyperphagia
    b. Rhinorrhea
    c. Constipation
    d. Photophobia
24. Naloxone is usually administered
    a. Orally
    b. By inhalation
    c. By injection
25. According to the text, the risk of dependence on narcotic analgesics is least likely when
    a. Escalation of dose is delayed as long as possible
    b. The client is taught to adapt to the pain with minimal medication
    c. Adequate medication is administered to control pain
26. Gradual weaning from narcotic analgesics ameliorates but does not abolish signs and symptoms of withdrawal. The amount of time required for elimination of physical dependence is usually a few
    a. Hours
    b. Days
    c. Weeks
    d. Months
27. Signs and symptoms of allergy to opioids are usually manifested by
    a. Bronchospasm
    b. Rhinorrhea
    c. Headache
    d. Skin rash
28. Treatment of opioid overdose is most likely to require
    a. Administration of norepinephrine to maintain blood pressure
    b. Hemodialysis to lower blood concentrations of the drug
    c. Mechanical ventilation to maintain respiration
    d. Cardiopulmonary resuscitation to maintain tissue perfusion
29. Which is more difficult to treat successfully, physical or psychologic dependence on opioids?
    a. Physical dependence
    b. Psychologic dependence
    c. Both are relatively easy to treat successfully
    d. Both are very difficult to treat successfully
30. The drug most likely to be used in the treatment of opioid dependence is
    a. Codeine
    b. Morphine
    c. Heroin
    d. Methadone
31. Before administering an opioid analgesic, the nurse should assess
    a. The pulse rate
    b. The blood pressure
    c. Respirations
    d. The client's level of dependence
32. Presence of residual opioids in a person with acquired tolerance to these drugs can be assessed most reliably by monitoring
    a. Respirations
    b. Blood pressure
    c. Level of consciousness
    d. Pupillary constriction
33. The drug(s) of choice for treating opioid overdose is (are)
    a. Amphetamine
    b. Xanthines
    c. Pentylenetetrazol (Metrazol)
    d. Naloxone (Narcon)
34. Opioid analgesics act by
    a. Entering the nuclei of nerve cells and changing the action of messenger RNA
    b. Occupying receptors on the membrane of nerve cells and influencing cytoplasmic enzymes
    c. Altering the structure of nerve cell membranes and inhibiting impulse transmission
    d. Blocking transmission of neurotransmitters across synapses

35. To be equipotent to parenteral doses, oral doses of opioid analgesics must usually be
    a. Larger than parenteral doses
    b. Smaller than parenteral doses
    c. Equal to parenteral doses
    d. Individually titrated
36. Abrupt withdrawal of drugs from dependent persons is likely to precipitate acute physiologic problems. The risk of death is greatest when the drug involved is
    a. An opioid
    b. Alcohol
    c. A barbiturate
    d. Cocaine
37. Legally, narcotics are defined as
    a. Derivatives of opium
    b. Strong analgesics likely to cause dependence
    c. Drugs designated as narcotics by federal legislation
    d. Class I drugs as defined by the Controlled Substance Act of 1970
38. Clients who use hypnotics over a long period of time should be monitored for
    a. Hypotension
    b. Respiratory acidosis
    c. Lethargy
    d. Personality change
39. The alcohol that is least toxic to humans is
    a. Ethyl (grain) alcohol
    b. Methyl (wood) alcohol
    c. Isopropyl alcohol
40. The brain tissue(s) most likely to be affected first by alcohol taken systemically is (are)
    a. The basal ganglia, which control gait
    b. The frontal lobes, which control inhibition of behavior
    c. The sensory cortex, which controls perception of pain
    d. The reticular formation, which controls sleep
41. How much energy is provided by metabolism of 1 ml of alcohol?
    a. 1 kcal
    b. 5 kcal
    c. 7 kcal
    d. 9 kcal
42. How much alcohol is metabolized by normal adults in 1 hour's time?
    a. 1 ml
    b. 10 ml
    c. 1 oz
    d. 4 oz
43. To avoid an escalating blood alcohol concentration, adults with normal liver and kidney function should not consume more than
    a. One typical "drink" (e.g., 10 oz beer)/hr
    b. 1 oz (30 ml) of alcohol/hr
    c. two typical "drinks"/hr
44. If a drinker wishes to maintain a low blood alcohol level, how long should a "happy hour" (double-sized) drink be "nursed"?
    a. ½ hour
    b. 1 hour
    c. 2 hours
    d. 3 hours
45. Alcohol will potentiate the action of
    1. Tranquilizers
    2. Over-the-counter sleeping pills
    3. Antidepressants
    4. Depressant analgesics
        a. 1, 2, 3
        b. 1, 2, 4
        c. 1, 3, 4
        d. 2, 3, 4
46. Disulfiram is used medicinally in the treatment of alcoholism for the purpose of
    a. Ameliorating the signs and symptoms of acute alcohol intoxication
    b. Monitoring the sobriety of those under treatment for chronic alcoholism
    c. Preventing habitual drinking
    d. Preventing impulse drinking
47. Acute alcohol toxicity that is life-threatening may require heroic measures to reduce alcohol concentration. The most likely treatment is
    a. Mechanical ventilation
    b. Rapidly flowing intravenous fluids
    c. Bowel cleansing with purgatives
    d. Hemodialysis
48. Nonfatal wood alcohol poisoning is most likely to cause permanent damage to
    a. Vision
    b. Hearing
    c. The liver
    d. The heart
49. A person with little or no tolerance to alcohol is likely to die if the blood alcohol concentration exceeds
    a. 0.15%
    b. 0.5%
    c. 1.5%
    d. 5%

Selection of Options

For each of the following, select *all* appropriate answers. Circle correct answers.

1. Central nervous system depressants likely to damage a developing fetus when taken by an expectant mother include
   a. Alcohol
   b. Benzodiazepines
   c. Tranquilizers
   d. Opioids

2. Opioid dependence during pregnancy is likely to cause
   a. Congenital defects in the baby
   b. Prolonged labor during parturition
   c. Opioid dependence in the newborn
   d. Apnea in the newborn

3. Local anesthetics may be administered
   a. By inhalation
   b. By injection into soft tissues
   c. Intravenously
   d. Intrathecally

4. Turning, coughing, and deep breathing are important nursing measures during the immediate postoperative period to prevent
   a. Prolongation of anesthesia
   b. Atelectasis
   c. Hemorrhage
   d. Phlebitis

5. Hospital personnel who work in the operating room or recovery room are exposed to anesthetics in the work environment. Adverse reactions to these drugs include
   a. Dizziness and fainting
   b. Nausea and vomiting
   c. Increased risk of abortion and congenital anomalies in offspring

6. Risk factors associated with adverse reactions to anesthesia include
   a. A high level of anxiety
   b. A history of abuse of central nervous system stimulants
   c. A history of heavy alcohol use
   d. Obesity

7. To detect progression from therapeutic anesthesia (plane 3 of stage III) to dangerously toxic anesthesia (plane 4 of stage III and stage IV), the anesthesiologist is most likely to monitor
   a. Level of consciousness
   b. Secretion of tears
   c. Respirations
   d. Pupillary dilation

8. In combination with certain drugs, opioids greatly increase the risk of toxicity. Some drugs that exhibit this synergism are
   a. Alcohol
   b. Analeptics
   c. Hypnotics
   d. Tranquilizers

9. What are the most likely effects when naloxone is administered to a person dependent on high doses of opioids?
   a. Any "high" persisting after the last opioid dose will be decreased or abolished
   b. Any "high" persisting after the last opioid dose will be enhanced
   c. Nausea, vomiting, diarrhea
   d. Miosis

10. The use of opioids in normal doses is likely to cause adverse physiologic reactions in clients with
    a. Myasthenia gravis
    b. Parkinson's disease
    c. Hyperthyroidism
    d. Multiple sclerosis
    e. Hypovolemia
    f. Marked obesity

11. Withdrawal of opioids from a dependent person is characterized by
    a. Rhinorrhea
    b. Midriasis
    c. Nausea and vomiting
    d. Diarrhea

12. Physiologic effects of opioid analgesics include
    a. A decrease in anxiety, fear, and pain
    b. Depression of mood and dysphoria
    c. Inhibition of sensory perception, especially that of pain

13. Gastrointestinal effects of opioids include
    a. Nausea
    b. Vomiting
    c. Diarrhea
    d. Biliary colic

14. Nursing measures to prevent or ameliorate headache following spinal anesthesia include
    a. Preventing rapid infusion of intravenous fluids
    b. Positioning the client with the head no higher than the body
    c. Promoting ample hydration
    d. Administering opioid analgesics

15. During normal sleep, REM sleep occurs
    a. Virtually continuously
    b. About every 15 to 30 minutes
    c. About every 90 to 120 minutes
    d. During the early hours of sleep
    e. During the later hours of sleep
16. Drugs that decrease REM sleep include
    a. Amphetamines
    b. Cocaine
    c. Barbiturates
    d. Flurazepam
17. Decisions made while under the influence of certain central nervous system drugs may not be legally enforceable. These drugs include
    a. Hypnotics
    b. Caffeine
    c. Opioids
    d. Tranquilizers
18. Use of which of the following combinations of drugs is likely to produce a life-threatening adverse reaction?
    a. Alcohol and caffeine
    b. Alcohol and tranquilizers
    c. Hypnotics and tranquilizers
    d. Alcohol and hypnotics
    e. Opioids and alcohol
    f. Hypnotics and opioids
19. What physiologic changes are most likely to occur during acute alcohol intoxication?
    a. Dehydration
    b. Hypoglycemia
    c. Water retention
    d. Depletion of B vitamins
20. By what routes may alcohol be absorbed by the body?
    a. PO
    b. SC
    c. IV
    d. Inhalation
    e. Topical
21. By what routes is alcohol administered for medicinal effect?
    a. PO
    b. Injection into soft tissues
    c. IV
    d. Inhalation
    e. Topical
22. Chronic use of alcohol markedly increases the risk of serious health problems. These include
    a. Teratogenic damage to a developing fetus
    b. Increased risk of cancer
    c. Progressive liver deterioration
    d. Peptic ulcers
    e. Loss of control of epilepsy and diabetes
    f. Brain degeneration
    g. Peripheral neuritis
    h. Pancreatitis
    i. Skeletal and cardiac muscle degeneration
    j. Hypertension
23. Health problems most likely to be associated with chronic alcoholism are
    a. Muscle weakness
    b. Malnutrition
    c. Vitamin A toxicity
    d. Frequent or serious infections
    e. Cirrhosis of the liver
24. Lay terms for alcohol withdrawal include
    a. The "shakes"
    b. "DTs"
    c. "Clap"
    d. Being "bombed"
25. Medications that help to control symptoms during alcohol withdrawal include
    a. Alcohol in progressively smaller dosages
    b. Tranquilizers
    c. Opioids
    d. Paraldehyde
26. Central nervous system drugs used most frequently in medical treatment are
    a. Central nervous system depressants
    b. Central nervous system stimulants
    c. Those with ascending action
    d. Those with descending action

25 Anticonvulsants

Seizures are uncontrollable physiologic responses to abnormal electrical discharges in the central nervous system. Responses are usually sporadic and self-limiting. Drug treatment is directed at preventing abnormal nerve activity.

Correct the False Statement

Indicate whether the following statements are true or false; if false, correct the underlined words or phrases.

1. If the aura preceding a seizure involves a visual hallucination, the focus at which the central nervous system impulses originate is likely to be located in the temporal lobe of the brain.

2. Full development of a seizure may be prevented if the affected person exerts voluntary control.

3. A diagnosis of seizure disorder can be made only when symptomatic episodes involve loss of consciousness.

4. The temporal lobe is usually the area of origin of impulse waves in psychomotor seizures.

5. Most drugs used as anticonvulsants act as synaptic transmitters.

6. In some people the use of phenytoin will increase the severity of diabetes mellitus.

7. Phenytoin is believed to be carcinogenic.

8. Phenobarbital and ethosuximide are frequently used in combination for the control of major motor seizures.

9. Phenobarbital is the drug of choice for initial treatment of petit mal seizures.

10. The initial treatment of status epilepticus usually involves the injection of diazepam.

11. The use of alcohol in moderation tends to improve the control of seizure disorders.

12. Phenobarbital can interact with other weak bases by competing with them for binding to plasma albumin.

13. The onset of action of phenobarbital is relatively rapid, with peak concentrations in the brain occurring 1 to 2 hours after oral doses.

14. Abrupt withdrawal of anticonvulsant drugs is likely to be followed by active seizures.

15. Valproic acid does not significantly bind to plasma proteins.

16. Carbamazepine is relatively less toxic than are other anticonvulsants.

_____ 17. When administered with meals, anticonvulsant drugs are less likely to cause gastrointestinal upset.

_____ 18. A diagnosis of seizure disorder does not carry a stigma similar to that of the old term "epilepsy."

Short Answer Questions

1. Define epilepsy.

2. Define seizure threshold.

3. Name three factors affecting the occurrence of seizures.

4. List at least seven hygienic measures that can decrease the risk of seizures.

5. Identify at least two techniques used to minimize undesirable changes in appearance caused by hirsutism.

Matching

Match the drug in the left-hand column with all of its adverse reactions in the right-hand column. Place your answers in the space provided.

_____ 1. Phenytoin
_____ 2. Phenobarbital
_____ 3. Trimethadione
_____ 4. Ethosuximide
_____ 5. Valproic acid
_____ 6. Clonazepam

a. Anemia
b. Nystagmus
c. Gastrointestinal upset
d. Hiccups
e. Lethargy and drowsiness
f. Cardiac arrhythmias
g. Liver abnormalities
h. Ataxia
i. Increased risk of fetal damage
j. Personality change
k. Muscle or joint pain
l. Psychologic depression
m. REM sleep deprivation
n. Visual disturbances
o. Gingival hypertrophy
p. Hirsutism
q. Alopecia
r. Blood dyscrasia
s. Irritability

Multiple Choice Questions

For each of the following, choose the one best answer.

1. A type of epilepsy for which phenytoin is *not* recommended is
   a. Grand mal seizures
   b. Jacksonian seizures
   c. Psychomotor seizures
   d. Petit mal seizures
2. Therapeutic blood concentrations of phenytoin range from
   a. 1 to 2 µg/ml
   b. 5 to 10 µg/ml
   c. 10 to 20 µg/ml
   d. 30 to 50 µg/ml
3. A drug frequently used in conjunction with phenytoin in the treatment of seizures is
   a. Ethosuximide
   b. Phenobarbital
   c. Trimethadione
   d. Valproic acid
4. When used to treat seizures, phenytoin is usually administered
   a. Four or five times a day
   b. One to three times a day
   c. Every 1 to 2 days
5. Intravenous solutions of phenytoin should be administered no faster than
   a. 5 g/minute
   b. 500 mg/minute
   c. 50 mg/minute
   d. 5 mg/minute
6. With which of the following solutions is phenytoin compatible?
   a. Normal saline solution
   b. Dextrose in water
   c. Acidic solutions
   d. None of the above
7. The usual dosage of phenytoin for the maintenance of control of seizures in adults is
   a. 100 µg twice a day
   b. 100 mg two or three times a day
   c. 1 g daily, divided into two or three doses
   d. 600 mg, administered in one dose daily
8. Early signs of phenytoin toxicity include
   a. Sluggishness or stupor
   b. Circulatory shock
   c. Nausea and vomiting
   d. Nystagmus and diplopia
9. Toxic doses of phenytoin may cause
   a. Lethargy and stupor
   b. Spontaneous abortion in pregnant women
   c. Osteomalacia
   d. Central nervous system excitation
10. Toxic effects of phenytoin appear in most people when the blood concentration reaches
    a. 25 µg/ml
    b. 50 µg/ml
    c. 100 µg/ml
    d. 200 µg/ml
11. To prevent and minimize gingival hyperplasia secondary to anticonvulsant medication, the nurse should
    a. Advise that the drug be taken with meals to prolong absorption time
    b. Teach meticulous oral hygiene and gum massage
    c. Refer the client to the physician for adjustment of the drug dosage
    d. Refer the client to a dentist for special treatments
12. Therapeutic plasma concentrations of phenobarbital range from
    a. 1 to 2 µg/ml
    b. 5 to 10 µg/ml
    c. 10 to 25 µg/ml
    d. 40 to 50 µg/ml
13. Phenobarbital is contraindicated for clients with
    a. Porphyria
    b. Phenylketonuria
    c. Glaucoma
    d. Benign prostatic hypertrophy
14. Clients receiving phenobarbital for control of seizures should be advised to discontinue the drug and contact the physician immediately if
    a. Lethargy develops
    b. Insomnia occurs
    c. Dreaming increases markedly
    d. Skin rash appears
15. Therapeutic serum concentrations of dimethadione range from
    a. 1 to 2 µg/ml
    b. 10 to 25 µg/ml
    c. 50 to 100 µg/ml
    d. 700 to 800 µg/ml
16. Initial doses of dimethadione are usually
    a. Carefully calculated for long-term maintenance effect
    b. Relatively low, with succeeding doses increasing gradually
    c. Relatively high, with succeeding doses decreasing in accordance with evidence of toxicity

17. Trimethadione is usually employed to treat
    a. Absence seizures
    b. Grand mal seizures
    c. Psychomotor seizures
    d. Jacksonian seizures
18. Toxic reactions commonly occur when the serum concentration of carbamazepine reaches or exceeds
    a. 2 µg/ml
    b. 5 µg/ml
    c. 10 µg/ml
    d. 50 µg/ml
19. When magnesium sulfate is administered as an anticonvulsant, it is usually given
    a. Orally
    b. Rectally, as an enema
    c. Intravenously
    d. Intrathecally
20. Magnesium sulfate is used most often as an anticonvulsant in the treatment of
    a. Major motor seizures of grand mal epilepsy
    b. Major motor seizures associated with toxemia of pregnancy
    c. Absence seizures (petit mal)
    d. None of the above; magnesium sulfate is not used as an anticonvulsant
21. Should women receiving anticonvulsants attempt to breast-feed their children?
    a. Yes, anticonvulsant drugs are not distributed in milk
    b. Sometimes, although a few anticonvulsant drugs are distributed in milk in high concentrations
    c. Usually not, because many anticonvulsant drugs are distributed in milk in high concentrations
    d. No, the drugs will be distributed in milk in high concentrations
22. During treatment of status epilepticus, anticonvulsant drugs are most likely to be administered
    a. By mouth
    b. Intramuscularly
    c. Intravenously
    d. By inhalation
23. The agent of choice for petit mal seizures is
    a. Phenytoin
    b. Phenobarbital
    c. Ethosuximide
    d. Diazepam
24. Which of the following anticonvulsants is employed for the treatment of status epilepticus rather than for maintenance therapy?
    a. Trimethadione
    b. Valproic acid
    c. Clonazepam
    d. Diazepam
25. A class of anticonvulsants that are used to treat petit mal but not grand mal seizures is
    a. The barbiturates
    b. The hydantoins
    c. Valproic acid
    d. The oxazolidinediones
26. Of the following anticonvulsant drugs, which is the most selective?
    a. Phenobarbital
    b. Phenytoin
    c. Valproic acid
    d. Trimethadione
27. An anticonvulsant that acts osmotically to decrease edema in the brain is
    a. Phenytoin
    b. Phenobarbital
    c. Magnesium sulfate
    d. Ethosuximide
28. The anticonvulsant drug that is used medicinally as a cardiac antiarrhythmic is
    a. Phenobarbital
    b. Phenytoin
    c. Ethosuximide
    d. Diazepam
29. The drug most likely to be prescribed to prevent recurrent seizures in children who have experienced febrile seizures is
    a. Phenobarbital
    b. Phenytoin
    c. Ethosuximide
    d. Diazepam
30. When counseling a young woman with a seizure disorder, who desires to start a family, you would inform her that
    a. Once pregnancy has begun, the anticonvulsant drug will be withdrawn to avoid adverse effects on the fetus
    b. The dosage of drugs should be reduced to a minimum by the physician before conception is attempted
    c. Seizures during pregnancy do not appreciably increase the risk of damage to or death of the fetus
    d. It is inadvisable to attempt to conceive until anticonvulsant drugs have been withdrawn completely
31. In the United States, many states have adopted laws that restrict certain activities for persons prone to seizure disorders. At present, the restriction imposed most often affects
    a. The right of the person to marry

b. The right of the person to have children
c. Entry into certain occupations
d. The privilege of driving a motor vehicle

32. A person with obvious gingival hypertrophy is likely to be receiving as a medication
    a. Phenytoin
    b. Phenobarbital
    c. Ethosuximide
    d. Valproic acid

33. What proportion of clients with seizure disorders achieve good control with anticonvulsant medications?
    a. About one out of five
    b. About half
    c. About three out of four
    d. About four out of five

34. Is lifelong anticonvulsant therapy required for all clients with seizure disorders?
    a. Yes; the seizure disorder recurs if medication is withdrawn
    b. By most clients, but not always by clients with childhood or posttraumatic epilepsy
    c. By most clients, but not always by clients with Jacksonian seizures
    d. No, weaning from the drugs may be attempted for most clients after a seizure-free period of 2 to 4 years

35. When anticonvulsant drugs must be discontinued abruptly, the most likely treatment plan is to
    a. Delay prescribing other anticonvulsant drugs until the person has been skin-tested for allergy to the new drug
    b. Discontinue all antigenic drugs for a week to suppress the allergic reaction quickly
    c. Initiate relatively low doses of an alternative anticonvulsant immediately
    d. Initiate relatively high doses of an alternative anticonvulsant immediately

36. Which of the following anticonvulsants is considered to be safe to administer during pregnancy?
    a. Phenobarbital
    b. Phenytoin
    c. Trimethadione
    d. Ethosuximide
    e. None of the above; all are reported to be teratogenic

Selection of Options

For each of the following, select *all* appropriate responses. Circle correct answers.

1. Among the physiologic effects of phenytoin are
   a. Decreased movement of calcium ions across cell membranes
   b. Decreased movement of sodium ions across cell membranes
   c. Decreased movement of potassium ions across cell membranes
   d. Increased movement of magnesium ions across cell membranes
   e. Increased stability of cell membranes

2. What routes of administration are recommended for phenytoin?
   a. PO
   b. SC
   c. IM
   d. IV

3. Advantages of using phenobarbital in controlling seizures include
   a. Economy
   b. Minimal sedative effect, as compared with other anticonvulsants
   c. Relatively few adverse reactions, as compared with other anticonvulsants
   d. Relatively high effectiveness in many types of seizure disorders

4. Contraindications for phenobarbital include
   a. Allergy to barbiturates
   b. Bronchopneumonia
   c. Central nervous system excitation
   d. Porphyria
   e. Acute depression

5. Generally, trimethadione is contraindicated for
   a. People with disease of the retina or of the optic nerve
   b. People with porphyria
   c. Pregnant women

6. Clients receiving valproic acid for the treatment of seizures should be cautioned
   a. To avoid chewing the capsules before swallowing
   b. To buy the same name brand consistently
   c. To avoid alcohol intoxication
   d. Not to discontinue the drug abruptly

7. Anticonvulsant drugs that do not bind significantly to plasma proteins include
   a. Phenobarbital
   b. Phenytoin
   c. Trimethadione
   d. Ethosuximide
8. Certain anticonvulsants are sometimes used in the treatment of
   a. Cardiac arrhythmias
   b. Neuralgia
   c. Myasthenia gravis
   d. Psychosis
   e. Minimal brain dysfunction
9. Abrupt discontinuation of an anticonvulsant drug is likely to increase the risk of
   a. Lethargy and stupor
   b. Status epilepticus
   c. Toxicity from the drug prescribed as a replacement

26
The Psychoactive Drugs

The use of psychoactive drugs is a valuable component in the treatment of the emotionally and mentally disturbed client. Drugs are classified as to the type of behavior affected. These drugs are used to alleviate disturbing symptoms so that the client can function more satisfactorily in everyday life.

Multiple Choice Questions

For each of the following, choose the one best answer.

1. The value of chemotherapy in the treatment of mental and emotional disturbance is based on its effectiveness in
   a. Modifying behavior
   b. Curing underlying causes
   c. Reducing sensory stimuli
   d. Altering the CNS
2. The most widely used antipsychotic drugs are the
   a. Benzodiazepines
   b. MAO inhibitors
   c. Rauwolfia alkaloids
   d. Phenothiazines
3. The antipsychotic agents are primarily used to
   a. Provide symptomatic relief of anxiety
   b. Alleviate extrapyramidal symptoms
   c. Prevent distortion of reality
   d. Alleviate psychotic activity
   e. a and c
4. The phenothiazines include the following compounds:
   a. Aliphatic, piperazine, piperadine
   b. Thioxanthenes, butyrophenones, dihydroindolones
   c. Benzodiazepines, propanediol, diphenylmethanes
   d. Amitriptyline, imipramine, maprotiline
5. The most common side effects of psychoactive medications are
   a. Orthostatic hypotension, feelings of restlessness, tremors
   b. Agranulocytosis, jaundice, diminished growth
   c. Respiratory distress, hypoglycemia, tardive dyskinesia
6. Chlorpromazine and fluphenazine are drugs in which class?
   a. Thioxanthene
   b. Phenothiazine
   c. Benzodiazepine
   d. Anticholinergic
7. An extrapyramidal effect that occurs later in the course of drug therapy and more frequently in the elderly is
   a. Parkinsonism
   b. Akathesia
   c. Dystonia
   d. Tardive dyskinesia
8. Nursing actions when administering antipsychotic agents include
   a. Observing for behavioral changes
   b. Accurately recording observations and actions taken
   c. Monitoring blood pressure
   d. Educating the client
   e. Prescribing antiparkinsonian agents for extrapyramidal symptoms
   f. a, b, c, d
9. Educating the client as to expected response and common side effects, dosages and time taken, interactions with food and other drugs has been found to
   a. Increase side effects
   b. Increase compliance with the drug regimen
   c. Decrease need for drugs
   d. Increase discontinuance of the medication as the client improves
10. Antianxiety agents are used to
    a. Alleviate muscle tension and moderate anxiety
    b. Modify psychotic activities
    c. Decrease phobias
    d. Prevent anxiety associated with psychoneurotic and psychosomatic conditions

11. Long-term use of the antianxiety agents results in
    a. Lowered intellectual capacity
    b. Depression
    c. Tolerance
    d. Increased seizure activity
12. The most widely prescribed antianxiety drugs are the
    a. Benzodiazepines
    b. Propanediols
    c. Diphenylmethanes
    d. Phenothiazines
13. Chlordiazepoxide is useful in treating symptoms of
    a. Paradoxic rage
    b. Confusion
    c. Decreased mental alertness
    d. Alcohol withdrawal
14. Meprobamate is used to relieve symptoms of
    a. Tension headaches, abnormal fears, psychosomatic disorders
    b. Bronchial spasm, respiratory depression, skin sensitivity
    c. Alcohol detoxification
    d. Parkinsonism
15. The drugs of first choice in treating depression are
    a. MAO inhibitors
    b. Psychomotor stimulants
    c. Tricyclic and heterocyclic compounds
16. Psychomotor stimulants used to elevate the mood in the relief of depression are the
    a. MAO inhibitors
    b. Tricyclics
    c. Antimanics
    d. Hydroxyzines
17. Foods that interact with the monoamine oxidase inhibitors to cause hypertensive crisis contain
    a. Sodium
    b. Potassium
    c. Lithium salt
    d. Tyramine
18. The MAO inhibitors are
    a. Marplan, Nardil, Parnate
    b. Eskalith, Lithate
    c. Vistaril, Atarax
    d. Equanil, Miltown
19. The drug(s) of choice for manic depressive illness is (are)
    a. Lithium carbonate
    b. Tricyclic compounds
    c. MAO inhibitors
    d. Benztropine mesylate
20. Early symptoms of lithium toxicity are
    a. Weight loss, ataxia, coarse tremors
    b. Blurred vision, slurred speech, tinnitus
    c. Nausea, polyuria, fine hand tremors, muscle weakness
    d. Confusion, muscle twitching, dizziness
21. The most effective serum lithium level is
    a. 0.5 mEq to 1.0 mEq/liter
    b. 1.0 mEq to 1.5 mEq/liter
    c. 1.5 mEq to 2.0 mEq/liter
22. Extrapyramidal symptoms are most commonly caused by the
    a. Antianxiety agents
    b. Antimanic agents
    c. Antipsychotic agents

Matching

A. Match the terms in the left-hand column with their definitions in the right-hand column. Place your answer in the space provided.

_____ 1. Parkinsonism
_____ 2. Akathesia
_____ 3. Dystonia
_____ 4. Tardive dyskinesia

a. Uncontrolled restlessness
b. Facial grimacing, torticollis, opisthotonus
c. Muscle rigidity, drooling, pill rolling, tremors
d. Rhythmic stereotyped motions of sucking, smacking lips, rocking, repetitive protrusion of the tongue

B. Match the generic names of the following antianxiety agents in the left-hand column with their trade names in the right-hand column.

_____ 1. chlordiazepoxide
_____ 2. alprazolam
_____ 3. chlorazepate
_____ 4. oxazepam
_____ 5. diazepam

a. Xanax
b. Serax
c. Valium
d. Librium
e. Tranxene

C. Match the generic names of the tricyclic and heterocyclic antidepressants in the left-hand column with their trade names in the right-hand column.

_____ 1. amitriptyline   a. Ludiomil
_____ 2. doxepin   b. Desyrel
_____ 3. maprotiline   c. Surmontil
_____ 4. trazodone   d. Elavil
_____ 5. trimipramine maleate e. Sinequan

D. Match the generic names in the left-hand column with their trade names in the right-hand column.

_____ 1. benztropine mesylate   a. Kemadrin
_____ 2. trihexyphenidyl hydrochloride b. Cogentin
_____ 3. biperiden   c. Artane
_____ 4. procyclidine   d. Akineton

Completion Exercises

Read each question carefully and place your answer in the space provided.
1. The psychoactive drugs inhibit the function of the _____ areas of the brain.
2. Inhibition in the function of this area of the brain specifically affects the following systems of the brain: _____ , _____ , and _____ .
3. It is believed that neurotransmitters play an important role in the behavioral changes of mental and emotional problems. Some of these are _____ , _____ , _____ , and _____ .
4. The major categories of the psychoactive drugs are _____ , _____ , and _____ .
5. The three categories of depression are _____ , _____ , and _____ .
6. Drugs used to alleviate the symptoms of depression and stabilize the mood are the _____ , _____ , _____ , and _____ .
7. Diuretics (should, should not) _____ be taken concurrently with lithium.

Correct the False Statement

Indicate whether the following statements are true or false; if false, correct the underlined words or phrases and place your answer in the space provided.

_____ 1. The antianxiety agents act by excitation of the polysynaptic reflexes of the spinal cord and the limbic structures.

_____ 2. Hydroxyzine is useful in treating clients with high levels of anxiety associated with psychoneuroses or organic problems.

_____ 3. Abruptly discontinuing use of the antianxiety agents will never result in withdrawal symptoms.

_____ 4. Antiparkinsonism agents control drug-induced extrapyramidal symptoms by relieving spasticity of involuntary muscles.

Short Answer Questions

1. The following statements define a word or phrase. Place your answer in the space provided.
   a. Controls the ANS and helps to regulate basic life functions: _____
   b. Monitors sensory input: _____
   c. Controls patterns of behavior and emotional response: _____
2. List seven conditions in which the benzodiazepines are effective.

3. Name at least six foods and beverages containing tyramine that interact with the MAO inhibitors.

4. Why is diet very important for clients on lithium and on MAO inhibitors?
    a. Lithium:

    b. MAO inhibitors:

UNIT SIX: DRUGS AFFECTING THE CARDIOVASCULAR SYSTEM

27 Cardiac Drugs

Cessation of circulation for even a few minutes causes immediate and widespread cell death. Therefore, as the moving force behind circulation, the heart is absolutely vital to life. Many chemical substances affect cardiac function.

PART 1: CARDIOTONIC GLYCOSIDES

Correct the False Statement

Indicate whether the following statements are true or false; if false, correct the underlined words or phrases and place your answer in the space provided.

_____ 1. Maintenance doses of digoxin are likely to be <u>considerably smaller</u> than are maintenance dosages of other cardiac glycosides.

_____ 2. Digitalizing dosages of cardiac glycosides are likely to be <u>considerably larger</u> than are maintenance dosages.

_____ 3. Digitalis preparations produce diuresis by <u>stimulating tubular secretions of electrolytes in the kidneys</u>.

_____ 4. The digitalis drug <u>digoxin</u> is extensively metabolized by the liver.

_____ 5. Hemodialysis <u>will</u> remove cardiac glycosides from the blood.

_____ 6. Cardiac glycosides are the drugs of choice for the treatment of <u>myocardial infarction</u>.

_____ 7. The actions of cardiac glycosides are <u>curative</u> in nature.

_____ 8. Serum concentration of digoxin is <u>an absolute</u> indicator of toxicity.

_____ 9. When a client exhibits signs and symptoms of digitalis toxicity, the nurse <u>may withhold one or more doses of digitalis</u>.

Crossword Puzzle

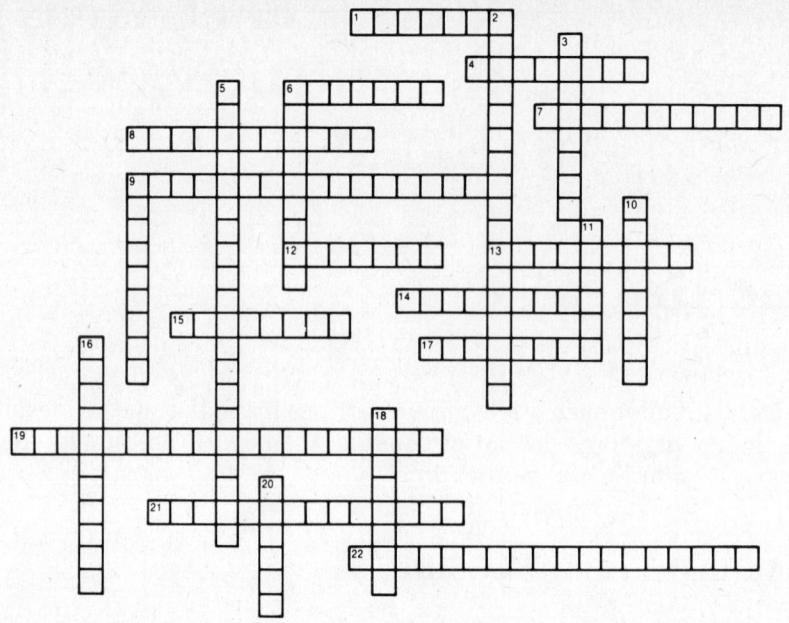

ACROSS

1. A cardiac condition treated with digitalis
4. A marine source of digitalis
6. A frequently prescribed digitalis drug
7. See 3 down
8. A drink rich in potassium
9. Effect of digitalis on cardiac contractility
12. An electrolyte that accentuates effects of digitalis
13. A cardiotonic drug eliminated by the liver
14. Chemical nature of digitalis
15. A food rich in potassium
17. Effect of digitalis on urinary output
19. Effect of digitalis on cardiac conductivity
20. The process of building up serum levels of digitalis
22. A cardiac arrhythmia treated with digitalis

DOWN

2. A record of cardiac function
3. A symptom of digitalis toxicity
5. Effect of digitalis on cardiac rate
6. Drugs that can increase toxic effect of digitalis
9. A nutrient antagonistic to digitalis
10. Plant source of digitalis
11. A psychosomatic reaction that contributes to digitalis toxicity
16. An index to digitalis toxicity
18. See 16 down
20. See 15 across

Multiple Choice Questions

For each of the following, choose the one best answer.

1. What is the chemical structure shared by most cardiotonic drugs?
   a. Alkaloid
   b. Aldehyde
   c. Glycoside
   d. Catecholamine
2. The natural source for digitalis drugs is
   a. Foxglove
   b. Periwinkle
   c. The poppy
   d. Willow bark
3. Digitalis drugs appear to act by
   a. Inhibiting the vagus nerve
   b. Blocking calcium channels in the myocardium
   c. Enhancing movement of sodium ions across the membranes of cardiac muscle cells
   d. Enhancing movement of calcium ions across membranes of cardiac muscle cells
4. Of the following digitalis drugs, which

is the most completely absorbed by the gastrointestinal tract?
   a. Digoxin
   b. Digitoxin
   c. Ouabain
   d. Deslanoside
5. What is the relationship between polarity and plasma protein binding of the digitalis drug?
   a. Direct relationship
   b. Inverse relationship
   c. No relationship
6. The digitalis preparation most likely to be ordered for patients with renal failure is
   a. Digoxin
   b. Digitoxin
   c. Deslanoside
7. The most effective tool for detecting early digitalis toxicity is
   a. The stethoscope
   b. The sphygmomanometer
   c. A blood test for serum concentration
   d. The cardiac monitor
8. The usual maintenance dosage of digoxin for adults is
   a. 0.125 mg to 0.25 mg/day
   b. 0.25 mg to 0.5 mg/day
   c. 1.25 mg to 2.5 mg/day
   d. 2.5 mg to 5 mg/day
9. A normal adult (maintenance) dosage of digitoxin could range from
   a. 0.125 mg to 0.25 mg/day
   b. 0.25 mg to 0.5 mg/day
   c. 0.5 mg to 0.75 mg/day
   d. 1.2 mg to 1.6 mg/day
10. The nutrient that acts as a physiologic antagonist to the action of digitalis is
    a. Calcium
    b. Potassium
    c. Protein
    d. Cholesterol
11. How safe is digitalis?
    a. Very safe—it has a wide safety margin
    b. Moderately safe—it has a therapeutic index of about 5
    c. Relatively risky—only careful management prevents toxicity
    d. Dangerous—most recipients exhibit chronic toxicity
12. A food that would help to reduce the risk of digitalis toxicity is
    a. Apple
    b. Banana
    c. Cranberry juice
    d. Pear
13. In most cases, digitalis drugs are withheld if the apical pulse in adults drops below
    a. 100/minute
    b. 80/minute
    c. 60/minute
    d. 50/minute
14. What is the relation of serum magnesium ion concentration and digitalis?
    a. Hypermagnesemia enhances the effects of digitalis
    b. Hypomagnesemia enhances the effects of digitalis
    c. Magnesium concentrations do not significantly alter the effects of digitalis
15. How does a recurrence of congestive heart failure influence response to digitalis?
    a. It makes the heart refractory to digitalis
    b. It makes the heart sensitive to digitalis
    c. It has little effect on cardiac response to digitalis

Matching

A. Match each chemical effect on the heart in the left-hand column with the property of the heart that is affected in the right-hand column. Place your answer in the space provided.

_____ 1. Inotropic   a. Conductivity
_____ 2. Dromotropic   b. Automaticity
_____ 3. Chronotropic   c. Strength of contraction
                            d. Rate of contraction

B. Match the portion of the ECG tracing affected in the left-hand column with the effect of digitalis in the right-hand column.

_____ 1. T wave   a. Depression or inversion
_____ 2. Heart rate   b. Acceleration
_____ 3. P–R interval   c. Deceleration
_____ 4. Q–T interval   d. Shortening
_____ 5. QRS complex   e. Prolongation
                            f. Narrowing

Selection of Options

For each of the following, select *all* appropriate responses. Circle correct answers.

1. The function of the heart is influenced by
   a. The cortex of the brain
   b. The autonomic nervous system
   c. Endocrine hormones
   d. The vagus nerve
   e. Electrolytes in body fluids
2. The effects of digitalis drugs on the heart include a
   a. Positive inotropic effect
   b. Positive chronotropic effect
   c. Negative dromotropic effect
3. Why is drug treatment sometimes initiated by administration of high ("loading") doses?
   a. To achieve a prompt therapeutic effect
   b. To saturate body tissue depots
   c. To raise serum concentrations quickly
   d. To stimulate metabolism and excretion of the drug
4. Factors influencing severity of toxicity from digitalis include
   a. Serum concentration of the drug
   b. Serum concentration of sodium ions
   c. Age of the recipient
   d. Pathologic status of the heart
   e. Ratio between serum concentration of calcium and potassium ions
   f. Level of stress response in the client
5. A drug considered to be "cumulative" is likely to exhibit the following characteristics:
   a. Extensive storage in the tissues
   b. Long serum half-life
   c. Narrow safety margin
6. Therapeutic uses for cardiotonic glycosides include treatment of
   a. Heart failure
   b. Atrial fibrillation
   c. Acute myocardial infarction
   d. Paroxysmal tachycardia
7. Before administering digitalis, the nurse should always
   a. Count the pulse
   b. Assess the client's appetite
   c. Measure the blood pressure
8. Signs and symptoms of *nontoxic* digitalis side effects include
   a. Local tissue irritation
   b. Postmedication nausea
   c. Heart block
   d. Skin rash
   e. Decrease in neutrophils
   f. Increase in eosinophils
   g. Breast enlargement in males
9. Contraindications for cardiotonic glycosides include
   a. Heart block
   b. Heart failure
   c. Hypertrophic subaortic stenosis
   d. Myocardial infarction with severe myocarditis
10. Among the factors that tend to increase the risk of digoxin toxicity are
    a. Immobility
    b. Nausea and vomiting
    c. Stress
    d. Diarrhea
    e. Renal impairment
11. Dietary changes most likely to be recommended to clients receiving digitalis drugs include
    a. Ample use of foods rich in fiber
    b. Limitation of foods rich in potassium
    c. Limitation of foods rich in sodium
    d. Ample use of foods rich in calcium
    e. Control of calories
12. In an adult client receiving digitalis, a pulse rate greater than 100/minute may signify
    a. Incomplete therapeutic response to the drug
    b. Beginning drug toxicity
    c. Severe drug toxicity
13. Among the signs and symptoms of digitalis toxicity are
    a. Anorexia
    b. Nausea
    c. Vomiting
    d. Constipation
    e. Bradycardia
    f. Tachycardia
    g. Changes in color vision

PART 2: ANTIARRHYTHMIC DRUGS

Correct the False Statement

Indicate whether the following statements are true or false; if false, correct the underlined words.

_____ 1. β-Adrenergic blocking agents can cause <u>transient hypertension when therapy is initiated</u>.

_____ 2. The antiarrhythmic drugs likely to cause a syndrome resembling Raynaud's disease are <u>quinidine and lidocaine</u>.

_____ 3. Drugs that are used to treat cardiac arrhythmias <u>may increase</u> the risk of other cardiac arrhythmias.

_____ 4. A complication that may follow cardioversion is <u>venous embolism</u>.

_____ 5. Treatment of cardiac arrhythmias by depressant drugs tends to <u>increase</u> the risk of congestive heart failure.

_____ 6. Adrenergic blocking agents and disopyramide tend to increase the risk of <u>hyperglycemia</u>.

_____ 7. Quinidine solutions that appear <u>cloudy</u> must be discarded.

_____ 8. Bretylium and amiodarone exert their antiarrhythmic action through <u>calcium channel blockade</u>.

Multiple Choice Questions

For each of the following, choose the one best answer.

1. A cardiac antiarrhythmic drug also used as a local anesthetic is
   a. Lidocaine
   b. Phenytoin
   c. Bretylium
   d. Propranolol

2. The cardiac antiarrhythmic drug that can cause cinchonism is
   a. Lidocaine
   b. Phenytoin
   c. Propranolol
   d. Quinidine

3. A drug that exerts anticholinergic effects is
   a. Propranolol
   b. Quinidine
   c. Lidocaine
   d. Phenytoin

4. An antiarrhythmic drug that tends to cause general tissue damage is
   a. Bretylium
   b. Nadolol
   c. Lidocaine
   d. Quinidine

5. Antiarrhythmic drugs that act as adrenergic blockers increase the risk of
   a. Tachycardia
   b. Hypertension
   c. Urinary retention
   d. Asthma

6. The antiarrhythmic drug lidocaine is used primarily for the treatment of
   a. Bradycardia
   b. Atrial fibrillation
   c. Heart block
   d. Premature ventricular contractions

7. Quinidine tends to increase the severity of the symptoms of the disease
   a. Malaria
   b. Hypertension
   c. Myasthenia gravis
   d. Multiple sclerosis

8. The antiarrhythmic drug most likely to be used for long-term control of chronic arrhythmias is
   a. Procainamide
   b. Quinine
   c. Bretylium
   d. Deslanoside

9. The drug of choice for the treatment of arryhthmias in digitalis toxicity is
   a. Procainamide
   b. Quinidine
   c. Lidocaine
   d. Phenytoin

10. The antiarrhythmic action of lidocaine is that of
    a. Beta-adrenergic blockade
    b. Calcium channel blockade
    c. Sodium channel blockade
    d. Prolongation of repolarization

Crossword Puzzle

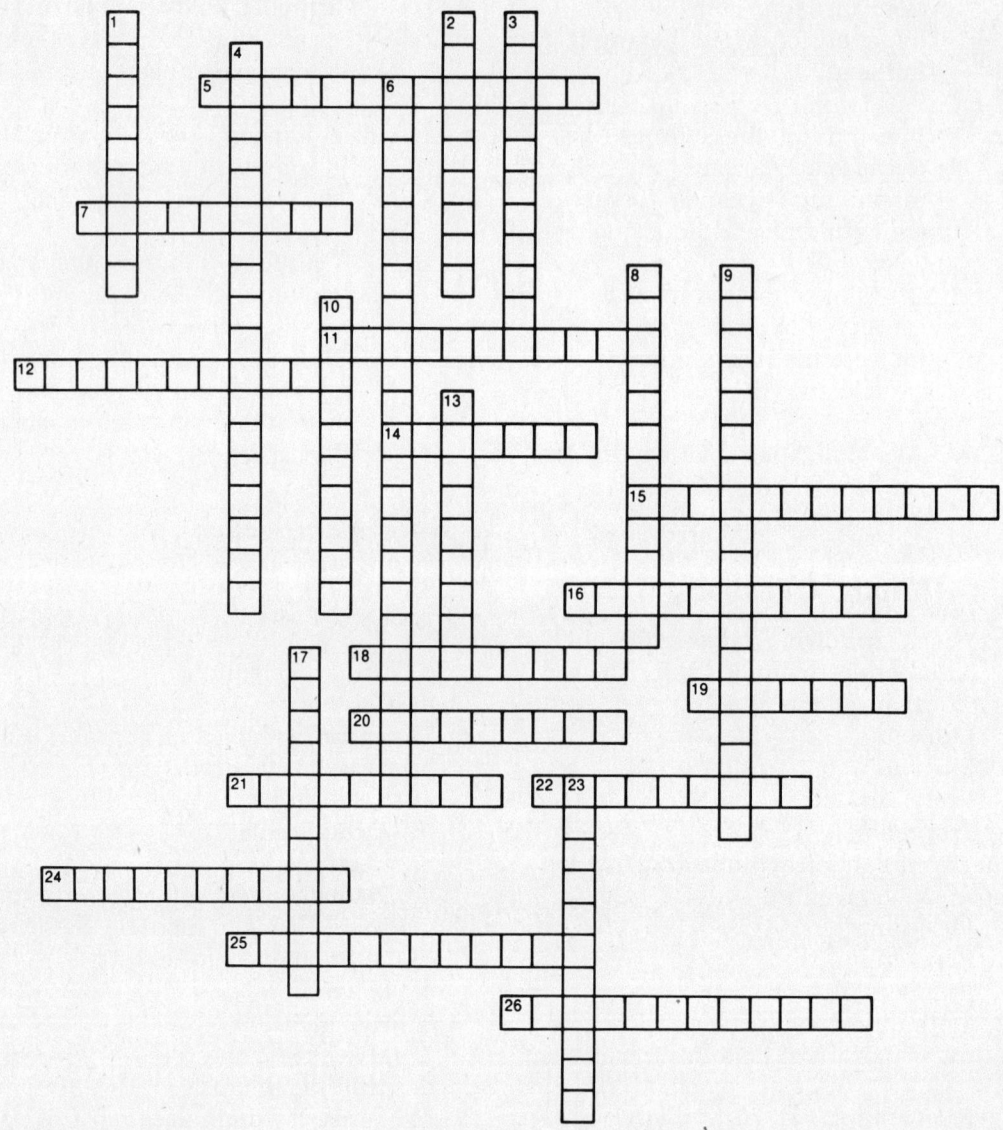

ACROSS

5. Successful treatment of atrial fibrillation
7. A cardiac antiarrhythmic drug often administered intravenously
11. A compensatory process that predisposes the heart to fibrillation
12. An abnormally rapid cardiac rate
14. Extremely rapid, inefficient contractions of the heart
15. A property of the heart that increases the risk of arrhythmias
16. Areas outside the conduction system that initiate stimuli
18. A mechanical means of stimulating the heart
19. An antiarrhythmic drug that is not significantly metabolized by the liver
20. An iatrogenic cause of heart block
21. An activity that increases vagal nerve stimulation

22. An antiarrhythmic drug also used as an anticonvulsant
24. A necrotic area of heart muscle
25. An antiarrhythmic drug that can cause a reaction resembling that of systemic lupus erythematosus
26. An antiarrhythmic drug that can cause urinary retention

DOWN

1. An antiarrhythmic drug whose use is confined to critical-care settings
2. A characteristic of the pulse in atrial fibrillation
3. A stress hormone that increases sinus tachycardia
4. The class of drugs used most often to correct arrhythmias
6. The most lethal of cardiac arrhythmias
8. The property of cardiac tissue that underlies spontaneous generation of impulses
9. An arrhythmia that predisposes to arterial embolism
10. A state in which sinoatrial impulses do not reach the ventricles
13. An antiarrhythmic drug that can cause cinchonism
17. An antiarrhythmic drug eliminated primarily by the liver
23. An adverse reaction common to many antiarrhythmic drugs

Selection of Options

For each of the following, select *all* appropriate responses. Circle correct answers.

1. Factors that increase the irritability of the myocardium include
   a. Ischemia
   b. Insomnia
   c. Anxiety
   d. Smoking
   e. Sedative drugs
2. Adverse reactions to antiarrhythmic drugs include
   a. Cardiac arrhythmias
   b. Hypotension
   c. Transient hypertension
   d. Cardiac arrest
   e. Mental changes
   f. Gastrointestinal upset
   g. Allergic manifestations
3. Drugs whose use is limited to acute care settings include
   a. Bretylium
   b. Propranolol
   c. Phenytoin
   d. Lidocaine
4. The families of clients receiving long-term antiarrhythmic therapy should be advised to
   a. Be prepared to call emergency medical services
   b. Become trained in emergency cardiopulmonary resuscitation
   c. Learn to assess the blood pressure
   d. Learn to assess pulses
5. Antiarrhythmic drugs that are used only in critical-care settings with continuous ECG monitors include
   a. Procainamide
   b. Lidocaine
   c. Phenytoin
   d. Bretylium

28
Vascular Drugs

Drugs that affect blood vessels, such as antilipemics, vasoconstrictors, vasodilators, and sclerosing agents, are used to enhance circulation. They may be used to correct temporary, acute conditions or to combat the slow, degenerative process of atherosclerosis.

Anagram–Scrabble

Unscramble the letters for the words below and enter them in the proper places in the scrabble grid, from top to bottom.

1.
OSTNIYOHEPN
MIBRHOT
PONGLOI
ROSSBIFI
ERLTOSSIOREARCIS
AFTICILANOCIC
UPSRESER
TROSEASHERLCOIS
SCUTBORNITO
AUPELQ
MAVSAPOSS

CERADSADE NETYCPA
SOLS FO CLASTITYEI
SOCHK
RETONSIPHYEN

2.
SESRTS
VACNIYTIIT
SEXECS SDLL
GIMOSKN
GIHH AFT TIDE
BAITEDES

HGHI DOBOL SOLTOHCEREL
OSHYMPYROTDIHI
OWL SHLD
RENPIYHOSETN
STYBEOI

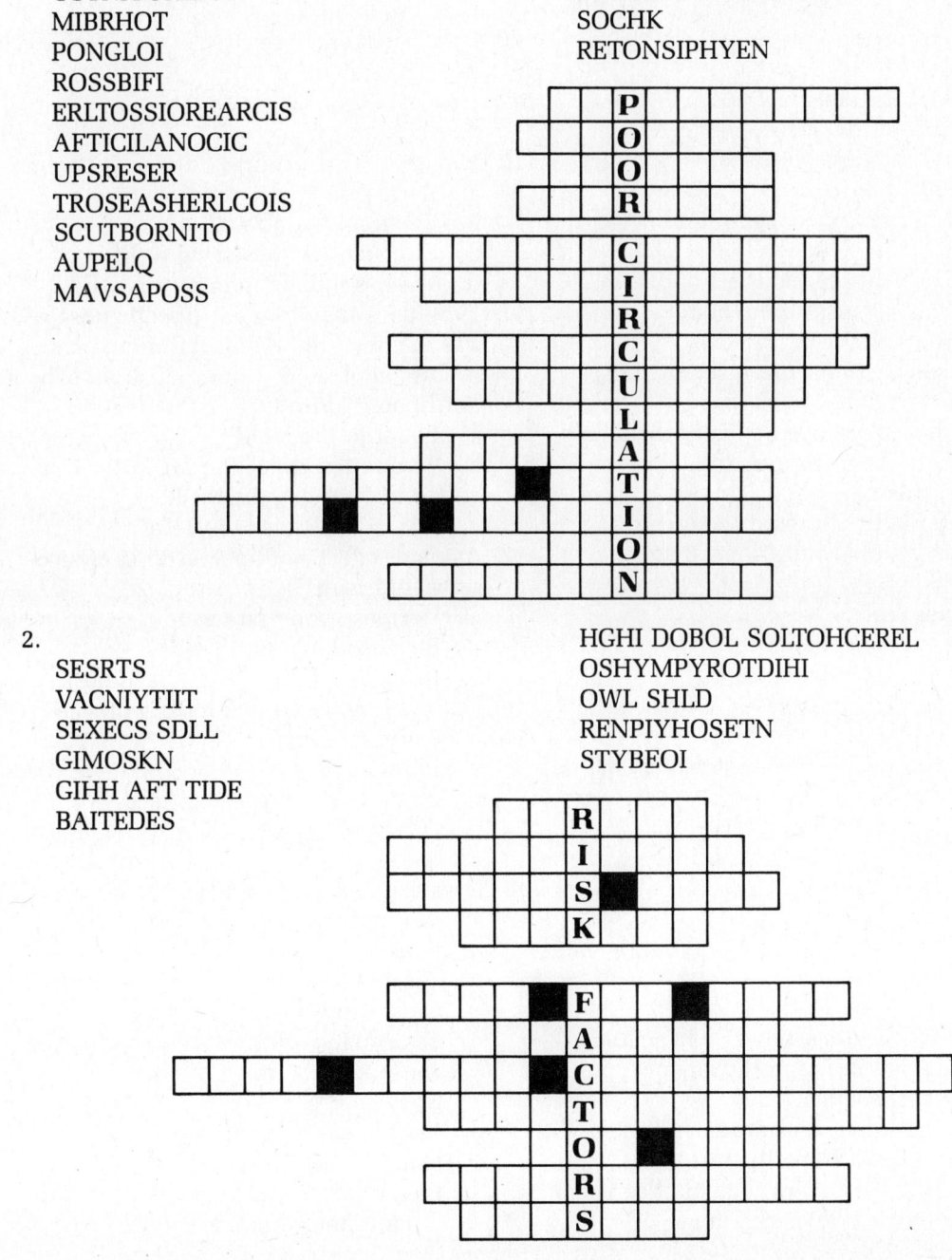

The remaining exercises are divided into sections as follows: Antilipemic Drugs, Vasodilators, Vasoconstrictors, and Sclerosing Agents.

PART 1: ANTILIPEMIC DRUGS

Multiple Choice Questions

For each of the following, choose the one best answer.

1. An iatrogenic disease likely to develop during clofibrate therapy is
   a. Intestinal obstruction
   b. Cholelithiasis
   c. Pulmonary embolism
   d. All of the above
2. Bile acid–sequestering resins are eliminated in
   a. The urine
   b. Feces
   c. Both of the above
   d. Neither of the above
3. Bile acid–sequestering resins interact with digitalis to
   a. Increase serum concentration of digitalis
   b. Increase physiologic effect of digitalis without altering serum digitalis concentrations
   c. Decrease serum concentration of digitalis
   d. Decrease physiologic effect of digitalis without altering serum digitalis concentrations
4. Therapy with bile acid–sequestering resins may cause a nutritional deficiency of
   a. Cholesterol
   b. Essential fatty acids
   c. Water-soluble vitamins
   d. Fat-soluble vitamins
5. It is likely that probucol acts
   a. Only locally in the gastrointestinal tract
   b. Only systemically
   c. Both locally and systemically
6. Probucol is stored in
   a. Bone
   b. Fat
   c. Plasma proteins
   d. Glandular tissue
7. Are antilipemic drugs selective in action?
   a. Yes, each drug is specific for one type of hyperlipemia
   b. Yes, to a degree; each drug is indicated for particular hyperlipemias
   c. No, all are effective to some degree in all types of hyperlipemias

8. (An) antilipemic drug(s) that can increase body odor is (are)
   a. Colestipol
   b. Clofibrate
   c. Probucol
   d. All of the above
9. An antilipemic drug likely to cause cardiac problems is
   a. Cholestyramine
   b. Clofibrate
   c. Colestipol
   d. Probucol
10. Nicotinic acid is a(n)
    a. Derivative of nicotine
    b. Essential amino acid
    c. Bile acid–sequestering resin
    d. Water-soluble vitamin
11. How does the daily antilipemic dose of niacin compare with the minimum daily requirement (MDR) for nutrition? The antilipemic dose is
    a. Equal to the MDR
    b. Five to ten times the MDR
    c. 40 to 50 times the MDR
    d. 100 to 400 times the MDR
12. As a side effect, antilipemic doses of nicotinic acid may
    a. Decrease body fat tissue
    b. Increase body fat tissue
    c. Increase the rate of LDL synthesis
    d. Increase the rate of HDL synthesis
13. Niacin is excreted
    a. In the urine
    b. By way of the bile into feces
    c. Unabsorbed, into feces
    d. All of the above
14. Does niacin have a wide margin of safety?
    a. Yes, even in large dosages it is virtually free of adverse reactions
    b. Yes, but in antilipemic dosages it can cause a few adverse reactions
    c. Yes, but in antilipemic dosages it can cause a wide range of adverse reactions
    d. Maintenance nutritional dosages are usually free of adverse reactions, but therapeutic nutritional supplementation often causes toxicity

15. An additive incorporated into some medications that can cause acute asthma in persons allergic to aspirin is
    a. Cornstarch
    b. Ink used for lettering tablets
    c. Enteric coatings
    d. Tartrazine

Correct the False Statement

Indicate whether the following statements are true or false; if false, correct the underlined words or phrases.

_____ 1. The oral antilipemic clofibrate acts systemically rather than locally.

_____ 2. The duration of action of clofibrate is prolonged in clients with hepatic impairment.

_____ 3. Clofibrate does not cross the placenta.

_____ 4. Anion exchange resins are absorbed from the gastrointestinal tract and act systemically.

_____ 5. Cholestyramine is used to treat pruritus associated with certain types of jaundice.

_____ 6. Clients receiving bile acid–sequestering resins should be taught how to prevent constipation.

_____ 7. To prevent esophageal irritation and obstruction, bile acid–sequestering resins should be taken in the dry form.

_____ 8. To increase systemic absorption, probucol should be administered on an empty stomach.

_____ 9. Research data indicate that lowering serum fat levels significantly decreases the risk of death from cardiovascular disease.

_____ 10. Research data on antilipemic drugs indicate that they are highly effective in delaying cardiovascular degeneration.

_____ 11. An immediate reaction to antilipemic doses of niacin is epigastric pain.

_____ 12. Thyroid extract is sometimes used as an antilipemic agent.

_____ 13. Dextrothyroxine is not very highly bound to plasma proteins.

_____ 14. Adverse reactions to antilipemics tend to be most severe when treatment is initiated and to subside with continued treatment.

Selection of Options

For each of the following, select *all* appropriate responses. Circle correct answers.

1. Among the hormones that tend to lower serum cholesterol and triglyceride concentrations are
   a. Glucocorticoids
   b. Estrogens
   c. Testosterone
   d. Thyroxine
   e. Catecholamines
2. The cardiac effects of clofibrate include reduction of
   a. Plasma triglyceride concentrations
   b. Serum VLDL concentrations
   c. Serum cholesterol concentrations
   d. Serum LDL concentrations
   e. Platelet adhesiveness
   f. Plasma fibrinolysis
3. Clofibrate therapy requires the following precautions to detect or prevent adverse reactions:
   a. Regular complete blood counts
   b. Regular liver function tests
   c. Regular kidney function tests
   d. Monitoring for gallbladder disease
   e. Avoidance of pregnancy (for women)

4. Bile acid–sequestering resins include
   a. Cholestyramine
   b. Colestipol
   c. Lactulose
   d. Kaolin
5. Adverse reactions to bile acid–sequestering resins include
   a. Gastrointestinal upset
   b. Acidosis
   c. Vitamin A toxicity
   d. Osteoporosis
   e. Central nervous system disturbance
   f. Arthritis
6. Which of the following drugs will be bound by anion exchange resins, with subsequent reduction in gastrointestinal absorption?
   a. Digoxin
   b. Dicumarol
   c. Vitamin C
   d. Penicillin G
   e. Thiazide diuretics
7. Probucol is excreted
   a. In urine
   b. By way of the bile into feces
   c. Unabsorbed into feces
8. Therapeutic actions of nicotinic acid include a decrease in serum
   a. Cholesterol concentrations
   b. HDL concentration
   c. Triglyceride concentration
9. The effect of antilipemic dosages of dextrothyroxine is to decrease
   a. Serum concentration of cholesterol
   b. Serum concentration of lipids
   c. Serum concentration of VLDLs
   d. Cholesterol synthesis in the liver
10. Side effects of dextrothyroxine include
    a. Hypothyroidism
    b. Nervousness
    c. Lethargy
    d. Insomnia
    e. Increased glucose tolerance
    f. Signs and symptoms of cardiac disease
11. Contraindications for dextrothyroxine include
    a. Heart disease
    b. Hypothyroidism
    c. Hypertension
    d. Pregnancy
    e. Lactation
12. Miscellaneous substances under investigation as antilipemic drugs include
    a. Progestogens
    b. Vitamin C
    c. Neomycin
    d. Aspirin
    e. Sitosterol
13. When taking a drug history prior to initiation of antilipemic drug therapy, the nurse should ask specifically about
    a. Alcohol
    b. Antilipemics
    c. Cardiovascular drugs
    d. Hormones
    e. Tobacco
    f. Xanthines

Short Answer Questions

1. By what route is dextrothyroxine administered?

2. By what route(s) is dextrothyroxine excreted?

3. How freely are antilipemic drugs prescribed in the treatment of cardiovascular disease?

4. Name at least three precautions necessary when bile acid–sequestering resins are administered.

PART 2: VASODILATORS

Find the Hidden Words

Hidden within the following letter grid are words from Chapter 28. They may be vertical, horizontal, or diagonal. Circle the letters as you find the hidden words.

LIST OF WORDS

amyl nitrate	guanethidine	Nitrobid	pindolol
atenolol	isoxsuprine	nitroglycerin	prazosin
captopril	mecamylamine	nitrates	propranolol
clonidine	methyldopa	nitroprusside	rauwolfia
cyclandelate	metoprolol	nylidrin	timolol
diazoxide	minoxidil	papaverine	tolazoline
diltiazem	nadolol	pargyline	trimethaphan
dipyridamole	nifedipine	Peritrate	verapamil

```
m i t o p r o p a m y l a e n i d i a z o x s u p r i n a d i a z n o l c
e e n i p i d i l t i m n n i f e d i l t r i m e t h y l d i l t i l o l
t p c l o l o c l o n i d i n e i a i r a d i a t a u w o a a e e o o l o
h i s a o i s o x s p r a z o s i n c l o n i t r o g u a n i f e d i l n
y n e t m l l s o i t o l a z o l i n e o e r i i v a n e t i m o c y c i
l d v e r y p i d i m l o l o n e t a a m i d i p y r a v n y l i d i l t
d i a n i p l e i n e e t a r t i r e p e n i d e h t e n a u g u a n i r
i p p i d o f n i f t p l r n a d o l o l n b i d i y d a i t u y t m o o
l y a t l i n e i t h i m d m i d g l d o l o l n t r i m e t h a p h a n
t r p r n e l o m a d a r y p i d l y l n i r e i r f s m e c r a u a m y
r a t a l l m t m e c a y h l i e y c y t a t a t l i s a m c o o l o l l
i u o u y i a l i m a p a r e v p c c h u a i i o n e u e r a p a b i i i
m w l m r t o t a a l o l i e o i e l t l n n w l t g r a v p i n d d o d
e o a t e e d i x o z a i d t i n r i e i m u y a p h p a h t e m i r t i
r l i n i v i m l i n e n i d i y i d m i a m r h y a o l o o r p i n r l
p r o p r a n o l o l i m a m y l n i t r a t e d t r r a r p y r s a i t
r a v e a r n l o l l y m a y m a f n i p i n e t a e t g u r a u o i m i
a d i r o r p o l o l o l t i l o l o d n i p r u h y i i i i u s x o e a
z y y i o u g l c l o y i h c a p t o p i n d o p h y n d n l g o s l t t
o h i t i m o y t e m t n y l i d r i n e o i i y h i a i o e n i t o h e
g t r i m e c a l a p a c l o l o l o l o r p o t e m i n o x i d i l y x
u e i m n i f a c i i m i n o x n i e n i r p u x o s i l g o r t i n l i
a m e e r i o e e e n i r e v a p a p r a z i g l o l i a r u r a i e t f
n i f t e e m v e r a e e n g u a h d i a l t e m i n i t r a u g h t i e
e d y h m m o w u a r e v o w u a r y p i d i l y n i r p u s x o z a i d
```

Multiple Choice Questions

For each of the following, choose the one best answer.

1. The main advantage of skin patches for administering nitroglycerin over nitroglycerin tablets given sublingually or orally is
   a. Avoidance of irritation to the oral and gastric mucosa
   b. Prompt therapeutic response
   c. Longer duration of action

2. When nitroglycerin is used regularly, headaches and flushing tend to
   a. Become more severe
   b. Persist at the level experienced initially
   c. Subside

3. Following regular exposure to nitrates, withdrawal tends to cause
   a. Flushing and throbbing headache
   b. A rise in blood pressure and anginal pain
   c. Postural hypotension
4. An adverse reaction to nitrates usually seen only in children is
   a. Weakness and dizziness
   b. Drug rash
   c. Paradoxic hypertension
   d. Methemoglobinemia
5. Clients beginning the use of nitroglycerin for the control of angina pectoris should be advised to
   a. Consult the physician for a change in medication if headaches occur
   b. Discontinue the drug and notify the physician if dizziness and weakness develop
   c. Take the medication only when pain is experienced
   d. Treat headache and postural hypotension symptomatically while continuing the medication for a trial period
6. Adverse reactions to nitroglycerin experienced during the early period of treatment can be minimized if the client avoids
   a. The use of alcohol
   b. The use of analgesics such as aspirin or acetaminophen
   c. Overhydration
   d. Inactivity
7. When administered sublingually, nitroglycerin has a duration of action of
   a. 5 minutes
   b. 30 minutes
   c. 1 hour
   d. 3 hours
8. When administered sublingually, nitroglycerin has an onset of action of about
   a. 30 seconds
   b. 2 minutes
   c. 5 minutes
   d. 10 minutes
9. When sublingual nitroglycerin is not effective the dose may be repeated in
   a. 3 to 5 minutes
   b. 15 to 20 minutes
   c. 30 to 60 minutes
   d. 60 to 90 minutes
10. When used to control or treat angina pectoris, transdermal preparations of nitroglycerin should be applied
    a. To the precordial area
    b. Somewhere on the anterior chest
    c. On areas in which anginal pain is experienced
    d. None of the above; the drug acts systemically and can be applied to many areas of the body
11. Peripheral vasodilators are contraindicated in
    a. Congestive heart failure
    b. Myocardial infarction
    c. Coarctation of the aorta
    d. Hypertension secondary to kidney disease
12. Most adrenergic blocking agents used as antihypertensive drugs are administered
    a. PO
    b. SC
    c. IM
    d. IV
13. The drug most likely to be employed in the treatment of renal hypertension is
    a. Propranolol
    b. Guanethidine
    c. Trimethaphan
14. Which of the following drugs is (are) administered intravenously?
    a. Diltiazem
    b. Nifedipine
    c. Verapamil
    d. All of the above
    e. None of the above
15. When clients receiving nifedipine for the treatment of hypertension are scheduled for surgery, it is likely that
    a. The nifedipine dosage will be maintained throughout the period of surgery
    b. The nifedipine dosage will be increased prior to the surgery
    c. The nifedipine dosage will be decreased prior to the surgery
    d. Nifedipine will be discontinued prior to the surgery
16. Dipyridamole is eliminated by way of the
    a. Urine
    b. Bile and feces
    c. Both of the above
    d. Neither of the above
17. A serious adverse reaction to captopril is
    a. Eighth cranial nerve toxicity and deafness
    b. Hepatotoxicity and liver impairment
    c. Nephrotoxicity and renal impairment
    d. Hypovolemia and hypotension

18. When pargyline dosage is determined, doses can be adjusted up to
    a. Bid
    b. Once a day
    c. Once a week
    d. Once in 2 weeks
19. In the United States, how many undiagnosed hypertensive adults are there for every 100 adults diagnosed as having the condition?
    a. Probably 5
    b. Probably 20
    c. Probably 50
    d. Probably 100
20. The percentage of adults in the United States with blood pressure above the "normal" range is probably
    a. 5%
    b. 20%
    c. 40%
    d. 50%
21. Of all the adults who have been told that they have hypertension, what percentage is adequately controlled?
    a. 5%
    b. 25%
    c. 50%
    d. 100%

Correct the False Statement

Indicate whether the following statements are true or false; if false, correct the underlined words or phrases.

_____ 1. In a normal healthy adult, hypertension may be defined as a systolic pressure greater than 150 mm Hg and a diastolic pressure greater than 100 mm Hg.

_____ 2. When used in the treatment of Raynaud's disease, nitroglycerin ointment may be applied to any area of the body, because the desired effect is systemic.

_____ 3. The action of nitroglycerin in angina pectoris is curative.

_____ 4. Clients using nitroglycerin sublingual tablets should be advised to store them on their person, where they will be readily available.

_____ 5. Many adverse reactions to vasodilator antihypertensive drugs tend to subside with continued use of the drug.

_____ 6. Sympatholytic vasodilators readily cross the blood–brain barrier.

_____ 7. Abrupt withdrawal of sympatholytic antihypertensive drugs can cause rebound hyperactivity of the sympathetic system.

_____ 8. Sympatholytic antihypertensive drugs increase the risk of shock from sudden stress.

_____ 9. Calcium channel blocking agents are well tolerated by most recipients.

_____ 10. Calcium channel blocking agents are usually administered only once a day.

_____ 11. When captopril is prescribed, clients should be advised to limit fluid intake to decrease the risk of water intoxication.

Selection of Options

For each of the following, select *all* appropriate responses. Circle correct answers.
1. Common adverse reactions to vasodilator antihypertensive drugs include
   a. Flushing
   b. Headache
   c. Bradycardia
   d. Postural hypotension
   e. Palpitation
   f. Renal losses of sodium and water
   g. Increased risk of angina pectoris
   h. Gastrointestinal upset

2. Advantages of Nitrobid adhesive patches over applications of nitroglycerin ointment using glassine paper include which of the following?
   a. The patches can be applied less frequently
   b. The glassine papers tend to become dislodged, facilitating inadvertent removal of medication from the skin
   c. The active ingredient in the patches has a longer serum half-life than does that in Nitrobid paste
3. Adverse reactions to antihypertensive drugs may be minimized by
   a. Taking the drugs with food or antacids
   b. Reducing fluid intake
   c. Increasing fiber in the diet
   d. Changing position slowly
4. Reserpine is administered
   a. PO
   b. SC
   c. IM
   d. IV
5. Trimethaphan is administered
   a. PO
   b. SC
   c. IM
   d. IV
6. Therapeutic uses for trimethaphan include
   a. Mainenance therapy for chronic hypertension
   b. Treatment of hypertensive crisis
   c. Producing controlled hypotension during surgery
   d. Control of angina pectoris
7. Calcium channel blocking agents act by
   a. Reducing serum levels of calcium ions
   b. Raising body pH and decreasing ionization of calcium
   c. Inhibiting flow of calcium ions into myocardial muscle cells
   d. Inhibiting flow of calcium ions into vascular smooth muscle cells
8. Therapeutic uses for calcium channel blocking agents include
   a. Management of mild hypertension
   b. Management of severe hypertension
   c. Control of angina pectoris
9. Caution should be exercised when calcium channel blocking agents are administered in conjunction with
   a. Quinidine
   b. Digitalis
   c. Basic salts
   d. Sympatholytic agents
10. When calcium channel blocking agents are used, the nurse should monitor the client for
    a. Blood pressure changes
    b. Anginal pain
    c. Changes in liver function tests
    d. Allergic reactions
    e. Any unusual developments that might indicate adverse reaction to the drugs
11. Appropriate advice for those on antihypertensive drugs who experience undesirable changes in sexual function includes telling the client that
    a. Sexual activity is risky in hypertension and decreased function is therapeutic
    b. Impairment of sexual function is sometimes unavoidable but will become less pronounced with continued therapy
    c. The physician should be consulted for changes in drug prescriptions that may eliminate the problem
    d. In men, the sexual problem can be treated by surgical implantation of a penile prosthesis
    e. The sexual problem can be ameliorated by counseling regarding alternative sexual expression
12. Clients with hypertension can enhance control of the condition by
    a. Reducing salt intake
    b. Reducing water intake
    c. Increasing physical activity as tolerated
    d. Achieving and maintaining a lean body weight
    e. Learning to manage stress well

Short Answer Questions

1. List at least three autocoids (endogenous biochemicals) believed to increase sympathomimetic vasoconstriction.

2. How often are transdermal nitroglycerin patches applied?

3. How often should nitroglycerin sublingual tablets be replaced?

4. Name at least five conditions whose risk is increased by the use of sympatholytic antihypertensive drugs.

5. List at least four precautions that are helpful when administering nitroprusside intravenously for hypertensive crisis.

PART 3: VASOCONSTRICTORS

Selection of Options

For each of the following, select *all* appropriate responses. Circle correct answers.

1. Vasoconstrictor drugs are useful in the treatment of
   a. Postural hypotension
   b. Hypotension related to anemia
   c. Hypotension related to spinal anesthesia
   d. Hypotension caused by emotional shock
2. Vasoconstrictor solutions are often combined with solutions used for
   a. Topical anesthesia
   b. Local anesthesia
   c. Spinal anesthesia
   d. General anesthesia
3. Therapeutic uses for vasoconstrictor drugs include treatment of
   a. Hypovolemic shock
   b. Cardiogenic shock
   c. Vasogenic shock
   d. Anaphylaxis
4. Over-the-counter drug preparations that are likely to contain vasopressors include
   a. Appetite suppressants
   b. Cold remedies
   c. Decongestant nose drops
   d. Sleeping pills
5. What kind(s) of dependence are usually seen when vasopressor decongestants are used repeatedly?
   a. Physical dependence manifested by systemic symptoms during withdrawal
   b. Physical dependence manifested by a local rebound effect as the drug wears off
   c. Psychologic dependence on the localized effects of the drug
   d. Psychologic dependence on the systemic effects of the drug

PART 4: SCLEROSING AGENTS

Multiple Choice Questions

For each of the following, choose the one best answer.

1. A diagnostic procedure useful in assessing varicose veins is the
   a. Angiogram
   b. Arteriogram
   c. Cardiogram
   d. Phlebogram
2. Sodium morrhuate is classified as a
   a. Sympatholytic vasodilator
   b. Peripheral vasodilator
   c. Vasopressor
   d. Sclerosing agent
3. The sclerosing agent used most often for the treatment of hemorrhoids is
   a. Sodium morrhuate
   b. Quinine and urea hydrochloride
   c. Sodium tetradecyl
4. Sclerosing agents are likely to cause
   a. Allergic anaphylaxis
   b. Hypertensive crisis
   c. Impaired clotting
   d. Severe headache

5. When sclerotherapy is undertaken, health-care personnel must be prepared to treat sudden
   a. Anaphylaxis
   b. Embolism
   c. Hemorrhage
   d. Thrombosis

6. The emergency drug most likely to be required for treatment of adverse reaction to sclerosing agents is
   a. Epinephrine
   b. Nifedipine
   c. Propranolol
   d. Phentolamine

Selection of Options

For each of the following, select *all* appropriate responses. Circle correct answers.

1. Risk factors for the development of varicose veins include
   a. Family history of varicose veins
   b. Obesity
   c. Pregnancy
   d. A vocation that involves prolonged sitting
   e. A vocation that involves prolonged standing
   f. A vocation that involves a lot of walking
   g. Abdominal tumors
   h. Smoking
   i. The use of circular elastic garters to support hose

2. Complications of varicose veins include
   a. Rash on the legs
   b. Leg ulcers
   c. Gangrene

3. Contraindications for sclerotherapy include
   a. Thrombophlebitis
   b. Previous vascular surgery
   c. Extensive deep vein varicosities
   d. Extensive superficial varicosities

4. Self-care measures for the relief of discomfort following sclerotherapy include
   a. Elevation of the legs
   b. Application of cold compresses
   c. Use of aspirin, acetaminophen, or ibuprofen

Short Answer Question

1. Identify at least three measures that tend to delay or prevent the development of varicose veins.

29
Drugs Affecting Coagulation

The blood's ability to coagulate is influenced by heredity, nutrition, hormone levels, and the function of certain body organs and systems. Although the complex mechanism is not completely understood, enough is known to correct some coagulation deficiencies and to manipulate coagulation to arrest or ameliorate certain disease conditions.

PART 1: HEMOSTATICS

Correct the False Statement

Indicate whether the following statements are true or false; if false, correct the underlined words or phrases.

_____ 1. The administration of <u>citrated blood</u> may correct all deficiencies of clotting factors.

_____ 2. Citrated blood contains all clotting factors except <u>prothrombin</u>.

_____ 3. The administration of large quantities of banked blood is likely to produce <u>an iatrogenic coagulation deficiency</u>.

_____ 4. Antihemophilic factor is administered intravenously <u>through standard tubing used for clear solutions</u>.

_____ 5. An overdose of protamine sulfate is likely to cause <u>intravascular thrombi</u>.

_____ 6. Aminocaproic acid is used in the treatment of bleeding caused by <u>overactivity of endogenous fibrinolytics</u>.

_____ 7. Aminocaproic acid is likely to be useful as an antidote for <u>heparin</u>.

_____ 8. Dosages of aminocaproic acid should be decreased for clients with <u>hepatic impairment</u>.

_____ 9. For rapid reversal of coumarin anticoagulation, <u>vitamin K</u> is administered.

_____ 10. Vitamin K is likely to cause a toxic reaction in <u>infants</u>.

_____ 11. Rapid administration of protamine sulfate may cause <u>acute hypertension</u>.

Multiple Choice Questions

For each of the following, select the one best answer.

1. Banked whole blood contains all clotting factors except
   a. Platelets
   b. Calcium
   c. Prothrombin
   d. Accelerator globulin

2. The clotting factor not found in plasma is
   a. Fibrinogen
   b. Calcium
   c. Stuart factor
   d. Platelets

3. The active ingredient in antihemophilia factor is
   a. Prothrombin
   b. Coagulation factor VIII
   c. Coagulation factor IX
   d. Coagulation factor X
4. Antihemophilia factor is used to treat bleeding episodes caused by
   a. Christmas disease
   b. Stuart disease
   c. Classic hemophilia
   d. Overdosage of the anticoagulant heparin
   e. Overdosage of the anticoagulant coumarin
5. When antihemophilia factor is infused intravenously, flow rates should be adjusted in accordance with changes in the
   a. Blood pressure
   b. Pulse rate
   c. Respiratory rate
   d. Visible bleeding
6. Factor IX complex is used to treat bleeding episodes caused by
   a. Christmas disease
   b. Stuart disease
   c. Classic hemophilia
   d. Overdosage of the anticoagulant heparin
   e. Overdosage of the anticoagulant coumarin
7. A drug used to treat hemorrhagic disease that acts as a vesicant is
   a. Blood plasma
   b. Antihemophilia factor
   c. Factor IX complex
   d. Menadione
8. Protamine sulfate is used in the treatment of hemorrhaging caused by
   a. Vitamin K deficiency
   b. Oral anticoagulants
   c. Heparin toxicity
   d. Classic hemophilia
9. Allergic reaction to protamine sulfate is most likely in persons with known sensitivity to
   a. Grains
   b. Fish
   c. Chocolate
   d. Nuts
10. Dosage of protamine sulfate is calculated in accordance with
    a. Body weight
    b. Severity of bleeding
    c. Estimated body residues of heparin
    d. Degree of liver impairment
11. When coagulants are used to treat clotting deficiencies, initial dosage is calculated
    a. To provide ample coagulation
    b. As exactly as possible to restore normal coagulation
    c. To err on the side of undercoagulation
12. A serious adverse reaction to protamine sulfate is
    a. Anaphylaxis
    b. Disseminated intravascular coagulation
    c. Severe hemorrhage
    d. Infection
13. Following administration of protamine sulfate, clients should be watched for signs and symptoms of
    a. Thrombophlebitis and peripheral embolism
    b. Anticoagulation caused by heparin rebound
    c. Hemolysis and renal impairment
14. Aminocaproic acid acts by
    a. Promoting prothrombin production by the liver
    b. Neutralizing coumarin
    c. Neutralizing heparin
    d. Inhibiting endogenous proteolytic enzymes
15. Aminocaproic acid is eliminated through the
    a. Urine
    b. Bile into feces
    c. Both of the above
    d. Neither of the above
16. The drug thrombin is derived from
    a. Animal tissues
    b. Human plasma
    c. Fish testes
    d. Chemical synthesis
17. An *early* sign or symptom of blood incompatibility reaction is
    a. Bradycardia
    b. Jaundice
    c. Backache
    d. Oliguria
18. To prevent deterioration, blood should be stored in a(n)
    a. Freezer
    b. Refrigerator
    c. Dry place at room temperature
    d. Incubator

19. Before removing dressings treated with topical hemostatics, the nurse should first
    a. Soak them in anticoagulant solution
    b. Soak them in saline solution
    c. Administer a coagulant
    d. All of the above
20. Because blood is now screened for human immunodeficiency virus (HIV), the chance of contracting AIDS from a transfusion is approximately
    a. 1 in 1000
    b. 1 in 10,000
    c. 1 in 100,000
    d. 1 in 1,000,000
21. Clients receiving tranexamic acid are most likely to react adversely by manifesting
    a. Multiple hemorrhages and hypovolemic shock
    b. Changes in vision
    c. Seizures
    d. Allergic hypersensitivity and anaphylactic shock
22. When a bleeding episode occurs, clients with coagulation deficiency are most likely to experience
    a. Anxiety and/or fear of death related to altered tissue perfusion due to hypovolemic shock
    b. Potential for altered perfusion related to myocardial ischemia due to coronary thrombosis
    c. Allergic hypersensitivity to drugs produced by recombinant DNA techniques
    d. Alteration in comfort: headache related to central nervous system irritation by hemostatic drugs

Selection of Options

For each of the following, select *all* appropriate responses. Circle correct answers.

1. Single clotting factors currently available as drug preparations include
   a. Calcium
   b. Factor VIII
   c. Thromboplastin
   d. Thrombin
2. Serious adverse reactions to whole blood administered to correct abnormal bleeding include
   a. Antigen–antibody reactions arising from incompatibility
   b. Infection caused by pathogens in the blood
   c. Circulatory overload
   d. Embolism of clots that form in the blood during storage
3. What are the sources from which clotting factors are manufactured?
   a. Animal tissues
   b. Human plasma
   c. Bacterial cultures
   d. Chemical synthesis
4. Adverse reactions to plasma administered to treat clotting deficiencies include
   a. Antigen–antibody reactions arising from incompatibility
   b. Increased risk of hepatitis A
   c. Increased risk of hepatitis B
   d. Increased risk of acquired immune deficiency syndrome (AIDS)
   e. Hypervolemia
5. Antihemophilia factor may be administered
   a. PO
   b. IM
   c. IV
   d. Topically
6. Thrombosis following administration of factor IX complex is most likely to occur in persons with blood types
   a. A
   b. B
   c. AB
   d. O
7. Vitamin K is effective in the reversal of impaired coagulation caused by
   a. Intestinal malabsorption
   b. Oral anticoagulant therapy
   c. Ingestion of certain rat poisons
   d. Impaired liver function
8. Protamine sulfate is administered
   a. PO
   b. SC
   c. IM
   d. IV
9. Aminocaproic acid is administered
   a. PO
   b. SC
   c. IM
   d. IV

10. Drugs applied topically to slow bleeding include
    a. Absorbable gelatin
    b. Epinephrine
    c. Fibrin foam
    d. Oxidized cellulose
    e. Protamine sulfate
    f. Thrombin
11. Foods that may help to correct vitamin K deficiency include
    a. Citrus fruits
    b. Green leafy vegetables
    c. Lactobacillus milk
    d. Vegetable oils
12. Tranexamic acid may be administered
    a. PO
    b. SC
    c. IM
    d. IV
    e. Intra-arterially
13. The risk of acquiring AIDS by using concentrated coagulation factors is
    a. High, because these products cannot be screened for HIV antibodies
    b. High, because these medications cannot be treated to kill or weaken viruses
    c. Low, because the blood from which these medications are made is screened for HIV antibodies
    d. Low, because these products are treated to weaken any viruses that may be present
    e. Nil, because these medications are sterilized

Short Answer Questions

1. List, in order, the major steps in the process by which blood clots.

2. Explain the mechanism of action of protamine sulfate in the reversal of heparin anticoagulation.

3. Which is more dangerous, hypocoagulability or hypercoagulability?

4. Give at least two reasons why antihemophilia factor is not administered routinely as a preventative.

PART 2: ANTICOAGULANTS

Correct the False Statement

Indicate whether the following statements are true or false; if false, correct the underlined words.

_____ 1. Anticoagulants prevent the formation and extension of clots <u>and dissolve clots already formed in the blood vessels</u>.

_____ 2. A natural source of warfarin is <u>moldy rye grain</u>.

_____ 3. The desired therapeutic result of coumarin anticoagulation is prothrombin time that is <u>about ten times</u> that of the normal control.

_____ 4. In small doses, aspirin acts as <u>an anticoagulant agent</u>.

_____ 5. When aspirin is used to decrease the risk of clot formation, <u>analgesic doses of the drug are contraindicated</u>.

_____ 6. High stress level in a client receiving anticoagulants is likely to <u>increase the risk of hemorrhage</u>.

_____ 7. Clients receiving low-dose heparin therapy who have had surgery should be watched for signs and symptoms of <u>formation of adhesions and keloid scars</u>.

_____ 8. The anticoagulant used to prevent clotting in heart–lung and artificial kidney machines is <u>sodium citrate</u>.

_____ 9. Massive blood transfusions are likely to cause coagulation deficiencies because banked blood is treated with the anticoagulant <u>heparin</u>.

_____ 10. An anticoagulant drug that can cause alopecia is <u>aspirin</u>.

_____ 11. To prevent rebound hypercoagulability, clients may be weaned off <u>heparin</u> instead of being withdrawn abruptly.

Multiple Choice Questions

For each of the following, choose the one best answer.
1. An *early* sign of coumarin toxicity is
   a. Visible blood in feces
   b. Visible blood in urine
   c. Disseminated petechiae
   d. Epistaxis
2. A tissue storage site for coumarin anticoagulant is
   a. Bone
   b. Fat
   c. Plasma proteins
   d. The liver
3. Clients on long-term oral anticoagulants should be cautioned against using
   a. Acetaminophen
   b. Aspirin
   c. Antacids
   d. One-a-day vitamin preparations
4. The most common side effect of heparin anticoagulation is
   a. Allergic rash
   b. Melena
   c. Ecchymoses in the antecubital space
   d. Suppression of normal intestinal flora

Selection of Options

For each of the following, select *all* appropriate responses. Circle correct answers.
1. Indications for anticoagulant therapy include
   a. Atrial fibrillation
   b. A history of coronary thrombosis
   c. Pregnancy
   d. Thrombophlebitis
2. Contraindications for anticoagulant therapy include
   a. Active hemorrhage
   b. Threatened abortion
   c. Thrombophlebitis
   d. Peptic ulcer
   e. Intracranial hemorrhage
   f. Eye surgery
   g. Brain surgery
3. The anticoagulant action of coumarin is often influenced by drugs that
   a. Are bound to plasma proteins
   b. Stimulate liver production of bile
   c. Alter function of liver microsomal enzymes
   d. Increase urinary output
4. Drugs that inhibit platelet aggregation include
   a. Aspirin
   b. Dextrans
   c. Phenindione
   d. Dipyridamole
5. Signs and symptoms of anticoagulant toxicity include
   a. Dark urine
   b. Tarry stools
   c. Bruising
   d. Cold, pale extremities
   e. Painful joints
   f. Epistaxis
6. Clients on long-term oral anticoagulant therapy should be advised to
   a. Avoid trauma
   b. Avoid marked fluctuation in vitamin C intake
   c. Avoid marked fluctuation in vitamin K intake
   d. Wear a medical identification device identifying the treatment regimen

Short Answer Questions

1. Is heparin effective when administered orally?

2. Why is heparin not administered intramuscularly?

3. Are oral anticoagulants used during pregnancy?

4. When both heparin and coumarin anticoagulants are administered concurrently, which drug is likely to be discontinued first?

5. What changes are necessary in subcutaneous injection technique when heparin is administered?

6. Is it necessary to restrict vitamin K in the diets of clients receiving oral anticoagulants?

7. Is it possible to administer concurrently with coumarin drugs that influence the physiologic action of the anticoagulant?

Completion Exercise

Read the following carefully and place your answers in the space provided. Compare and contrast heparin and coumarin anticoagulants.

	COUMARIN	HEPARIN
Mechanism of action		
Route(s) of administration		
Unit of measurement of doses		
Frequency of dosage		
Onset of action		
Antidote(s)		
Laboratory test for monitoring response		
Toxic reaction		
Other adverse reaction(s)		

PART 3: FIBRINOLYTICS

Matching

For each fibrinolytic drug in the left-hand column, choose its source(s) from the column on the right.

DRUG	SOURCE
1. Plasmin	a. Natural production in the human body
2. Tissue plasminogen activator	b. Bacterial cultures
3. Streptokinase	c. Recombinant DNA techniques
4. Urokinase	d. Laboratory synthesis

Correct the False Statement

Indicate whether the following statements are true or false; if false, correct the underlined words.

_____ 1. Fibrinolytics are <u>vitamin K analogs</u>.

_____ 2. To effectively dissolve intravascular clots, fibrinolytic therapy must begin within <u>3 to 5 hours</u> of formation of the clot.

_____ 3. When used to treat coronary thrombosis, fibrinolytic drugs are likely to be administered <u>orally</u>.

Multiple Choice Questions

For each of the following, choose the one best answer.

1. A client, hospitalized for treatment of thrombophlebitis of the deep veins of his right leg, is receiving both heparin and warfarin. He tells you he is afraid of bleeding to death "because the medications may thin my blood too much." Your best reply would be
   a. He is in no danger of sudden death.
   b. The drugs do not really "thin" the blood.
   c. The two drugs antagonize each other, reducing the risk of severe hemorrhage.
   d. The drugs slow clotting but do not abolish it.

2. During the natural process of clot dissolution, fibrin is degraded by
   a. Plasminogen activator
   b. Plasmin
   c. Urokinase
   d. Fibrin degradation products

3. A procedure used to deliver a fibrinolytic drug directly into the coronary artery is
   a. Intravenous
   b. Cardiac catheterization
   c. Arteriovenous shunt
   d. Coronary bypass

4. A client under treatment for myocardial ischemia is most likely to experience a cardiac arrhythmia when
   a. The fibrinolytic medication is first administered
   b. Perfusion is restored to the myocardium
   c. The heparin is discontinued to allow withdrawal of the arterial sheath
   d. Fibrinolytic therapy is discontinued

5. Intracoronary infusion of streptokinase has been ordered for an emergency room client with a diagnosis of myocardial ischemia and impending MI (myocardial infarction). Consent for treatment was secured from his wife. When should he be told about the procedure?
   a. As soon as the order is written, to give him time to prepare himself
   b. As close to the time of the procedure as possible, to prevent him from becoming extremely anxious
   c. The client need not be told; he can be anesthetized in his bed before the procedure
   d. The timing of the disclosure is irrelevant as long as the client is informed

Selection of Options

For each of the following, select *all* appropriate responses. Circle correct answers.

1. Adverse reactions to fibrinolytics include
   a. Increased risk of hemorrhage
   b. Allergic reactions
   c. Local tissue reactions
   d. Nausea and vomiting

2. Contraindications for fibrinolytics include
   a. Hemorrhage
   b. Cellulitis
   c. Coagulation deficiencies
   d. Renal impairment
   e. Severe liver disease

3. Fibrinolytic treatment increases the risk of
   a. Hemorrhage
   b. Thromboembolus
   c. Fistula formation
   d. Scarring of the thrombosed veins
   e. Infarction

4. Which of the following fibrinolytic drugs produces a systemic anticoagulation?
   a. Streptokinase
   b. Urokinase
   c. Tissue plasminogen activator
   d. Alpha protease

Short Answer Question

1. How must fibrinolytic drugs be stored and handled to preserve their efficacy?

PART 4: DRUGS THAT ENHANCE PERIPHERAL CIRCULATION

Selection of Options

For each of the following, select *all* appropriate responses. Circle correct answers.
1. Probable reactions to pentoxifylline include
   a. Increased deformation of red blood cells
   b. Increased viscosity of the blood
   c. Anticoagulation
   d. Decreased systemic vascular resistance
   e. Decreased fertility in men

PART 5: EXERCISES RELATING TO THE ENTIRE CHAPTER

Multiple Choice Questions

For each of the following, choose the one best answer.
1. What kind of drug is tranexamic acid?
   a. Hemostatic
   b. Anticoagulant
   c. Fibrinolytic
   d. Both fibrinolytic and anticoagulant
2. When an arteriovenous cannula becomes obstructed by a clot, the physician will probably
   a. Irrigate the cannula with heparin until the clot dissolves or can be aspirated
   b. Irrigate the cannula with streptokinase until the clot dissolves and can be aspirated
   c. Irrigate the cannula with tranexamic acid until the clot can be pushed through the cannula
   d. Remove the cannula and establish another at a new vascular site
3. The agent most likely to restore all coagulation factors to a normal level is
   a. Fresh uncitrated blood
   b. Blood that has been processed by a blood bank
   c. Plasma
   d. Packed red blood cells
4. Of the following drugs, which is most likely to cause adverse interaction with other drugs?
   a. Thrombin
   b. Heparin
   c. Warfarin
   d. Urokinase

Short Answer Questions

1. List at least three nursing behaviors that promote trust by clients in life-threatening situations such as hemorrhage or coronary thrombosis.

2. Name at least five nursing actions likely to lower clients' stress levels.

UNIT SEVEN: DRUGS AFFECTING THE GASTROINTESTINAL SYSTEM

30
Agents Affecting the Upper Gastrointestinal Tract

Large quantities of nonprescription drugs for self-treatment of problems of the upper gastrointestinal tract are purchased over the counter. This fact makes consumer education very important. Nurses must be familiar with nonprescription drugs so that they can help clients use them safely. In addition they must understand prescription drugs in order to assist with medical treatment.

Matching

A. Match the agent in the left-hand column with the actions or properties it exhibits in the right-hand column.

_____ 1. Sodium perborate
_____ 2. Hydrogen peroxide
_____ 3. Potassium permanganate

a. Causes toxicity when ingested
b. Acts as an oxidizing agent
c. Discolors the membranes
d. Must be used while solutions are fresh
e. Can cause "hairy tongue" when used for a prolonged period

B. Match the metallic ion contained in antacids in the left-hand column with all of its appropriate adverse effects in the right-hand column.

_____ 1. Sodium
_____ 2. Calcium
_____ 3. Magnesium
_____ 4. Aluminum

a. Diarrhea
b. Constipation
c. Water retention
d. Neurotoxicity
e. Potentiation of digitalis
f. Gastrointestinal or renal concretions
g. Hypertension

Crossword Puzzle

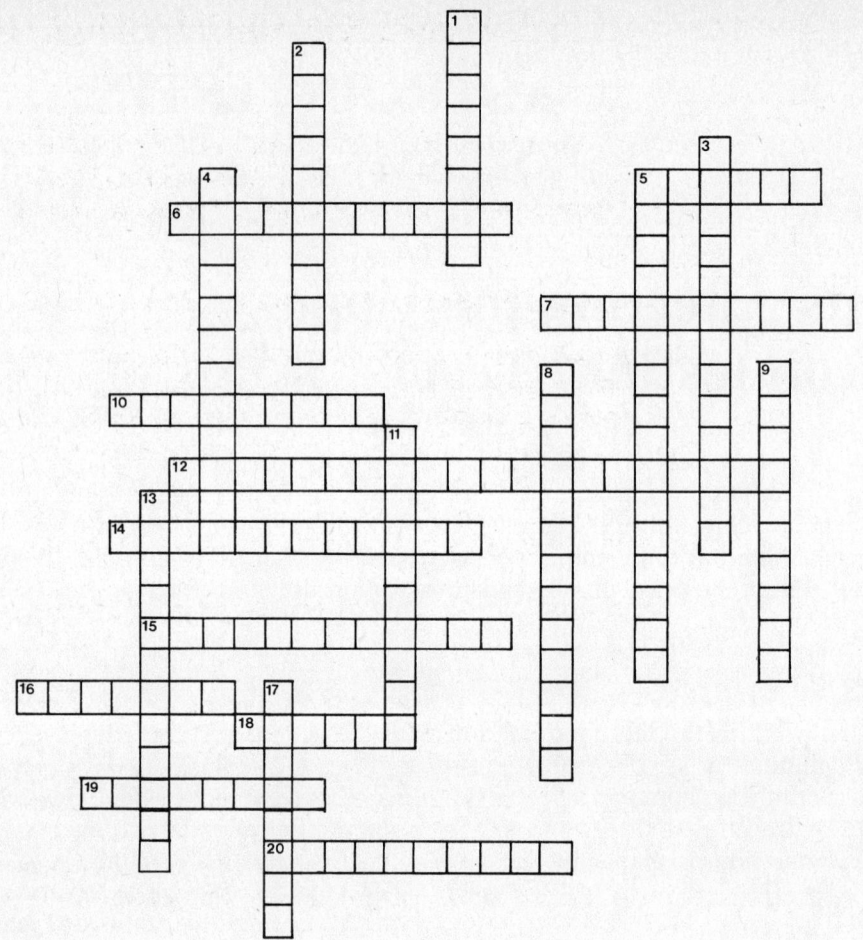

ACROSS

5. The trade name for ranitidine
6. An erosion of gastrointestinal mucosa that is exposed to gastric secretions
7. Generic name of the newest histamine-2 receptor antagonist
10. Frequency of ranitidine dosage
12. The site of action of ranitidine and cimetidine
14. A condition treated by both antacids and histamine-2 receptor antagonists
15. A side effect of ranitidine
16. The trade name for cimetidine
18. A gastric enzyme that is most active in an acid medium
19. Drugs used to neutralize hydrochloric acid in the stomach
20. The first histamine-2 receptor antagonist approved for medical use

DOWN

1. An adverse reaction to cimetidine
2. The generic name for Zantac
3. A form of medication that may be prematurely released when taken with antacids
4. A medication that forms a nonabsorbable complex when taken with calcium antacids
5. A syndrome treated by histamine-2 receptor antagonists
8. Usual timing of cimetidine dosage for treatment of peptic ulcer
9. A drug that forms a mechanical barrier between peptic ulcer sites and gastric secretions
11. The effect of cimetidine on liver microsomal enzymes
13. A side effect of cimetidine in men
17. An undesirable side effect caused by all three histamine-2 receptor antagonists

Correct the False Statement

Indicate whether the following statements are true or false; if false, correct the underlined words or phrases.

_____ 1. In people with normal dietary intake and good habits of hygiene, offensive breath odors are most likely to be caused by systemic conditions.

_____ 2. Fluorides are incorporated into the crystalline structure of tooth enamel only when they are ingested for systemic effect.

_____ 3. Fluoride rinses are recommended for children age 3 years and older.

_____ 4. Foods most likely to promote tooth decay are those containing fatty acids.

_____ 5. A good mouthwash will mask breath odor for 3 hours.

_____ 6. Clients using oral lozenges should be advised to remove the lozenge from the mouth as soon as discomfort subsides.

_____ 7. Digestants are essential for the breakdown of food into insoluble particles.

_____ 8. Pepsin facilitates the breakdown of protein in the stomach.

_____ 9. Pancreatin contains the enzymes lipase, amylase, and trypsin.

_____ 10. Pancreatic enzymes are taken on an empty stomach.

_____ 11. 10% hydrochloric acid solution is diluted during its administration.

_____ 12. Bile aids in the digestion of fats.

_____ 13. Digestive enzymes can be easily destroyed by a basic environment.

_____ 14. Bile is secreted by the duodenum.

_____ 15. Emulsification reduces surface tension of foods.

_____ 16. Vitamin K is water soluble.

_____ 17. The ingestion of food stimulates hydrochloric acid secretion.

_____ 18. An autogenous biochemical that directly stimulates gastric acid secretion is epinephrine.

_____ 19. Histamine-2 receptor antagonists act in the same way as antihistamines.

_____ 20. Histamine-2 receptor antagonists inhibit gastric acid secretion in response to food as much as they inhibit basal secretion of hydrochloric acid.

_____ 21. In persons with normal liver function, oral doses of both cimetidine and ranitidine undergo first-pass metabolism of half or more of the dose.

_____ 22. Histamine-2 receptor antagonists readily cross the blood–brain barrier.

_____ 23. Both cimetidine and ranitidine are distributed to milk.

_____ 24. Dosage of histamine-2 receptor antagonists should be reduced for clients with renal impairment.

_____ 25. In clients with renal failure, histamine-2 receptor antagonists should be administered after the hemodialysis treatments.

_____ 26. Ranitidine does not exert the same antiandrogenic effects that are seen with cimetidine.

_____ 27. A therapeutic response to histamine-2 receptor antagonists rules out gastric malignancy.

_____ 28. Histamine-2 receptor antagonists are considered safe for use during pregnancy.

_____ 29. Antacids sold over the counter are considered nontoxic and free from serious adverse side effects.

_____ 30. Liquid preparations of oral antacids are generally more effective than are tablets.

_____ 31. In the treatment of peptic ulcers, a disadvantage of antacids not shared by histamine-2 receptor antagonists is a shorter duration of action.

_____ 32. The use of antacids in the treatment of hiatal hernia is primarily a comfort measure.

_____ 33. The action of sucralfate is systemic rather than local.

_____ 34. Apomorphine exerts a weaker analgesic action than does morphine.

_____ 35. The effects of apomorphine can be reversed by administering the morphine antagonist naloxone (Narcon).

_____ 36. Apomorphine is not contraindicated for patients who are allergic to opioids.

_____ 37. Following oral administration of ipecac, it is likely that the drug will be absorbed in appreciable amounts by approximately 90% of recipients.

_____ 38. If ipecac fails to produce emesis after two doses, an antidote should be administered.

_____ 39. After a prompt and complete emptying of the stomach for the treatment of accidental ingestion of an overdose of medicine, follow-up care is usually unnecessary.

_____ 40. Before an emetic is administered, nothing should be given by mouth.

_____ 41. Adverse reactions to trimethobenzamide occur infrequently and seldom require discontinuation of the drug.

_____ 42. When antiemetics are ordered to be given PRN, the nurse may administer the drug prophylactically to prevent vomiting.

Multiple Choice Questions

For each of the following, choose the one best answer.

1. Halitosis ("bad breath") may arise from
   a. Inability to eat and drink
   b. Lack of rudimentary oral hygiene
   c. Ingestion of strong-flavored foods or alcoholic drinks
   d. Systemic disease
   e. All of the above
2. An ingredient of toothpaste that can reduce the incidence of tooth decay is
   a. Calcium carbonate
   b. Alcohol
   c. Propylene glycol
   d. Stannous fluoride
3. The authority that endorses fluoride toothpastes as effective deterrents to dental decay is the
   a. Food and Drug Administration
   b. Council on Drugs of the American

Medical Association
c. Council on Dental Therapeutics of the American Dental Association
d. The United States Public Health Department

4. Salt and soda bicarbonate toothpowder should *not* be recommended to clients
   a. Prone to respiratory acidosis
   b. Prone to metabolic alkalosis
   c. On restricted fluid intake
   d. On restricted sodium intake

5. All oxidizing agents used to clean the mouth act by
   a. Sterilizing the mouth
   b. Breaking down foreign material in the mouth
   c. Effervescing and mechanically washing away debris
   d. All of the above

6. A sodium perborate solution suitable for use as a mouthwash would have the following concentration:
   a. 0.2%   c. 2%
   b. 1%   d. 5%

7. To prepare a hydrogen peroxide mouthwash from 3% hydrogen peroxide solution, you should
   a. Mix one part of 3% peroxide with two parts of water
   b. Mix one part of 3% peroxide with one part of water
   c. Use the 3% peroxide undiluted
   d. Obtain a stronger solution; hydrogen peroxide mouthwash should be a 5% solution

8. The mouth cleaners most likely to reduce the normal flora of the mouth significantly are
   a. Solutions of sodium perborate
   b. Lozenges containing antiseptics
   c. Rinses containing potassium permanganate
   d. Solutions of hydrogen peroxide

9. A substance used to treat small razor cuts is
   a. Styptic pencil
   b. Potassium permanganate
   c. Hydrogen peroxide
   d. All of the above

10. When administered as a digestant, hydrochloric acid is prepared from a
    a. 0.9% solution   d. 5% solution
    b. 1% solution   e. 10% solution
    c. 1.5% solution

11. When administered orally, hydrochloric acid should be given
    a. At least 1 hour before meals
    b. Just before meals
    c. With meals
    d. After meals

12. When administered as a digestant, the usual adult dosage range for 10% hydrochloric acid is
    a. 1 ml to 2 ml   c. 15 ml to 30 ml
    b. 4 ml to 8 ml   d. 30 ml to 50 ml

13. When administered orally, hydrochloric acid solutions should be diluted to a strength of about
    a. 0.5%   c. 5%
    b. 1%   d. 10%

14. When administered as a digestant, pepsin elixir is given in doses of
    a. 4 ml once a day
    b. 8 ml tid pc
    c. 15 ml bid ac
    d. 1 oz with each meal or snack

15. What is the source of pancreatin?
    a. Chemical synthesis
    b. Animal tissue
    c. Plant extract
    d. Bacterial culture

16. The usual dosage of pancreatic enzymes is defined in terms of
    a. Trypsin
    b. Amylase content
    c. Lipase content
    d. All of the above

17. What is the chemical structure of most enzymes?
    a. Acid   c. Steroid
    b. Base   d. Protein

18. Digestive enzymes should be administered
    a. Before meals with cold fluids
    b. Before meals with hot fluids
    c. After meals with cold fluids
    d. After meals with hot fluids

19. Bile and bile acids act as
    a. Acids
    b. Enzymes
    c. Active transport carriers
    d. Surfactants

20. Bile salts are most important to the digestion of
    a. Sugars   c. Proteins
    b. Starches   d. Fats

21. The source of bile acids used medicinally is
    a. Chemical synthesis
    b. Animal tissue
    c. Plant extract
    d. Bacterial culture

22. What type of substance is dehydrocholic acid?
    a. An inorganic acid
    b. A bile acid
    c. A bile salt
    d. An enzyme
23. Ox bile extract is administered
    a. Between meals   c. After meals
    b. Before meals   d. At bedtime
24. The conversion of pepsinogen to active pepsin is most rapid at a pH of
    a. 2   c. 7
    b. 5   d. 8
25. Gastric pH normally ranges between
    a. 0 and 2   c. 5 and 7
    b. 2 and 5   d. 7 and 8
26. The main protection for the gastric mucosa against acid secretions is
    a. The buffering action of food
    b. The buffering action of saliva
    c. Thin mucus
    d. Viscid mucus
27. A secondary effect of histamine-2 antagonists is
    a. Stimulation of gastric mucosa secretion
    b. Stimulation of gastric pepsin secretion
    c. Inhibition of gastric mucus secretion
    d. Inhibition of gastric pepsin secretion
28. If cimetidine is administered to clients receiving opioid analgesics, the nurse should observe the clients carefully for
    a. Hypotensive shock
    b. Respiratory depression
    c. Jaundice
    d. Restlessness and hyperactivity
29. An adverse reaction to long-term use of ranitidine that has not been seen with long-term use of cimetidine is
    a. Headache
    b. Respiratory depression
    c. Vitamin B_{12} deficiency
    d. Impaired sexual response
30. When cimetidine therapy is reduced or withdrawn, the dose that is likely to be the last one discontinued is the
    a. Morning dose
    b. Noon dose
    c. Late afternoon dose
    d. Bedtime dose
31. Antacids administered orally tend to cause
    a. Respiratory acidosis
    b. Respiratory alkalosis
    c. Metabolic acidosis
    d. Metabolic alkalosis
    e. Little change in acid-base balance, unless they are absorbed systemically
32. The antacid most likely to cause acute gastric distention is
    a. Calcium carbonate
    b. Aluminum hydroxide
    c. Magnesium hydroxide
    d. Sodium bicarbonate
33. At the present time, the incidence of adverse reactions to sucralfate is believed to be
    a. Less than 5%
    b. About 10% to 15%
    c. About 20% to 25%
    d. About 30% to 50%
34. What percentage of sucralfate is absorbed systemically from the gastrointestinal tract?
    a. Less than 1%
    b. 3% to 5%
    c. Approximately 50%
    d. 70% to 90%
35. Two classes of drugs with useful antiemetic properties are
    a. Opioids and barbiturates
    b. Anticholinergics and antihistamines
    c. Sympathomimetics and xanthines
36. The most common adverse reaction to benzquinamide is
    a. Hyperphagia   c. Myoclonus
    b. Drowsiness   d. Pallor
37. An antiemetic likely to be used in the treatment of Ménière's disease is
    a. Benzquinamide
    b. Diphenidol
    c. Metoclopramide
    d. Scopolamine
38. An antiemetic that sometimes causes visual and auditory hallucinations is
    a. Benzquinamide
    b. Diphenidol
    c. Metoclopramide
    d. Atropine
39. An antiemetic that acts as a dopamine receptor antagonist is
    a. Benzquinamide
    b. Diphenidol
    c. Metoclopramide
    d. Scopolamine
40. An antiemetic whose use is limited to acute care settings is
    a. Diphenidol
    b. Metoclopramide
    c. Scopolamine
41. An antiemetic used for the management of gastrointestinal motility disorders is

a. Benzquinamide
   b. Diphenidol
   c. Metoclopramide
   d. Scopolamine
42. An antiemetic likely to be used for the control of chronic nausea and vomiting is
   a. Benzquinamide
   b. Diphenidol
   c. Metoclopramide
   d. Trimethobenzamide
43. To decrease the morning sickness of pregnancy, the nurse may recommend
   a. Eating dry crackers before arising
   b. Drinking effervescent beverages
   c. Drinking large amounts of water
   d. The use of over-the-counter antiemetics
44. Dosages of over-the-counter antiemetics used to prevent carsickness should be taken
   a. Immediately prior to starting the trip
   b. At least 15 minutes before beginning the trip
   c. At least 30 minutes before beginning the trip
   d. At least 1 hour before beginning the trip
45. Following administration, apomorphine usually induces vomiting within
   a. 15 minutes   c. 60 minutes
   b. 30 minutes   d. 2 hours
46. Apomorphine is used therapeutically to
   a. Prevent vomiting of caustic poisons
   b. Prevent vomiting of nonvolatile poisons
   c. Induce vomiting of volatile or caustic poisons
   d. Induce vomiting of noncaustic nonvolatile poisons
47. Following oral administration, ipecac usually produces emesis within
   a. 1 minute   c. 15 minutes
   b. 5 minutes   d. 30 minutes
48. The ipecac preparation recommended for first aid in the treatment of poisoning is
   a. Oral tincture of ipecac
   b. Oral ipecac fluidextract
   c. Oral ipecac syrup
   d. 10% solution for injection
49. The recommended dosage of ipecac used to treat poisoning is
   a. A single dose of up to 30 ml
   b. A single dose of up to 60 ml
   c. Up to two doses of 15 ml to 30 ml each
   d. Up to two doses of 30 ml to 50 ml each
50. How many doses of apomorphine may be given to treat overdose or poisoning?
   a. Only one
   b. Up to two, 30 minutes apart
   c. Up to three, 15 minutes apart
   d. Any number, provided they are given at least 1 hour apart
51. The antidote for apomorphine is
   a. Compazine
   b. Caffeine
   c. Naloxone
   d. Gastric lavage to recover the dose before intestinal absorption
52. Ipecac should not be used to treat children younger than
   a. 6 months   c. 3 years
   b. 1 year   d. 6 years

Selection of Options

For each of the following, select *all* appropriate responses. Circle correct answers.
1. Abrasives used in toothpastes include
   a. Pumice
   b. Calcium carbonate
   c. Finely ground glass
   d. Milk of magnesia
2. Cleansing ingredients in toothpastes include
   a. Soap
   b. Glycerin
   c. Pumice
   d. Alcohol
3. Fluoride preparations are applied topically to the teeth to
   a. Make the tooth enamel whiter
   b. Render the tooth enamel resistant to acids
   c. Desensitize exposed root surfaces of teeth
4. Fluoride compounds for dietary supplementation are available in the form of
   a. Bulk chemicals to be added to the public water supply
   b. Salt to be sprinkled on food
   c. Tablets for oral ingestion
   d. Solutions for injection
5. Allergy to fluorides is likely to cause
   a. Skin rash
   b. Sore mouth
   c. Gastrointestinal upset
   d. Respiratory distress

6. After ingesting a dose of liquid hydrochloric acid, the client should
    a. Ingest a small dose of sodium bicarbonate
    b. Rinse the mouth with a bicarbonate solution
    c. Drink an acid fruit juice
    d. Consume food
7. What type of drug is pepsin?
    a. An aromatic oil
    b. A carminative
    c. A digestant
    d. An enzyme
8. What types of drugs are in pancreatin?
    a. Inorganic acid
    b. Enzyme
    c. Lipase
    d. Amylase
    e. Protease
    f. Emulsifier
9. Ox bile extracts should not be given to clients with
    a. Jaundice
    b. Complete biliary obstruction
    c. Incomplete biliary obstruction
10. Mechanical barriers to migration of hydrochloric acid to inappropriate parts of the digestive tract include
    a. Esophageal sphincter of the stomach
    b. Cardiac sphincter of the stomach
    c. Pyloric sphincter of the stomach
    d. Reflux of bile and pancreatic secretions from the duodenum
11. Drugs that decrease gastric acid production by inhibiting stress responses include
    a. Barbiturates
    b. Tranquilizers
    c. Anticholinergics
12. Histamine-2 receptor antagonists include
    a. Cimetidine
    b. Tagamet
    c. Ranitidine
    d. Zantac
    e. Chlor-Trimeton
13. Histamine-2 receptor antagonists are used medicinally in the treatment of
    a. Peptic ulcer
    b. Gastric cancer
    c. Gastritis
    d. Allergic reactions
    e. Zollinger–Ellison syndrome
14. The nurse should observe the client receiving either cimetidine or ranitidine for
    a. Change in the degree of epigastric distress
    b. Headache
    c. Hypotension
    d. Rash
    e. Joint pain
15. Because it inhibits liver microsomal enzymes, cimetidine increases the physiologic effects of a given dose of
    a. Chlordiazepoxide
    b. Diazepam
    c. Lidocaine
    d. Penicillin
    e. Phenytoin
    f. Salicylates
    g. Theophylline
16. Known adverse reactions to ranitidine include
    a. Headache
    b. Leukocytosis
    c. Impaired sexual function in men
    d. Malaise
    e. Diarrhea
    f. Rash
    g. Tachycardia
    h. Anaphylaxis
17. Nursing measures that may result in reduced secretion of gastric acid are
    a. Assisting the client to reduce smoking
    b. Assisting the client to reduce the ingestion of alcohol
    c. Promoting the use of whole milk in the diet
    d. Actions to eliminate stressors affecting the client
    e. Assisting the client to improve stress management
18. Sucralfate has an affinity for
    a. Parietal cells of the gastric mucosa
    b. Histamine-2 receptor sites
    c. Pepsin molecules
    d. Peptic ulcer sites
19. Adverse reactions to sucralfate include
    a. Constipation
    b. Nausea
    c. Pruritic rash
    d. Insomnia
    e. Dizziness and vertigo
20. Antiemetics used specifically for the prevention or treatment of nausea or vomiting associated with surgery include
    a. Benzquinamide
    b. Diphenidol
    c. Metoclopramide
    d. Scopolamine
21. Benzquinamide may be administered
    a. Orally

    b. Intramuscularly
    c. Subcutaneously
    d. Rectally
22. The effects of metoclopramide include
    a. Antiemesis
    b. Stimulation of dopamine receptors
    c. Stimulation of gastrointestinal motility
    d. Accelerated transit of the contents of the stomach and small intestine
23. Rapid intravenous injection of metoclopramide is likely to cause
    a. Cardiac arrhythmias
    b. Distressing changes in mood
    c. Nausea and vomiting
    d. Hypotensive shock
24. Metoclopramide tends to enhance the effects of
    a. Alcohol
    b. Amphetamines
    c. Barbiturates
    d. Opioids
25. Trimethobenzamide is administered by the following routes:
    a. PO
    b. SC
    c. IM
    d. IV
26. Beverages that help to alleviate nausea include
    a. Fruit juices
    b. Ginger ale
    c. Tea
    d. Water
27. Contraindications to the use of metoclopramide include
    a. A history of seizure
    b. Intestinal obstruction
    c. Intestinal perforation
    d. Procainamide allergy
28. Probable mechanisms of action of the emetic apomorphine include
    a. Irritation of the gastric mucosa
    b. Direct stimulation of the chemoreceptor trigger zone
    c. Indirect stimulation of the chemoreceptor trigger zone through excitation of the vestibular centers
    d. Induction of a nauseating olfactory hallucination
29. Adverse reactions to apomorphine include
    a. Excitation
    b. Flushing
    c. Circulatory failure
    d. Respiratory failure
    e. Involuntary muscle movements
30. Contraindications for the use of apomorphine include
    a. Age extremes
    b. Cardiovascular disease
    c. Coma
    d. Presence of a gag reflex
    e. Ingestion of a corrosive poison
31. Mechanisms of action of ipecac include
    a. Irritation of the gastric mucosa
    b. Induction of a nauseating olfactory hallucination
    c. Stimulation of the chemoreceptor trigger zone
32. Advantages of ipecac over apomorphine for the treatment of poisoning are that ipecac
    a. May be administered orally
    b. Is safe to use during pregnancy
    c. May be given safely to clients allergic to opioids
    d. Does not produce central nervous system depression
    e. Does not produce respiratory depression
33. Emetine that is absorbed systemically tends to cause
    a. Central nervous system disruption
    b. Cardiotoxicity
    c. Neuromuscular abnormalities
    d. Bone marrow depression
34. Tissue sites at which antiemetics act include the
    a. Vestibule of the inner ear
    b. Chemoreceptor trigger zone
    c. Gastrointestinal mucosa
    d. Vomiting center

Short Answer Questions

1. How would you prepare an effective, low-cost tooth powder?

2. Using household measures, how would you prepare 100 ml of the following?
   a. 2% solution of sodium perborate

   b. 1% solution of sodium bicarbonate

   c. 0.9% solution of sodium chloride?

3. What concentration of sodium chloride in water would be isotonic? _____

4. Define the term "digestant."

5. Name four major categories of digestants.

6. Briefly describe instructions that you would give to the patient receiving 10% hydrochloric acid solution.

7. List at least five factors predisposing to problems associated with "hyperacidity."

8. Name at least six mechanisms by which the genetic predisposition to "hyperacidity" may be expressed.

9. What is "acid rebound"?

10. Why should clients receiving histamine-2 receptors be observed closely for changes in physiologic, intellectual, and affective status?

11. Identify at least four environmental factors that increase the risk of problems attributed to "hyperacidity."

12. Should water be administered with liquid antacids? Why or why not?

13. How frequently are oral antacids usually administered?

14. Are over-the-counter antacids cheaper overall than the legend drug cimetidine for the treatment of peptic ulcer?

15. Is it advisable to leave antacid medications at the bedside for clients to administer to themselves?

16. May one over-the-counter antacid be substituted for another?

17. How is sucralfate eliminated from the body?

18. How should oral antacids in tablet form be administered?

19. Define "emetic."

20. Define "antiemetic."

21. The anticholinergic most often used as an antiemetic is _____.

22. Name three signs or symptoms that require immediate discontinuation of diphenidol.

23. How can vomiting be differentiated from regurgitation?

24. Is the use of antiemetics recommended for the treatment of nausea and vomiting of pregnancy?

25. Name at least three types of poisoning in which the use of emetics is contraindicated or controversial.

26. What can the nurse do when a drug overdose or a noncorrosive nonlipid poison has been taken, and no emetic is available for first aid?

Personal Exercise: Self-Medication

Common drug advertisements deal with the signs and symptoms of indigestion. How do *you* decide which remedy is best for you?

31
Agents Affecting the Lower Gastrointestinal Tract

The following exercises relate to the material in the textbook on antiflatulents, laxatives, and antidiarrheals.

Correct the False Statement

Indicate whether the following statements are true or false; if false, correct the underlined words or phrases.

_____ 1. Flatulence and abdominal cramping caused by lactulose <u>tend to subside</u> with continued administration of the drug.

_____ 2. Hyperosmotic laxatives containing magnesium <u>are preferred for</u> treating constipation in clients with renal failure.

_____ 3. The laxatives whose actions mimic most closely the physiologic process of fecal elimination are <u>the surfactant laxatives</u>.

_____ 4. The use of psyllium hydrophilic mucilloid <u>tends to reduce</u> plasma cholesterol concentrations.

_____ 5. The use of laxatives <u>tends to be</u> habit-forming.

_____ 6. An initial defecation reflex tends to persist for <u>5 to 10 minutes</u>.

_____ 7. Reducing stress levels may help to correct constipation in persons in whom stress increases <u>parasympathetic nervous activity</u>.

_____ 8. For the treatment of recurrent chronic constipation, the nurse may recommend regular long-term use <u>of lubricant laxatives</u>.

_____ 9. Phenolphthalein sometimes changes <u>the color</u> of urine or stools.

_____ 10. Aloin is an herbal remedy that is <u>effective and safe</u> for use as a laxative.

_____ 11. Mineral waters <u>are effective</u> laxatives.

_____ 12. Adsorbent antidiarrheals act by <u>neutralizing irritants and toxins in the intestine</u>.

Crossword Puzzle

ACROSS

3. A laxative food
4. A type of drug likely to be used to treat diarrhea during narcotic withdrawal
8. Term used for the strongest type of laxative
9. A chemical reaction in the intestine that generates gas
10. A food substance that promotes intestinal fermentation and flatus
12. Chemical nature of most antiflatulents
15. A nutrient likely to become deficient when mineral oil is used regularly

ACROSS (continued)

17. A folk remedy that is effective in relieving flatulence
21. A laxative that is absorbed and subsequently secreted in breast milk
23. An organism in the normal gastrointestinal flora that protects against some kinds of diarrhea
25. A laxative food enjoyed by most children
26. Drugs that act as antiflatulents

DOWN

1. A folk remedy for diarrhea
2. A potentially lethal result of careless handling of dry bulk laxatives
5. A defoaming antiflatulent
6. Term used for a strong laxative
7. A food component that promotes fecal elimination
11. A food component that promotes fermentation in the gut
13. A nonnutritive lubricating laxative
14. A beverage that is useful for diarrhea
16. A nursing measure to relieve gas in the colon
18. A food that acts as a laxative
19. The black drug in a "black and white" laxative
20. A food useful in reducing diarrhea caused by broad-spectrum antibacterial anti-infectives
22. The chemical formed from castor oil that produces its laxative effect
24. Pain in newborns associated with flatulence

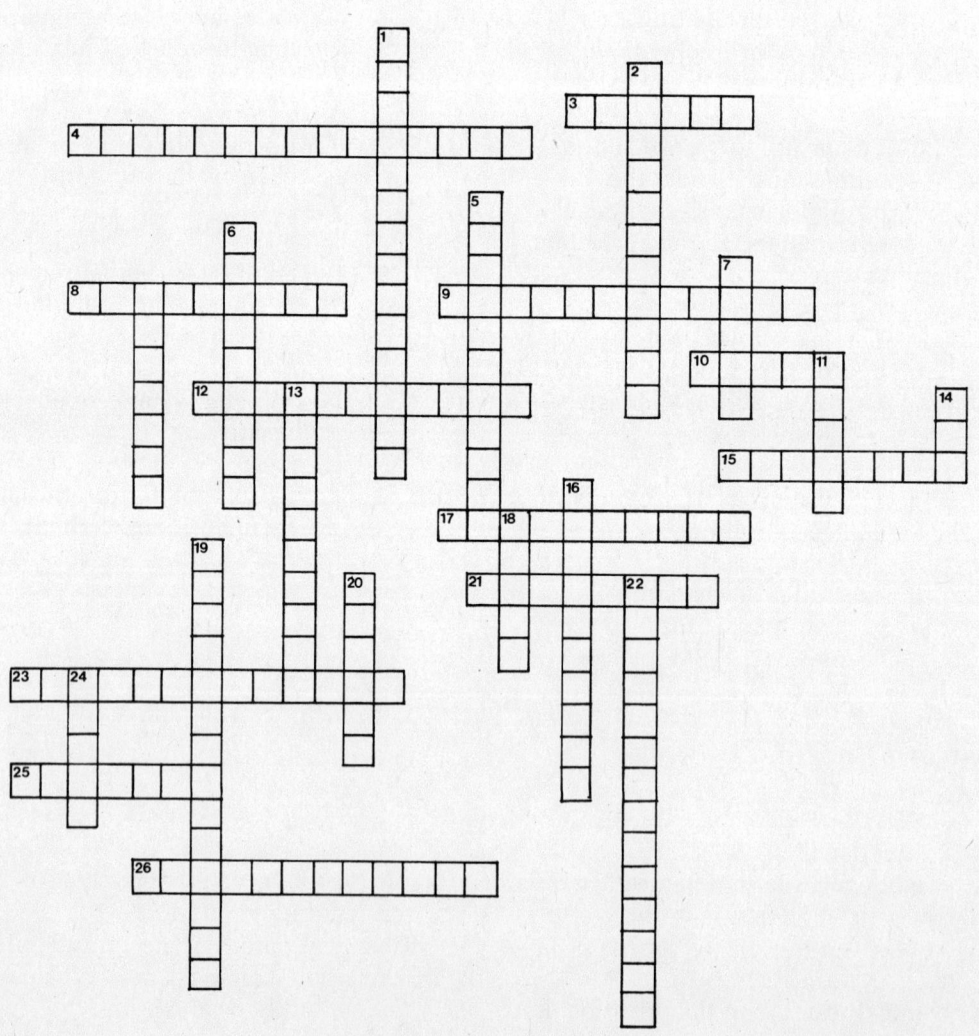

Multiple Choice Questions

For each of the following, choose the one best answer.

1. The chemical nature characteristic of most carminatives is
   a. Aromatic oil
   b. Inorganic salt
   c. Protein
   d. Steroid
2. A home remedy used as a carminative is
   a. Oil of cloves
   b. Lemon extract
   c. Peppermint
   d. Wintergreen
3. The mechanism of action of peppermint when used as a carminative is
   a. Adsorption
   b. Demulcent
   c. Irritant
   d. Laxative
4. A common effect of carminative medications is
   a. Anorexia or nausea
   b. Eructation
   c. Constipation
   d. Alcoholic intoxication
5. An autogenous chemical that increases the tone and action of the intestines is
   a. Acetylcholine
   b. Epinephrine
   c. Norepinephrine
   d. Atropine
6. The laxative ingredient in rhubarb is
   a. Acetylcholine
   b. Oxalic acid
   c. Senna
   d. Tannin
7. The laxative most likely to be administered prior to x-ray examination of the gastrointestinal tract is
   a. Cascara
   b. Castor oil
   c. Castoria
   d. Milk of magnesia
8. An herbal remedy that acts as a laxative is
   a. Aloin
   b. Comfrey tea
   c. Willow bark tea
   d. Elderberry wine
9. Which of the following types of laxatives produce physical dependence?
   a. Bulk-forming
   b. Hyperosmotic
   c. Irritant
   d. Lubricant
10. A laxative contraindicated for use by lactating women is
    a. Castor oil
    b. Danthron
    c. Milk of magnesia
    d. Psyllium hydrophilic mucilloid
11. Use of the diphenylmethane laxative phenolphthalein may increase the risk of developing
    a. Appendicitis
    b. Hepatitis
    c. Serious skin eruptions
    d. Ulcerative colitis
12. Stimulant laxatives such as phenolphthalein should not be used by children younger than
    a. 6 months
    b. 1 year
    c. 3 years
    d. 6 years
13. Dehydrocholic acid is related chemically to the endogenous chemical(s)
    a. Acetylcholine
    b. Bile acids
    c. Histamine
    d. Lipase
14. A laxative that stimulates the flow of bile is
    a. Dehydrocholic acid
    b. Milk of magnesia
    c. Senna
    d. Mineral oil
15. A laxative likely to be used to prevent constipation caused by the use of sodium polystyrene is
    a. Cascara
    b. Milk of magnesia
    c. Psyllium hydrophilic mucilloid
    d. Sorbitol
16. When administering bulk laxatives, the nurse should be sure to
    a. Follow the dry drug with ample amounts of fluid
    b. Mix the dry drug thoroughly with fluid before administration
    c. Caution the client against excessive fluid intake
17. Dysphagia is a contraindication for
    a. Irritant laxatives
    b. Hyperosmotic laxatives
    c. Bulk-forming laxatives
    d. Lubricant laxatives

18. Most lubricant laxatives are
    a. Irritants
    b. Mucilloids
    c. Oils
    d. Surfactants
19. A laxative used as a retention enema, but not administered orally, is
    a. Magnesium sulfate
    b. Mineral oil
    c. Sodium phosphate
    d. Vegetable oils
20. The enema solution that is least irritating is
    a. Tap water
    b. Normal saline
    c. Sodium phosphate
    d. Soap suds
21. When is the best time to administer mineral oil?
    a. On arising
    b. With meals
    c. 2 hours before bedtime
    d. At bedtime
22. The laxatives that are least harmful when used in conjunction with weight reduction regimens are
    a. Bulk-forming laxatives
    b. Hyperosmotic laxatives
    c. Irritant laxatives
    d. Lubricants
23. Is daily defecation a desirable health habit?
    a. Yes, a short intestinal transmit time appears to be beneficial
    b. No, daily defecation tends to deplete the body of nutrients
    c. No, a standard pattern should not be recommended
24. In most diarrheas, the most important therapeutic measure in treatment is
    a. Adsorption of the intestinal irritants
    b. Inhibition of peristalsis
    c. Reduction of the frequency of stools
    d. Replacement of fluid and electrolyte loss
25. A contraindication for the use of kaolin
    a. Cramping abdominal pain
    b. Fever
    c. Watery stools
    d. A positive stool culture
26. Most antidiarrheal foods act as
    a. Adsorbents
    b. Anticholinergics
    c. Astringents
    d. Demulcents
27. Excessive loss of intestinal contents caused by diarrhea, laxatives, or enemas tend to cause serious depletion of body
    a. Calcium
    b. Carbohydrates
    c. Sodium
    d. Potassium
28. An adverse reaction likely to develop when astringent antidiarrheals are employed is
    a. Constipation
    b. Central nervous system depression
    c. Central nervous system stimulation
    d. Overhydration
29. Opioids are most useful for the treatment of diarrhea caused by
    a. Diverticulosis
    b. Intestinal infections
    c. Overuse of laxatives
    d. Hyperkalemia
30. The most urgent need of a client with acute severe diarrhea is
    a. Correction of the underlying pathology
    b. Correction of the fluid and electrolyte imbalance
    c. Reduction in the frequency of stools
    d. Relief of pain
31. Clients at greatest risk for rapid dehydration and electrolyte depletion from diarrhea are
    a. Infants and small children
    b. Pubescent youngsters
    c. Young adults
    d. Adults 40 to 60 years of age
    e. Adults older than 60 years of age

Selection of Options

For each of the following, select *all* appropriate responses. Circle correct answers.

1. Measures that tend to reduce flatulence include
    a. Increased rest
    b. Increased fiber in the diet
    c. Parboiling of beans before final preparation
    d. Ice packs to the abdomen
    e. Intermittent use of a rectal tube

2. According to the text, antiflatulents the nurse may recommend include
   a. Alcohol
   b. Peppermint
   c. Simethicone
   d. Sodium bicarbonate
   e. Turpentine
3. Peristalsis is stimulated by
   a. Distention of the bowel
   b. Irritation of the wall of the intestine
   c. Parasympathetic nervous activity
   d. Sympathetic nervous activity
4. Laxative foods stimulate defecation by
   a. Increasing the water content of the stool
   b. Irritating the intestinal wall
   c. Increasing the bulk in the stool
   d. Lubricating the colon
5. Laxative foods that contain irritants should not be given to clients with
   a. Chronic constipation
   b. Crohn's disease
   c. Spasticity of the colon
   d. Ulcerative colitis
6. Contraindications for castor oil include
   a. Crohn's disease
   b. Extremes of age
   c. Intestinal obstruction
   d. Intestinal perforation
   e. Obstructive jaundice
   f. Ulcerative colitis
7. Anthraquinone cathartics include
   a. Aloe
   b. Cascara
   c. Castor oil
   d. Senna
8. Occupational illnesses that may occur in nurses caused by exposure to bulk-forming laxatives include
   a. Allergic reactions
   b. Irritable bowel
   c. Physical dependence
   d. Suffocation
9. Nutritional problems that may be caused by injudicious use of laxatives include
   a. Deficiencies of vitamins A and D
   b. Fluid deficit
   c. Hypercholesterolemia
   d. Hypokalemia
10. Ample fluids are required for effective action of
    a. Bulk-forming laxatives
    b. Hyperosmotic laxatives
    c. Lubricant laxatives
    d. Stool softeners
11. Constipation may be an early sign of
    a. Depression
    b. Hiatal hernia
    c. Intestinal malignancies
    d. Intestinal obstruction
    e. Intestinal ulceration
12. Clinical situations characterized by increased risk of diarrhea include
    a. Constipation
    b. Excessive use of tea
    c. Hypothyroidism
    d. Intestinal infection
    e. Narcotic withdrawal syndrome
    f. Use of cholinergic drugs
13. General dietary recommendations appropriate for clients with diarrhea include
    a. Limiting diet to clear fluids
    b. Increasing use of coffee
    c. Increasing use of Gatorade
    d. Increasing use of prune juice
    e. Increasing use of tea
14. Opium is contraindicated for the treatment of diarrhea caused by
    a. Diverticulitis
    b. Infections of the gastrointestinal tract
    c. Ingestion of intestinal irritants
15. Foods that are useful in the prevention and treatment of diarrhea caused by the use of broad-spectrum antibiotics include
    a. Elderberry wine
    b. Cheese
    c. Natural buttermilk
    d. Tea
    e. Yogurt
    f. Sweet milk
16. Assessment of a client presenting with acute diarrhea as a chief complaint must include a careful appraisal of
    a. Level of consciousness
    b. Fluid and electrolyte status
    c. Characteristics and frequency of stools
    d. Usual dietary practices
17. Assessment data of particular importance for monitoring clients with persistent diarrhea include
    a. Body weight
    b. Tissue turgor
    c. Level of consciousness
    d. Skeletal muscle strength
    e. Blood pressure

18. Disease conditions that increase the risk of constipation include
    a. Diabetes mellitus
    b. Gastroenteritis
    c. Multiple sclerosis
    d. Peptic ulcer
    e. Spinal cord injuries
    f. Stroke
19. Fecal impaction in clients with cardiovascular disease increases the risk of
    a. Heart block
    b. Hypertension
    c. Right-sided heart failure
    d. Stroke
20. Signs and symptoms of adverse reactions to repeated enemas include
    a. Diaphoresis
    b. Weakness
    c. Cardiac arrhythmias
    d. Prolonged cardiac diastole
    e. ECG changes indicative of hypokalemia

Short Answer Questions

1. Define the following terms:
   a. Diarrhea:

   b. Constipation:

   c. Laxative:

   d. Adsorbent:

2. How do the terms "purgative," "laxative," and "cathartic" differ?

3. List at least three characteristics of the ideal laxative.

4. Name at least four laxative foods.

5. Because it is inactive until changed chemically by the body, castor oil may be considered to be a prodrug. How does the body "activate" castor oil, and what chemical is produced by this process?

6. Name at least four hyperosmotic laxatives.

7. Identify four hygienic measures that help to reduce constipation.

8. List at least five factors that increase the risk of constipation in institutionalized populations.

9. Name at least three foods that can contribute to constipation.

10. Name at least three adsorbent antidiarrheals.

11. Identify one undesirable side effect of adsorbent antidiarrheals.

12. What is the effect of artificial sweeteners (saccharin and cyclamates) on the colon?

13. Name at least four foods that should be avoided by clients prone to chronic diarrhea.

UNIT EIGHT: DRUGS AFFECTING THE ENDOCRINE SYSTEM

32
Steroid Hormones and Their Antagonists

Hormones are glandular secretions, produced by organs and tissues, that are transported through the bloodstream to other tissues, in which they alter the rate of cellular processes. Steroid hormones help maintain blood volume and blood pressure, influence metabolic processes, and determine sexuality and sexual function. The following exercises deal with corticosteroids and sex hormones.

Matching

Match each therapeutic use listed in the left-hand column with the appropriate glucocorticoid dosage schedule in the right-hand column.

_____ 1. Treatment of severe acute allergic reactions
_____ 2. Replacement therapy
_____ 3. Treatment of collagen diseases
_____ 4. Prevention of cerebral edema
_____ 5. Prevention of sympathetic ophthalmia

a. Dosage at fixed intervals around the clock
b. Administration of doses every other day
c. Administration of a dose daily on arising
d Administration of a dose daily at the hour of sleep

Correct the False Statement

Indicate whether the following statements are true or false; if false, correct the underlined words or phrases.

_____ 1. In most treatment situations, the drug action of the glucocorticoids is palliative rather than curative.

_____ 2. Allergic reactions to the glucocorticoids rarely, if ever, occur because these drugs suppress the immune system.

_____ 3. Persons receiving glucocorticoid replacement therapy should increase their drug dosage twofold or more when experiencing unusual stress.

_____ 4. When glucocorticoids are prescribed once daily, or once every other day, the drugs should be given after breakfast.

_____ 5. Glucocorticoid therapy may produce psychological dependence because of its stimulant and euphorigenic properties.

_____ 6. When long-term therapy with prednisone is prescribed, for anti-inflammatory effect, antirheumatic drugs such as phenylbutazone are contraindicated for all members of the family.

_____ 7. Clients receiving high doses of glucocorticoids are likely to experience daytime drowsiness.

_____ 8. The likelihood of systemic reaction to over-the-counter ointments and creams containing cortisone is minimized because cortisone is not absorbed transdermally.

_____ 9. When therapeutic glucocorticoids are prescribed for persons with a history of tuberculosis, antimycobacterial drugs are very likely to be prescribed also.

_____ 10. Mineralocorticoids probably alter kidney function by enhancing the effects of antidiuretic hormone.

_____ 11. Mineralocorticoids such as aldosterone affect renal function by promoting potassium reabsorption and sodium excretion.

_____ 12. Clients receiving parenteral mineralocorticoids should be monitored for irritation or inflammation at injection sites.

_____ 13. A diagnostic test that is unlikely to be ordered for clients receiving mineralocorticoids is fasting blood sugar.

_____ 14. When mineralocorticoid therapy is initiated for the treatment of Addison's disease, clients are apt to exhibit a high sensitivity to the drugs.

_____ 15. High doses are avoided when mineralocorticoid therapy is initiated because of a high risk of hypotensive shock.

_____ 16. Desoxycorticosterone should usually be given with a fine-gauge needle.

_____ 17. A mineralocorticoid preparation that also has glucocorticoid properties is desoxycorticosterone.

_____ 18. In general, clients receiving glucocorticoids for replacement therapy are less likely to recover endocrine function than are those receiving replacement mineralocorticosteroids.

_____ 19. Sex hormones are produced endogenously only by the gonads.

_____ 20. Normal genital development in utero is dependent in part on testosterone in both sexes.

_____ 21. Production of androgens in males is higher in utero than is production of the hormones during prepubescent childhood.

_____ 22. Sex hormones generally enhance catabolism.

_____ 23. In both sexes, high levels of sex hormones tend to stimulate epiphyseal closure and halt growth.

_____ 24. Androgens prescribed for anabolic effects are free of masculinizing properties.

_____ 25. The addition of androgens to drug regimens of clients receiving anticoagulants tends to cause decreased therapeutic response to the anticoagulant.

_____ 26. The hormones most often used in the treatment of cancer of the prostate are androgens.

_____ 27. Oral administration of natural androgens is more effective than is oral administration of synthetic androgens.

_____ 28. Adverse reactions to buccal or sublingual administration of androgens include tissue irritation at the site of administration.

_____ 29. A promising antiandrogen now under investigation for use as a drug is chlorotrianisene.

_____ 30. The production of sex hormones in the body fluctuates more markedly in young men than it does in young women.

_____ 31. In a young adult woman with adequate estrogen concentrations, the skin is thicker than it is in estrogen-deficient women.

_____ 32. Estrogens can function as both estrogenic and antiestrogenic substances.

_____ 33. An estrogen that is stored in large amounts in fatty tissue is estriol.

_____ 34. Estrogens applied topically do not exert systemic effects.

_____ 35. Risks of adverse effects of hormone contraceptives are usually as high as those stemming from pregnancy.

_____ 36. Estrogen therapy is contraindicated during pregnancy and lactation.

_____ 37. During menopause, hot flashes tend to subside as time passes.

_____ 38. Following menopause, most women will need to use more soap for skin care than they did at younger ages.

_____ 39. Clomiphene is used therapeutically as a contraceptive.

_____ 40. Natural progesterone is metabolized more rapidly by the liver than are synthetic or semisynthetic progestogens.

_____ 41. Contraindications for progesterone are similar to those for estrogens.

_____ 42. The use of progestogen contraceptives tends to decrease the incidence and severity of acute asthma.

Short Answer Questions

1. List at least four signs or symptoms of primary corticosteroid deficiency.

2. When cortisone ointments or creams are administered topically, are the drugs absorbed systemically?

3. List at least ten adverse signs or symptoms of high doses of cortisone.

4. Identify at least eight baseline data parameters that should be assessed before glucocorticoid therapy is begun.

5. Why is stress management important for clients receiving glucocorticoids?

6. What effects do mineralocorticoids have on fluid and electrolyte balances?

7. Identify at least ten signs or symptoms of mineralocorticoid toxicity.

8. List at least six parameters that should be monitored in clients receiving mineralocorticoids.

9. What risks are imposed by the use of androgens in young males?

10. How useful are androgens in the treatment of delayed maturation in young males?

11. Are anabolic androgens safe for use by male athletes to enhance muscular development?

12. What type of diet should be given to clients receiving anabolic androgens?

13. Which hormones have stronger anabolic effects, estrogens or androgens?

14. Which sex hormones are considered to be diabetogenic?

15. Is impotence an unavoidable consequence of effective estrogen therapy for cancer of the prostate?

16. Are estrogens used to treat acne in pubescent women?

17. Name three factors usually considered to be indications for the use of estrogen replacement therapy in postmenopausal women.

18. List three conditions whose risks appear to be increased by ample estrogen levels in postmenopausal women.

19. Identify two recommendations appropriate for women who wish to correct postmenopausal hirsutism.

20. Name two antiestrogenic drugs currently available for clinical use.

Multiple Choice Questions

For each of the following, choose the one best answer.

1. Glucocorticoid secretion is stimulated by
   a. Hypokalemia
   b. Hypervolemia
   c. Hypernatremia
   d. Stress
2. Mineralocorticoid secretion is stimulated by
   a. Hypokalemia
   b. Hypovolemia
   c. Hypernatremia
   d. Hypertension
3. How do glucocorticoids affect the immune response?
   a. They enhance it
   b. They inhibit it
   c. They enhance production of antitoxins but not of antibodies
   d. They increase the tendency toward allergic reactions
4. A chronic inadequacy of corticosteroid secretion may cause
   a. Hypertension
   b. Inhibition of adrenocorticotropin secretion
   c. Signs and symptoms of pregnancy
   d. Masculinization in females
5. Does the use of glucocorticoids produce dependence?
   a. Prolonged use or high dosages usually produce physical dependence
   b. They often produce psychologic dependence but rarely cause physical dependence
   c. They produce pronounced dependence that is both physical and psychologic
   d. No, they are not habituating
6. Maintenance doses of corticosteroids used to treat Addison's disease
   a. Should be maintained at a steady level
   b. Are adjusted in relation to changes in blood pressure
   c. Are adjusted in relation to changes in stress level
   d. Are adjusted in relation to changes in blood sugar levels
7. Glucocorticoids used as antineoplastics are most effective in the treatment of
   a. Solid tumors
   b. Genital malignancies
   c. Skin cancer
   d. Lymphomas

8. The response to glucocorticoids that is most therapeutic for persons with brain injury is
   a. Immunosuppression
   b. Reduction of inflammation
   c. Hypervolemia
   d. Hyperglycemia
9. Clients treated with glucocorticoids for drug effect, who receive large doses or prolonged therapy, should be told
   a. To omit one or more doses when specific symptoms of toxicity develop
   b. To be sure to take the drug every day at bedtime
   c. That discontinuing the drug abruptly can be harmful
   d. To increase intake of dietary salt or of other sodium compounds
10. Abrupt withdrawal of high doses of glucocorticoids is likely to cause
    a. Hypertensive crisis
    b. Hypotension and a tendency toward shock
    c. Formation of abnormal clots and emboli
    d. Inhibition of pituitary secretion of corticotropin
11. The glucocorticoid preparation most likely to be used to prevent cerebral edema is
    a. Cortisone
    b. Dexamethasone
    c. Hydrocortisone
    d. Prednisone
12. In most people, serum concentration of endogenous glucocorticoids is highest
    a. At the end of the normal sleep period
    b. Midway through the normal day-long activity period
    c. At the beginning of the normal sleep period
    d. None of the above; serum concentration of the hormone does not fluctuate significantly diurnally
13. If pharmacologic doses of glucocorticoids are prescribed for persons receiving phenytoin for control of a seizure disorder, the doses are likely to be
    a. Higher than usual
    b. Lower than usual
    c. Administered every other day rather than daily
    d. Administered parenterally rather than orally
14. The major role of the glucocorticoids in normal physiology is
    a. Maintaining strong bones
    b. Maintaining adequate immune response
    c. Moderating coagulation to prevent abnormal clots
    d. Assisting the body to adapt to stress
15. Persons receiving glucocorticoid replacement therapy should be taught the importance of
    a. Eating regular meals with moderate carbohydrate intake
    b. Consistent routines for sleep and activity
    c. Cleanliness and special foot care
    d. Reducing sodium intake in the diet
16. What effect do the glucocorticoids have on wound healing?
    a. They accelerate it by promoting cell division
    b. They delay it by inhibiting cell division
    c. They prevent delay in wound healing caused by inflammation
    d. They prevent delay in wound healing caused by infection
17. Clients receiving long-term therapy with glucocorticoids need special protection from
    a. Trauma likely to cause hemorrhage
    b. Trauma likely to cause bone fracture
    c. Abnormal sodium loss and fluid depletion
    d. Foods likely to cause diarrhea caused by irritation of the colon
18. During long-term therapy with high dosages of glucocorticoids, clients are likely to experience
    a. A high level of physical health
    b. Mild to moderate psychologic depression
    c. Some degree of hypoadrenocorticism (Addison's disease)
    d. Some degree of toxicity (Cushing's syndrome)
19. When used in the treatment of adrenogenital syndrome, mineralocorticoids reduce the signs and symptoms of masculinization by
    a. Inactivating androgens in the body
    b. Enhancing estrogenic responses in the body
    c. Inhibiting pituitary secretion of adrenocorticotropin
    d. Inhibiting androgen production in the testes

20. Mineralocorticoids are most likely to be prescribed for persons with
    a. Addison's disease
    b. Cushing's syndrome
    c. Heat exhaustion
    d. Diarrhea
21. A mineralocorticoid preparation that is effective when given orally is
    a. Cortisone
    b. Desoxycorticosterone
    c. Fludrocortisone
    d. Prednisone
22. When expectant mothers with Addison's disease have received hormones for replacement therapy, the newborn baby should be monitored for signs and symptoms of
    a. Corticosteroid imbalance
    b. Hyperinsulinism
    c. Masculinization
    d. Thyroid imbalance
23. Desoxycorticosterone should be administered
    a. Orally
    b. Subcutaneously
    c. Intramuscularly
    d. Intravenously
24. Desoxycorticosterone pellets should be administered
    a. Orally
    b. Buccally
    c. By a special intramuscular injection device
    d. By surgical implantation
25. Therapeutic response to mineralocorticoids is apt to be decreased by
    a. Exposure to cold, dry environments
    b. Exposure to hot, humid environments
    c. Alleviation of stress
    d. Increased sodium and water intake
26. When signs and symptoms of mineralocorticoid toxicity develop, the client should
    a. Reduce sodium, potassium, and water intake
    b. Increase sodium, potassium, and water intake
    c. Increase sodium and water intake but reduce potassium intake
    d. Increase potassium intake but reduce sodium and water intake
27. A potentially fertile female baby may be born with external genitalia that appear to be male if, *in utero*,
    a. Estrogen levels were deficient
    b. Progesterone levels were deficient
    c. Androgen levels were deficient
    d. Androgen levels were excessive
28. What effect do androgens have on body lipids?
    a. They increase LDH and VLDL serum concentrations
    b. They increase HDL serum concentrations
    c. They increase subcutaneous fat deposits
    d. They increase body stores of cholesterol
29. Sex hormones are normally deactivated in the body by
    a. Metabolism for energy through the Krebs cycle
    b. Chemical transformation by the target cells
    c. Liver enzyme metabolism
    d. Urinary excretion
30. Anabolic androgenic hormones are used therapeutically to treat
    a. Postpubertal cryptorchidism
    b. Aplastic anemia
    c. Male impotence
    d. Postpartum breast engorgement
31. Androgen therapy in women can cause
    a. Urinary incontinence
    b. Male pattern baldness
    c. Temporary huskiness of the voice
    d. Osteoporosis
32. Young men who receive androgen replacement therapy are likely to experience
    a. Toxic reactions to the drugs
    b. Impaired self-image
    c. Delayed epiphyseal closure
    d. Urinary incontinence
33. Vaginal atrophy in postmenopausal women is usually treated with
    a. Low-dose oral estrogens
    b. Subcutaneous estrogen injections
    c. Sustained-release intramuscular estrogen injections
    d. Topical applications of estrogen creams
34. Topical estrogen cream should be administered
    a. On arising
    b. Daily at bedtime
    c. Prior to intercourse
    d. After intercourse
35. Tamoxifen is used therapeutically as a(n)
    a. Contraceptive
    b. Fertility drug
    c. Estrogen replacement
    d. Antineoplastic

36. An adverse reaction to clomiphene is
    a. Permanent impairment of fertility
    b. Increased risk of pregnancy
    c. Multiple births
    d. Accelerated growth of genital malignancies
37. The physiologic effects of progesterone are dependent in part on adequate tissue concentrations of
    a. Androgens
    b. Estrogens
    c. Cell membrane receptors
    d. Somatotropin
38. Hormones useful in the treatment of postpartum afterpains are
    a. Estrogens
    b. Antiestrogens
    c. Androgens
    d. Progestogens

Selection of Options

For each of the following, select *all* the appropriate responses. Circle correct answers.

1. The effects of glucocorticoids on the central nervous system include
    a. General stimulation
    b. Blunting of sensory perception
    c. Inhibition of antidiuretic hormone secretion
    d. Inhibition of somatotropin secretion
2. Glucocorticoid therapy is often employed in the treatment of
    a. Autoimmune diseases
    b. Atherosclerosis
    c. Hypertension
    d. Acute allergic reactions
    e. Malignant neoplasms
    f. Transplant rejection
    g. Infections
    h. Intracranial trauma
3. Although the general action of glucocorticoids is to increase water retention and edema, their anti-inflammatory action effectively reduces harmful edema in persons with
    a. Brain trauma
    b. Intracranial metastases
    c. Lymphatic metastases
    d. Pyelonephritis
    e. Glomerulonephritis
4. Drugs that should be avoided when glucocorticoids are administered for drug effect include
    a. Antihistamines such as Chlor-Trimeton
    b. Histamine-2 receptor antagonists such as cimetidine
    c. Antirheumatics such as aspirin or phenylbutazone
    d. Potassium-sparing diuretics such as spironolactone
    e. Vaccines and toxoids
    f. Anticoagulants
5. The use of pharmacologically active doses of glucocorticoids is likely to be associated with increased need for
    a. Antacids such as aluminum hydroxide
    b. Antimycobacterials such as isoniazid
    c. Antibiotics such as penicillin
    d. Hemostatic agents such as clotting factor VIII
    e. Sodium in the diet
    f. Calcium in the diet
    g. Potassium in the diet
6. Caution must be exercised when glucocorticoids are prescribed for
    a. Postmenopausal women and elderly men
    b. Persons with seizure disorder
    c. Persons with liver impairment
    d. Persons with renal impairment
    e. Persons with osteoporosis
7. Relative contraindications for glucocorticoid therapy include
    a. Childhood
    b. Pregnancy
    c. Lactation
    d. Advanced age
    e. Positive tuberculin reaction
8. Persons receiving glucocorticoids should be monitored for signs and symptoms of
    a. Hypertension
    b. Hypotension
    c. Infection
    d. Delayed healing
    e. Inflammation
    f. Peptic ulcer
    g. Thromboemboli
    h. Diabetes mellitus
    i. Sodium imbalance
    j. Potassium imbalance
    k. Abnormal moods
    l. Drowsiness
    m. Weight gain
    n. Cardiac abnormalities
9. Clients receiving pharmacologic doses of glucocorticoids should be advised to take a diet that is

a. Low in sodium
   b. Low in potassium
   c. High in calories
10. The addition of prednisone to drug regimens increases the risk of toxicity from
   a. Antibiotics
   b. Digitalis
   c. Potassium-sparing diuretics
   d. Potassium-wasting diuretics
11. What effect do estrogens have on body lipids?
   a. They decrease LDH and VLDH serum concentrations
   b. They decrease HDL serum concentrations
   c. They increase biliary excretion of cholesterol
   d. They increase subcutaneous fat deposits
   e. They increase body stores of cholesterol
12. Functions of androgens in females include
   a. Normal reproductive development in utero
   b. Enhancement of anabolic processes such as muscle building
   c. Enhancement of libido
   d. Stimulation of gonadotropin secretion by the pituitary
13. What drugs are likely to be prescribed to alleviate postpartum breast engorgement in nonnursing mothers?
   a. Estrogens
   b. Progestogens
   c. Androgens
   d. Glucocorticoid antagonists
14. Androgen therapy in men can cause
   a. Gynecomastia
   b. Urinary retention
   c. Priapism
   d. Permanent elevation of the voice register
   e. Impaired sexual response
15. Young men receiving androgen replacement therapy should immediately report the development of
   a. Sudden spurts in growth
   b. High fever
   c. A deepening of the voice
   d. Priapism
   e. Gynecomastia
   f. Increased libido
16. Cyproterone acetate has been used investigationally in the treatment of
   a. Acne
   b. Male pattern baldness
   c. Dwarfism
   d. Precocious puberty in males
   e. Excessive masculinization in males
   f. Severe sexual deviance in males
17. Normal young adult women who take exogenous estrogens are at increased risk for
   a. Hypercholesterolemia
   b. Cholelithiasis
   c. Thrombophlebitis and thromboembolism
   d. Hemorrhage
18. Body storage depots for estrogens include
   a. Serum proteins
   b. The gonads
   c. Fatty tissue
   d. The enterohepatic circulation
19. Estrogens are eliminated from the body by
   a. Metabolism for energy through the Krebs cycle
   b. Fecal elimination through bile
   c. Excretion in urine
   d. Chemical destruction by the target cells
20. Currently, estrogens are often used therapeutically
   a. To alleviate acute symptoms of menopause
   b. To prevent development of estrogen deficiency in postmenopausal women
   c. To stimulate sexual maturation in girls with primary gonadal failure
   d. As contraceptives
   e. To treat hormone-dependent breast cancers in postmenopausal women
   f. To treat cancer of the prostate in men
21. Risks of adverse reactions to estrogen therapy are increased in women who
   a. Smoke cigarettes
   b. Drink alcoholic beverages
   c. Are more than 35 years of age
   d. Are less than 20 years of age
   e. Have never had children
22. Estrogen therapy may increase the severity of
   a. Hypercholesterolemia
   b. Thromboemboli
   c. Migraine
   d. Manic depressive psychosis
   e. Seizure disorders
   f. Peptic ulcer disease
   g. Diabetes mellitus
   h. Cholelithiasis

23. Women at high risk for estrogen deficiency after menopause tend to
    a. Be more obese than their age peers
    b. Have smaller bones than their age peers
    c. Weigh less than their age peers
24. Young women at high risk for postmenopausal estrogen deficiencies may reduce the eventual need for high-dose estrogen therapy by
    a. Increasing their consumption of protein
    b. Increasing their consumption of calcium
    c. Engaging in active weight-bearing exercise
    d. Restricting vitamin D intake
25. Signs and symptoms that should be reported immediately when they occur in women receiving estrogen therapy include
    a. Nausea
    b. Tenderness in the calf
    c. Bloating
    d. Pain on dorsiflexion of the foot
    e. Sudden neurologic deficit (paralysis, aphasia)
26. Side effects of progesterone include
    a. Breakthrough vaginal bleeding
    b. Suppression of part of the immune response
    c. Enhancement of the effects of prolactin
    d. Formation of a mucous plug in the cervix
    e. A rise in body temperature

33
Protein Hormones: Insulin and Other Drugs Affecting Blood Glucose

The following exercises deal with substances used pharmacologically to control blood sugar.

Correct the False Statement

Indicate whether the following statements are true or false; if false, correct the underlined words or phrases.

_____ 1. Protein hormones tend to act <u>more rapidly than</u> do steroid hormones.

_____ 2. Protein hormones are degraded <u>at the receptor site by the target tissue</u>.

_____ 3. The effects of insulin are <u>anabolic rather than catabolic</u>.

_____ 4. Insulin is <u>frequently</u> administered orally.

_____ 5. Insulin preparations require <u>constant</u> refrigeration.

_____ 6. Porcine insulin is generally <u>less antigenic</u> than is bovine insulin.

_____ 7. Insulin has a <u>relatively low</u> therapeutic index.

_____ 8. Hyperglycemic ketoacidosis usually develops <u>more rapidly than</u> does hypoglycemic insulin reaction.

_____ 9. If solid deposits are visible in an insulin solution, the vial should be <u>rotated gently to redissolve the precipitate</u>.

_____ 10. The action of glucagon is <u>generally similar to</u> that of insulin.

_____ 11. The structure of glucagon of animal origin <u>differs somewhat from</u> that of human glucagon.

_____ 12. Glucagon has a <u>wide</u> margin of safety.

Short Answer Questions

1. Name at least two hormones with simple protein structures.

2. Protein hormones and their metabolites are excreted _____ .
3. Identify the physiologic change that stimulates insulin secretion.

4. Identify two factors that are associated with allergy to insulin.

5. Why is it desirable to warm refrigerated insulin prior to injection?

175

6. Is it advisable for a newly diagnosed diabetic to be refracted for corrective eyeglasses?

7. Name at least five effects of insulin.

8. List at least three conditions required for proper storage of the insulin bottle in current use.

9. Name two antidotes for insulin toxicity.

10. When preparing mixtures of regular and modified insulin, which type of insulin should be drawn into the syringe first?

11. How frequently can successive doses of glucagon be administered?

12. How long does it take for injected glucagon to exert peak action?

13. How long does the blood sugar level remain elevated following onset of action of glucagon?

Multiple Choice Questions

For each of the following, choose the one best answer.

1. The mechanism of action of some protein hormones involves
   a. Interaction with a membrane receptor and subsequent migration of the hormone-receptor complex to the cytoplasm of the cell
   b. Interaction with a membrane receptor and subsequent migration of the hormone-receptor complex to the nucleus of the cell
   c. Interaction with an intracellular protein and subsequent migration of the hormone-receptor complex to the nucleus of the cell
   d. Interaction with a cell membrane receptor without penetration of the hormone to the interior of the cell

2. A mineral incorporated into medicinal insulin compounds is
   a. Cobalt   c. Magnesium
   b. Iron   d. Zinc

3. When given once a day, insulin is most often administered
   a. On arising
   b. Before breakfast
   c. After the midday meal
   d. At bedtime

4. Within the body, insulin molecules are commonly bound to
   a. Fatty tissue
   b. Plasma proteins
   c. Insulin antibodies
   d. Islet cells of the pancreas

5. The major therapeutic use for insulin is the treatment of
   a. Anorexia nervosa
   b. Malnutrition
   c. Diabetes insipidus
   d. Diabetes mellitus

6. Most parenteral solutions of insulin contain drug concentrations of
   a. 40 U/ml

b. 80 U/ml
  c. 100 U/ml
  d. 200 U/ml
7. The insulin preparation prescribed most often at present is
  a. Crystalline zinc insulin
  b. Isophane insulin
  c. Lente insulin
  d. Protamine zinc insulin
8. A drug that masks the symptoms of insulin reaction is
  a. Aspirin
  b. Vitamin C
  c. IV saline solution
  d. Propranolol
9. After initial resolution of acute hypoglycemia in an insulin-dependent diabetic, recurrent insulin toxicity may be prevented by
  a. Alleviating the client's stress
  b. Feeding the client
  c. Having the client exercise
  d. Withholding food from the client
10. In acutely ill diabetic clients, when differentiation between hyperglycemic ketoacidosis and insulin reaction is difficult, what treatment should be given?
  a. Treatment appropriate for diabetic ketoacidosis
  b. Treatment appropriate for hypoglycemic insulin reaction
  c. Treatment should be delayed until the diagnosis is clear
11. To treat insulin reaction in a conscious client, the nurse should administer
  a. Unsweetened orange juice
  b. Sweetened orange juice
  c. A protein food
  d. Gatorade
12. To prevent recurrent hypoglycemia after initial resolution of an insulin reaction, it would be best to give the client
  a. Rapidly assimilable carbohydrates (sweets)
  b. Starch–protein combinations such as crackers and cheese
  c. Fats such as cream or butter
  d. Bouillon or other salty foods
13. To correct hypoglycemia, glucagon is usually administered
  a. Orally
  b. Subcutaneously
  c. Intramuscularly
  d. Intravenously
14. The most critical need of the client in hypoglycemic insulin reaction is correction of
  a. Glucose deprivation in the brain
  b. Fluid volume deficit
  c. Acid–base imbalance
  d. Central nervous system depression
15. The most critical need of the client in hyperglycemic ketoacidosis is correction of
  a. Glucose deprivation in the brain
  b. Fluid volume deficit
  c. Metabolic alkalosis
  d. Central nervous system depression
16. During diabetic ketoacidosis, clients are at increased risk for
  a. Acute infections
  b. Cerebral hemorrhage
  c. Severe edema
  d. Respiratory alkalosis
17. Insulin "coverage" (intermittent doses prescribed for high blood sugar concentrations) rarely exceeds
  a. 5 U/dose
  b. 25 U/dose
  c. 50 U/dose
  d. 100 U/dose
18. Insulin used for "coverage" is usually
  a. Isophane insulin
  b. Lente insulin
  c. Protamine zinc insulin
  d. Regular (crystalline zinc) insulin
19. A likely sequela of diabetic ketoacidosis is
  a. Permanent neurologic deficit secondary to stroke
  b. Increased dependence on insulin for control of diabetes mellitus
  c. Persistent abnormality of behavior
  d. Increased resistance to insulin caused by high levels of insulin antibodies
20. Clients receiving daily doses of long-lasting insulin in the morning are most likely to experience hypoglycemia
  a. Before breakfast
  b. Before lunch
  c. Before supper or at bedtime
  d. During sleep
21. Hypoglycemia during night hours is most likely to be manifested by
  a. Convulsions
  b. Diaphoresis
  c. Coma
  d. Hyperpnea (Kussmaul breathing)

22. When insulin syringes are used for more than one injection, their use should be limited to
    a. A period not exceeding 3 days
    b. A maximum of five injections
    c. Injection of regular (crystalline zinc) insulin
    d. Doses that do not exceed 0.5 ml in volume
23. Bizarre or socially unacceptable behavior is a likely effect of
    a. Diabetic ketoacidosis
    b. Hyperventilation syndrome
    c. Hypoglycemic insulin reaction
    d. Nonketotic hyperosmotic syndrome
24. Of frequently used tests for glucose imbalance, the most reliable one is the
    a. Urine test for glucose using Benedict's solution
    b. Urine test for glucose using an enzyme-impregnated color-reactive paper
    c. Blood sugar test performed on venous blood specimens
    d. Finger stick test for blood glucose
25. Sulfonylurea hypoglycemics reduce blood sugar concentrations by
    a. Directly stimulating movement of glucose into cells
    b. Directly enhancing glucose uptake by skeletal muscles
    c. Inhibiting glucagon release by the pancreas
    d. Stimulating insulin release by the pancreas
26. Hypoglycemic insulin reaction may be difficult to detect because some symptoms are suppressed in clients receiving
    a. Adrenergic blocking agents
    b. Glucocorticoids
    c. Oral hypoglycemics
    d. Regular insulin
27. Use of alcohol by clients receiving oral hypoglycemics may cause
    a. A disulfiramlike reaction
    b. Severe gastric irritation
    c. Excessive sedation
    d. An increased risk of hyperglycemia
28. During the early weeks of therapy with oral hypoglycemics, clients should promptly report
    a. All hypoglycemic reactions
    b. Excessive sedation
    c. Hyperglycemia, however slight
    d. Signs and symptoms of infection
29. Glucagon is not administered orally because
    a. Its onset of action by this route is too slow
    b. It is highly irritating to the gastric mucosa
    c. Its structure is destroyed by digestive enzymes
    d. It is metabolized in high quantities by first pass through the liver
30. Glucagon injections to correct a hypoglycemic episode may be repeated
    a. Once only
    b. Up to 3 times
    c. Up to 5 times
    d. Not at all; only one dose is used
31. Doses of glucagon are measured in
    a. Grams
    b. Milligrams
    c. Micrograms
    d. Units
32. Following successful treatment with glucagon of hypoglycemia caused by exogenous insulin, clients should be given
    a. A sweet food
    b. Starches and proteins
    c. Fats such as cream or butter
    d. Ample fluids

Selection of Options

For each of the following, select *all* of the appropriate responses. Circle correct answers.
1. Chemical structures of nonsteroidal endocrine hormones include
    a. Simple proteins
    b. Glycoproteins
    c. Lipoproteins
    d. Amino acid derivatives
2. Hormones derived from amino acids include
    a. Epinephrine
    b. Luteinizing hormone
    c. Norepinephrine
    d. Thyrotropin
    e. Thyroxine
    f. Triiodothyronine
3. Physiologic effects of insulin include
    a. Decrease in blood sugar levels
    b. Decrease in glycogen stores
    c. Decrease in fat deposition

d. Increased energy production
   e. Increased protein and nucleic acid synthesis
   f. Ketoacidosis
4. Therapeutic effects of insulin in persons with diabetes mellitus include
   a. Decrease in blood sugar levels
   b. Increased energy production from carbohydrate metabolism
   c. Increased energy production from protein metabolism
   d. Decreased breakdown of fatty tissue for energy
   e. Decreased ketoacidosis
   f. Enhanced growth in children
   g. A slowing of cardiovascular degeneration
5. Factors that enhance the action of insulin include
   a. Active exercise
   b. Reduction in adiposity
   c. Limitation of vitamin C intake
   d. Reduction in stress
6. Of the following insulins, which may be administered intravenously?
   a. Crystalline zinc insulin
   b. Isophane insulin
   c. Lente insulin
   d. Protamine zinc insulin
   e. Regular insulin
7. Drugs that tend to reverse the acute effects of insulin reaction include
   a. Cortisone
   b. Epinephrine
   c. Glucagon
   d. Sugar
8. Hypoglycemia can be differentiated from hyperventilation syndrome because hypoglycemia is characterized by
   a. Central nervous system stimulation
   b. Little change in respirations
   c. Headache
   d. Flushing of the skin
9. Serious physiologic imbalances characteristic of diabetic acidosis include
   a. Hyperosmolarity of body fluids
   b. Dehydration
   c. Metabolic acidosis
   d. Glucose deprivation in the brain
   e. Hyperkalemia with depletion of body stores of potassium
   f. General tissue malnutrition
10. During titration of insulin dosages, clients should
    a. Avoid excessive stress
    b. Avoid active exercise
    c. Maintain a normal diet
11. When using insulin, clients should
    a. Keep all bottles of insulin refrigerated
    b. Rotate the bottle gently to ensure even distribution of the drug in the solution
    c. Warm the insulin bottle in warm water before drawing up the dose
    d. Avoid injecting bubbles of air into the insulin solution
12. Insulin doses can be measured precisely with
    a. Insulin syringes with scales marking even-numbered units of dosage
    b. Insulin syringes with scales marking single units of dosage
    c. Tuberculin syringes
    d. Subcutaneous syringes with scales marking dosages in tenths of a milliliter
13. When administering insulin, the angle of insertion of the needle varies with
    a. The needle gauge
    b. The needle length
    c. The thickness of the client's skin
    d. The client's adiposity
14. Insulin preparations are produced by
    a. Extraction from animal tissues
    b. Chemical alteration of animal hormones
    c. Genetic recombination techniques
    d. Chemical synthesis
15. Oral hypoglycemics in current use include
    a. Acid-resistant insulin
    b. Biguanide compounds
    c. Sulfonamides
    d. Sulfonylureas
16. Clinical indications for the use of oral hypoglycemics include
    a. Insulin-dependent diabetes mellitus
    b. Non-insulin-dependent diabetes mellitus
    c. Inability to control diabetes mellitus by diet
    d. Presence of cardiovascular pathology
    e. Pregnancy
17. Drugs that interact with oral hypoglycemics to enhance their effects include
    a. Anti-inflammatory steroids
    b. Oral anticoagulants
    c. Sulfonamides
    d. Salicylates

18. Serious adverse reactions to sulfonylurea drugs include
    a. Agranulocytosis
    b. Cardiovascular disease
    c. Stroke caused by severe hypoglycemia
    d. Jaundice
19. Clients receiving sulfonylurea hypoglycemics should avoid the use of
    a. Alcohol
    b. Antibiotics
    c. Glucocorticoids
    d. Salicylates
20. The effects of glucagon on glucose balance include
    a. Increased blood concentration of glucose
    b. Increased glycogenesis
    c. Increased glycogenolysis
    d. Increased gluconeogenesis
21. Because glucagon maintains a steady supply of glucose to tissues that are obligate users of this nutrient, it protects energy metabolism in the
    a. Brain
    b. Gonads
    c. Skeletal muscles
    d. Retina
22. An excess of glucagon would cause
    a. Decreased severity of diabetes mellitus
    b. Increased severity of diabetes mellitus
    c. Impairment of brain metabolism
    d. Decreased glycogenesis
23. Therapeutic uses of glucagon include
    a. Treatment of hypoglycemia
    b. Treatment of hyperglycemia
    c. Preparation for intestinal x-ray examination
    d. Stimulation of intestinal motility

34
Thyroid, Parathyroid, Pituitary, and Hypothalamic Hormones

The following exercises are divided into parts:
1. Questions specific to the proteinaceous hormones of the thyroid, parathyroid, pituitary, and hypothalamus glands and antithyroid compounds.
2. Questions relating to all three chapters on endocrine drugs (to be done after study of Chapters 32, 33, and 34 is completed).

PART 1: THYROID, PARATHYROID, PITUITARY, AND HYPOTHALAMIC HORMONES

Correct the False Statement

Indicate whether the following statements are true or false; if false, correct the underlined words or phrases.

_____ 1. The structure of parathormone is <u>steroid</u> in nature.

_____ 2. The chemical structure of animal parathormone <u>differs somewhat</u> from that of human parathormone.

_____ 3. Reconstituted solutions of calcitonin <u>require</u> refrigeration for proper storage.

_____ 4. Calcitonin is most often used therapeutically for the treatment of <u>osteoporosis</u>.

_____ 5. Clients receiving calcitonin therapy are likely to develop acute <u>hyperglycemia</u>.

_____ 6. Iodinated thyroid hormones are derivatives of the amino acid <u>tryptophan</u>.

_____ 7. Iodinated thyroid hormones are <u>catabolic</u> in effect.

_____ 8. Onset of action of iodinated thyroid hormones occurs within <u>minutes to hours</u>.

_____ 9. The effects of iodinated thyroid hormones <u>tend to be cumulative</u>.

_____ 10. Iodinated thyroid hormones <u>are used in</u> the medicinal treatment of obesity.

_____ 11. The administration of thyroxine can be dangerous in clients with <u>cardiac disease</u>.

_____ 12. A contraindication for antithyroid drugs is <u>lactation</u>.

_____ 13. Oral iodide medications should be administered <u>on an empty stomach</u>.

_____ 14. Clients using iodides may need instruction in nonpharmacologic measures to control <u>nasal stuffiness</u>.

_____ 15. <u>In therapeutic doses,</u> radioiodine has no discernible effect on cells or tissues.

_____ 16. The therapeutic effect of radioiodine is caused by the presence of <u>alpha particles</u>.

_____ 17. In therapeutic doses, radioiodine <u>produces fibrosis</u> of the thyroid gland.

_____ 18. The pharmacokinetics of radioiodine <u>do not differ</u> from those of nonradioactive iodine.

_____ 19. The volume or weight of drug required for a given dose of radioiodine <u>decreases</u> as the drug ages.

_____ 20. A therapeutic dose of radioiodine will be approximately <u>10 times</u> as large as a tracer dose.

_____ 21. Radioiodine is an effective treatment for <u>all types of thyroid malignancies</u>.

_____ 22. When radioiodine is employed to treat a radiosensitive thyroid malignancy, the drug destroys the primary tumor <u>but is not effective against metastases</u>.

_____ 23. The adverse reaction most likely to occur when therapeutic doses of radioiodine are employed is <u>rash in persons with iodine allergy</u>.

_____ 24. Special precautions are required to protect health-care personnel from radioactivity <u>when therapeutic doses of radionucleides are employed</u>.

_____ 25. The duration of action of a given dose of radioiodine in the body is <u>shorter than</u> the duration of its radioactivity.

_____ 26. Anterior pituitary hormones <u>are effective</u> when administered orally.

_____ 27. Adrenocorticotropin acts by <u>reacting with a protein in the cytoplasm of target cells</u>.

_____ 28. The site of strongest action of corticotropin is <u>the zona reticularis</u> of the adrenals.

_____ 29. Therapeutic doses of adrenocorticotropin are usually administered <u>once a week for several weeks</u>.

_____ 30. Somatotropin is <u>an anabolic</u> hormone.

_____ 31. Before administering vasopressin tannate, the nurse should <u>shake the vial vigorously</u>.

Short Answer Questions

1. List at least three physiologic effects of calcitonin.

2. Name at least six signs and symptoms of thyroid toxicity.

3. Identify three conditions in which thyroid hormones are used as replacement therapy.

4. Do clients who have received radioiodine pose a risk to public health? If so, why?

5. Name two antithyroid drugs marketed in the United States.

6. Identify at least two effects of iodine on the thyroid gland.

7. For how long is iodine administered preoperatively to clients scheduled for thyroidectomy?

8. Identify an area in the United States that is a "goiter belt."

9. Name three atomic particles emitted by radioiodine.

10. Two units used to measure radioactivity are _____ and _____ .

11. What type of health problems are likely to affect clients who receive therapeutic doses of adrenocorticotropin?

12. Name three factors that tend to degrade adrenocorticotropin solutions.

13. Is growth hormone necessary for normal health in adults?

14. Is thyrotropin dangerous in diagnostic doses?

15. Identify two body tissues known to contain receptors for antidiuretic hormone.

Multiple Choice Questions

For each of the following, choose the one best answer.

1. Parathormone is administered
   a. Orally
   b. Topically
   c. By injection
   d. By inhalation
2. A contraindication for administration of parathormone is
   a. Acute tetany
   b. Hypercalcemia
   c. Concurrent use of calcium gluconate
   d. Previous exposure to parathormone
3. The therapeutic effects of parathormone may be enhanced by
   a. Hyperventilation
   b. Bag rebreathing
   c. Limitation of vitamin D intake
   d. Administration of oxygen
4. Iodinated thyroid hormones are usually administered
   a. Orally
   b. Topically
   c. By injection
   d. By inhalation
5. Medicinal iodinated thyroid hormones are stored in the body
   a. In the thyroid gland
   b. Bound to plasma proteins
   c. In fatty tissue
   d. In bones

6. Daily doses of thyroid hormones should be taken
   a. Before breakfast
   b. After lunch
   c. At bedtime
   d. None of the above; because of its slow onset of action, timing of doses within the diurnal cycle is not critical
7. Most antithyroid drugs act by
   a. Suppressing synthesis of thyroid hormone
   b. Inhibiting release of thyroid hormone
   c. Inhibiting pituitary secretion of thyrotropin
8. Antithyroid drugs are most often administered
   a. Orally
   b. Subcutaneously
   c. Intramuscularly
   d. Intravenously
9. Clients receiving antithyroid drugs should promptly report
   a. Swelling in the neck
   b. Symptoms of a head cold
   c. Symptoms of a sore throat
   d. Symptoms of gastrointestinal upset
10. When antithyroid drugs are required during pregnancy, the client is apt to receive, in addition,
    a. Glucocorticoids
    b. Growth hormone
    c. Thyroid hormone
    d. Iodine supplements
11. Courses of antithyroid treatment usually last several
    a. Days
    b. Weeks
    c. Months
12. Over-the-counter drugs that are contraindicated when clients are receiving antithyroid medications are
    a. Antacids   c. Laxatives
    b. Decongestants d. Salicylates
13. A substance available over the counter that can be used to prevent iodine deficiency is
    a. Iodized salt
    b. Potassium iodide
    c. Tincture of iodine
14. Tissue depots for storage of iodine include
    a. Bones and the thyroid gland
    b. Fatty tissue and the liver
    c. Plasma proteins and fatty tissue
    d. Plasma proteins and the thyroid gland
15. A common adverse reaction to iodine is
    a. Allergic rash
    b. Thickening of pulmonary secretion
    c. Acute iodine poisoning
    d. Anaphylaxis
16. A contraindication for iodide therapy is history of
    a. Goiter
    b. Thyrotoxicity
    c. Tuberculosis
    d. Cardiovascular disease
17. Which of the following represents a tracer dose of radioiodine?
    a. 10 pc   c. 10 c
    b. 10 mc   d. 10 picograms
18. What is the action of therapeutic doses of radiodine?
    a. Destruction of malignant cells in the thyroid gland without injury to normal cells in that gland
    b. Destruction of thyroid tissue, whether malignant or normal, active or inactive
    c. Destruction of cells in the body that concentrate iodine, whether normal or malignant
    d. Destruction of malignant cells of the body, whether thyroid in origin or not
19. The half-life of ^{131}I is approximately
    a. 8 hours   c. 1 week
    b. 1 day   d. 1 month
20. Radioiodine will lose 99% of its radioactivity by the end of approximately
    a. 56 hours   c. 1 month
    b. 2 weeks   d. 8 weeks
21. The main physiologic function of corticotropin is stimulation of
    a. Catecholamine production by the adrenal medulla
    b. Sex hormone production by the adrenal cortex
    c. Glucocorticoid production by the adrenal cortex
    d. Mineralocorticoid production by the adrenal cortex
22. ACTH is most likely to be used therapeutically for treatment of acute exacerbations of
    a. Arthritis   c. Multiple sclerosis
    b. Peptic ulcers d. Ulcerative colitis
23. How is ACTH measured?
    a. In units
    b. In grains
    c. In milligrams
    d. Animal preparations are measured in units and synthetic preparations are measured in milligrams

24. Signs and symptoms of ACTH toxicity resemble those of
    a. Addison's disease
    b. Cushing's syndrome
    c. Graves' disease
    d. Malignant hypertension
25. Common adverse reactions to ACTH are
    a. Allergic reactions
    b. Diabetes mellitus and diabetes insipidus
    c. Acne and dermal atrophy
    d. Increased sodium excretion and hypovolemia
26. Control of the underlying disease condition in clients receiving therapeutic courses of ACTH can be enhanced if clients learn how to
    a. Avoid infections
    b. Avoid trauma
    c. Control pain perception
    d. Control stress
27. In children, the primary function of somatotropin is
    a. Promotion of growth
    b. Stimulation of closure of the epiphyses
    c. Prevention of hyperglycemia
    d. Sexual maturation
28. In adults, somatotropin acts primarily to
    a. Maintain bone and muscle mass
    b. Enhance adaptation to the stress of fasting
    c. Promote healing of fractures
    d. Promote healing of wounds
29. Somatotropin is most likely to be useful in the treatment of
    a. Addison's disease
    b. Pituitary dwarfism
    c. Refractory hyperinsulinism
    d. Acromegaly
30. Thyrotropin is used therapeutically for
    a. The definitive diagnosis of thyroid hypofunction
    b. Treatment of cretinism
    c. Treatment of myxedema
    d. Treatment of Graves' disease
31. The source of thyrotropin is
    a. Animal tissues
    b. Chemical synthesis
    c. Human cadaver tissues
    d. Recombinant DNA techniques
32. The physiologic function of vasopressin (ADH) is to control
    a. Blood volume
    b. Glucose concentration in body fluids
    c. Osmolarity of body fluids
    d. Sensitivity to stimulation of the uterus
33. The primary therapeutic use of vasopressin is
    a. Stimulation of labor
    b. Treatment of hypertension
    c. Treatment of diabetes mellitus
    d. Treatment of diabetes insipidus
34. A side effect of antidiuretic hormone in women is
    a. Abnormal lactation
    b. Improvement of premenstrual tension
    c. Uterine atony
    d. Uterine cramps
35. Delay in administering maintenance doses of ADH may result in exacerbation of signs and symptoms of diabetes insipidus. The client may ameliorate the physiologic imbalances by
    a. Taking extra sodium in the diet
    b. Drinking Gatorade
    c. Taking an herbal tea containing belladonna
    d. Drinking extra water

Selection of Options

For each of the following, select *all* of the appropriate responses. Circle correct answers.

1. Physiologic effects of parathormone include
    a. Weakening of the bones
    b. Decreased serum calcium ion concentration
    c. Increased intestinal absorption of calcium
    d. Increased reabsorption of calcium by the kidneys
2. Medicinal uses of parathormone include
    a. Initial treatment of hypoparathyroidism
    b. Maintenance treatment for control of hypoparathyroidism
    c. Treatment of osteoporosis
    d. Experimental orthodontics
3. Adverse reactions that are likely to occur in parathormone toxicity include
    a. Diarrhea
    b. Decreased cardiac output
    c. Increased appetite
    d. Peptic ulcers
    e. Stones in the urinary tract
    f. Changes in emotional affect

4. Adverse reactions to calcitonin include
   a. Allergic hypersensitivity
   b. Gastrointestinal upset
   c. Pallor
   d. Swelling and tenderness of the hands
5. Calcitonin is administered
   a. Orally
   b. Topically
   c. Subcutaneously
   d. Intramuscularly
6. When thyroid hormone therapy is instituted for the treatment of myxedema, clients are at risk for development of
   a. Addisonian crisis
   b. Congestive heart failure
   c. Hypocalcemic tetany
   d. Severe hypoglycemia
7. Iodinated thyroid hormones used for the treatment of thyroid deficiencies include
   a. Dextrothyroxine
   b. Levothyroxine
   c. Thyroglobin
8. Foods containing goitrogens include
   a. Brassica vegetables
   b. Meat from kale-fed cattle
   c. Infant formulas made from soybeans
   d. Strawberries and peaches
9. Adverse reactions to antithyroid drugs include
   a. Increased production of thyrotropin
   b. Goiter
   c. Nasal congestion
   d. Skin rash
10. Foods likely to be rich in iodine include
    a. Upland vegetables
    b. Seafood
    c. Foodstuffs grown in coastal regions
    d. Milk
11. Tests of thyroid function that employ radioiodine are not accurate if the client has recently used or ingested
    a. A diet high in iodine
    b. An iodine disinfectant
    c. Antithyroid drugs
    d. Colestipol
12. Radioiodine may be administered
    a. Orally
    b. Subcutaneously
    c. Intramuscularly
    d. Intravenously
13. Radioiodine is employed medicinally
    a. To treat cancer of the thyroid
    b. To treat Graves' disease
    c. To treat simple goiter
    d. To diagnose thyroid pathology
14. Radioiodine is absolutely contraindicated for clients
    a. With iodine allergy
    b. During the growth years
    c. During pregnancy
15. The structures of anterior pituitary hormones include
    a. Amino acid derivatives
    b. Proteins
    c. Glycoproteins
    d. Steroids
16. By what routes is ACTH administered?
    a. Orally
    b. Subcutaneously
    c. Intramuscularly
    d. Intravenously
17. Clients who undergo diagnostic tests using ACTH usually have health problems characterized by
    a. Weakness
    b. Depression
    c. Hypertension
    d. Decreased resistance to stress
    e. Hyperglycemia
18. Before ACTH therapy is initiated, the potential recipient should be screened for
    a. Allergic hypersensitivity to the drug
    b. Diabetes mellitus
    c. History of tuberculosis
    d. Hypotension
    e. Infection
    f. Malignancies
    g. Peptic ulcer disease
19. Thyrotropin is administered
    a. Orally
    b. Topically
    c. By injection
    d. By inhalation
20. Thyrotropin can cause
    a. Tachycardia
    b. Nausea and vomiting
    c. Subnormal temperature
    d. Allergic reactions
21. Following hypophysectomy (surgical removal or ablation of the pituitary), clients are likely to produce little or no
    a. Oxytocin
    b. Vasopressin
    c. Thyrotropin
    d. Adrenocorticotropin
    e. Somatotropin
    f. Gonadotropins
    g. Thyroid hormone
    h. Parathormone
    i. Calcitonin

j. Glucocorticoids
k. Mineralocorticoids
l. Sex hormones
m. Insulin
n. Glucagon
22. Following hypophysectomy, clients are usually given, as replacement therapy, drug preparations of
a. Adrenocorticotropin
b. Thyrotropin
c. Gonadotropins
d. Somatotropin
e. Mineralocorticoids
f. Glucocorticoids
g. Thyroid hormone
h. Sex hormones
i. Insulin
23. Vasopressin is administered
a. Orally
b. Topically
c. By injection
d. By inhalation

PART 2: EXERCISES RELATING TO HORMONES IN GENERAL

The following exercises are designed for use after completion of Chapters 32, 33, and 34.

Matching

A. Match the disease or condition in the left-hand column with the hormone imbalance most likely to be present in the right-hand column. Place your answer in the space provided.

_____ 1. Acromegaly
_____ 2. Adrenogenital syndrome
_____ 3. Cushing's syndrome
_____ 4. Diabetes mellitus
_____ 5. Dwarfism
_____ 6. Graves' disease
_____ 7. Eunuchoidism
_____ 8. Menopause
_____ 9. Myxedema
_____ 10. Reactive hypoglycemia

a. Excessive estrogen effect
b. Deficiency of female hormones
c. Excessive androgen effect
d. Deficiency of male hormone
e. Hypocortism
f. Hypercortism
g. Excessive somatotropin
h. Deficiency of somatotropin
i. Excessive thyroid hormone
j. Deficiency of thyroid hormone
k. Excess insulin effect
l. Inadequate insulin effect

B. Match the hormone in the left-hand column with the most likely long-term dosage regimen in the right-hand column.

_____ 1. Androgens
_____ 2. Estrogens
_____ 3. Glucocorticoids
_____ 4. Insulin
_____ 5. Mineralocorticoids
_____ 6. Thyroxine

a. Initial doses tend to be high, with subsequent reduction to maintain effective levels
b. Initial doses tend to be low, with subsequent increases to achieve optimal response
c. Doses are modified frequently in accordance with results of laboratory tests
d. Doses used are only high enough to alleviate distressing symptoms

C. Match the hormone in the left-hand column with the antagonistic drug that produces *opposite* physiologic actions in the right-hand column.

_____ 1. Insulin
_____ 2. Parathormone
_____ 3. Thyroxine

a. Calcitonin
b. Cortisone
c. Glucagon
d. Prophylthiouracil

D. Match the hormone in the left-hand column with the function or factor that *inhibits* its production, thus completing a negative feedback mechanism, in the right-hand column.

_____ 1. Thyrotropin
_____ 2. ACTH
_____ 3. ADH
_____ 4. Gonadotropins
_____ 5. Mineralocorticoids
_____ 6. Calcitonin
_____ 7. Parathormone

a. Increased concentration of sex hormones
b. Increased serum concentration of glucocorticoids
c. Decreased osmolarity of body fluids
d. Increased serum concentration of thyroid hormone
e. Increased blood pressure
f. Decreased sodium concentration in body fluids
g. Increased calcium ion concentration in the serum
h. Decreased calcium ion concentration in the serum

Crossword Puzzle

ACROSS

3. A glucocorticoid drug used to prevent cerebral edema
6. One name for ACTH
8. A drug that inhibits synthesis of thyroid hormones
11. A hormone that increases calcium concentration in body fluids
13. The metabolic process of body tissue breakdown
16. The hormones that exert the greatest effect on renal reabsorption of sodium and potassium
17. An antiestrogenic drug used as a fertility drug
18. The pituitary hormone that stimulates thyroid gland function
20. A radionuclide used to diagnose and treat thyroid pathology
23. A common adverse reaction to antithyroid drugs
25. Abbreviation for a trophic pituitary hormone
26. A drug preparation used to treat diabetes insipidus
29. A substance that causes thyrotropin secretion because of its inhibition of thyroid gland function
30. The hormones responsible for male secondary sex characteristics
31. An antiestrogenic drug used to treat cancer of the breast

DOWN

1. A disease characterized by deficiency of ADH
2. A hormone that increases basal metabolism
3. Abbreviation for a synthetic estrogen associated with increased risk of vaginal cancer in women exposed to it *in utero*
4. The metabolic process of building up body tissue
5. The pituitary hormone that stimulates glucocorticoid production by the adrenals
6. A unit for measuring radioactivity
7. A goitrogenic substance found in infant formulas
8. Abbreviation of the name of a long-lasting insulin
9. A thyroid hormone used as a drug
10. A class of drug used to diagnose and treat thyroid pathology
12. A hormone that decreases calcium concentration in body fluids
14. The most frequently prescribed preparation of insulin
15. A pituitary hormone used medicinally to stimulate labor
19. The amino acid incorporated into thyroid hormone molecules
21. Growth hormone
22. A hormone whose actions reverse the effects of insulin
24. The hormone responsible for female secondary sex characteristics
27. A glucocorticoid drug used to treat chronic collagen disease
28. A nutrient that functions as an antidote for insulin toxicity

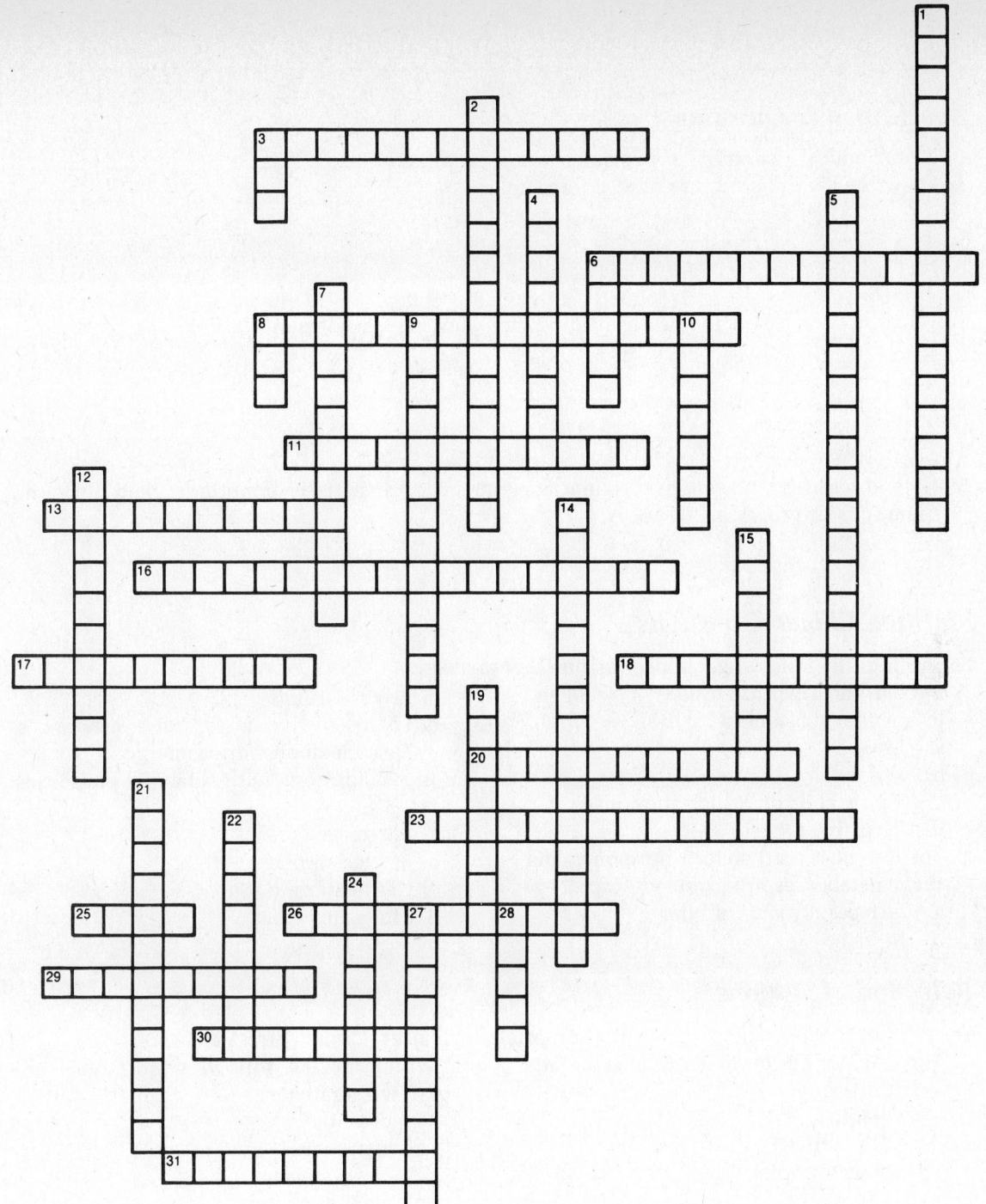

Correct the False Statement

Indicate whether the following statements are true or false; if false, correct the underlined words or phrases.

_____ 1. The effects of hormones used as drugs are <u>highly specific</u>, with a single hormone usually <u>producing a single effect</u> in the body.

_____ 2. <u>Steroid hormones</u> are destroyed by digestion and are usually administered parenterally.

189

_____ 3. Exogenous protein hormones <u>rarely</u> produce allergic reactions.

Short Answer Questions

1. The chemical structures of hormones are most often either _____ or _____ .
2. Draw the central structure of a steroid molecule.

3. What biochemical is the basic building block for steroid hormones?

4. Define Addison's disease.

5. Give at least two reasons why client assessment is particularly important when hormone therapy is in progress.

Multiple Choice Questions

For each of the following, choose the one best answer.

1. Steroid hormones are usually metabolized to inactive substances by the
   a. Liver
   b. Kidneys
   c. Target cells on which they act
   d. Digestive process
2. For the most part, steroid hormones and their metabolites are excreted
   a. In feces, by way of bile
   b. In urine
   c. By the lungs
   d. None of the above; these substances are metabolized for energy
3. A sex hormone with catabolic properties is
   a. Estrone
   b. Progesterone
   c. Testosterone
   d. Insulin

Selection of Options

For each of the following, select *all* appropriate responses. Circle correct answers.

1. Hormones with steroid structures include
   a. Cortisone
   b. Insulin
   c. Thyroxine
   d. Somatotropin
   e. Aldosterone
   f. Estrogen
   g. Progesterone
   h. Androgens
2. Hormones that are usually considered to be essential for survival include
   a. Sex hormones
   b. Glucocorticoids
   c. Mineralocorticoids
   d. Thyroid hormone
   e. Insulin
   f. Antidiuretic hormone
   g. Somatotropin
3. Which of the following hormones are known teratogens?
   a. Androgens
   b. Estrogens
   c. Progestogens
   d. Somatotropin
   e. Thyroxine
   f. ADH
4. The mechanism of action of steroid hormones usually involves
   a. Interaction with a receptor site on the membrane of the target cell
   b. Penetration of the cell membrane by the hormone molecule
   c. Interaction with a cytoplasmic receptor protein
   d. Alteration of the function of nuclear chromatin

e. Alteration of the nature of cell function
   f. Alteration of the rate of cell function
5. Which of the following statements is (are) true of cholesterol?
   a. It is a toxic biochemical that performs no useful biologic function
   b. When blood concentrations of cholesterol are high, there is an increased risk of cardiovascular degeneration
   c. It is essential to life (in mammals)
   d. For humans, it is an essential dietary component
   e. The body can make cholesterol from many other nutrient substances
6. Hormones that are destroyed by digestive enzymes include
   a. Androgens
   b. Antidiuretic hormone
   c. Epinephrine
   d. Estrogens
   e. Luteinizing hormone
   f. Norepinephrine
   g. Thyroxine

UNIT NINE: DRUGS AFFECTING SPECIFIC BODY SYSTEMS

35
Drugs Affecting the Respiratory Tract

A patent airway is the number one priority in nursing care. However, many general nursing measures also involve respiratory care of clients. Nurses are important in assisting clients to manage their respiratory disorders and to lead productive lives.

Short Answer Questions

1. Identify the following:
   a. P
   b. PO_2
   c. PCO_2
   d. PaO_2
   e. $PaCO_2$
2. Define the following:
   a. Oxygen tension:

   b. Oxygen saturation:

   c. Airway resistance:

   d. Bronchospasm:

   e. Carbon dioxide narcosis:

   f. Surfactant:

   g. Hypoxia:

   h. Hyperpnea:

   i. Hypocapnea:

   j. Diffusion capacity:

   k. Cyanosis:

   l. Anoxia:

   m. Cor pulmonale:

3. Why is the nose important?

4. Describe why the nurse must be concerned if the nose is bypassed (i.e., in a mouth breather or a person with an endotracheal tube or tracheostomy tube).

5. Describe the action and importance of the mucociliary system and the mucous blanket.

6. List etiologic factors that inhibit mucociliary transport.

7. Explain the physiology of breathing.

8. Diagram in equation form an allergic person's response to an antigen leading to bronchospasm and bronchoconstriction.

9. Explain how theophylline produces bronchodilation.

10. Describe the pathophysiology seen with emphysema.

11. Discuss the relationship of hydration and sputum viscosity.

12. What is the effect of expectorants on the mucous blanket?

13. Describe the factors that inhibit or prevent learning in clients with respiratory dysfunctions.

14. List at least five goals for the client with a nursing diagnosis of respiratory impairment.

Sequences

Arrange the following parts of the body in the order in which air from the atmosphere passes through in the breathing process by numbering each in sequence.

_____ Trachea
_____ Nose
_____ Pharynx
_____ Alveoli
_____ Bronchi
_____ Bronchial tree
_____ Larynx

Completion Exercise

Read each question carefully and place your answer in the space provided.
1. Complete the following table on sympathomimetic drugs.

DRUG	RECEPTOR	ACTION	ADVERSE REACTIONS
Epinephrine			
Isoproterenol			
Metaproterenol			
Terbutaline			

Using the following word list, identify the parts of the upper and lower respiratory system shown in the two figures below.

Nasal concha
Glottis
Bronchiole
Paranasal sinuses
Trachea

Bronchus
Larynx
Epiglottis
Alveolus
Pharynx

2. a. _____
   b. _____
   c. _____
   d. _____
   e. _____
   f. _____

3. a. _____
   b. _____
   c. _____
   d. _____

195

4. Complete the table of drug–drug interactions for theophylline.

DRUG	EFFECT ON THEOPHYLLINE
Cimetidine	
Allopurinol	
Furosemide	
Propranolol	
Digoxin	
Phenytoin	
Lithium carbonate	

Situational Exercises

What would you do in the following situations? Write your answer in the space provided.
1. Mr. P's blood gases are as follows: pH, 7.31; PaO_2, 38; $PaCO_2$, 105; bicarbonate, 36.
   a. Postulate what stimulates this person's respiratory drive.

   b. Compare with a normal person's respiratory drive.

   c. List six symptoms that you would expect to find with Mr. P, based on the above blood gases.

2. Mrs. G is receiving theophylline. Her blood level is 25 μg/ml. What adverse reactions would you anticipate?

3. Mrs. S has a diagnosis of asthma. She is being started on cromolyn sodium. What should this person be taught with respect to its use prophylactically in contrast to use of other drugs for acute attacks?

4. Mr. T, who has long-standing emphysema, is cyanotic and dyspneic, and his blood gases reveal a PO_2 of 40 and a PCO_2 of 110. Why would oxygen be used with extreme caution?

Personal Exercises: Respiratory System

Read each question carefully and write your answers on a separate sheet of paper.
1. Try an intermittent positive breathing machine in a pulmonary laboratory. What does it feel like? Try a spirometer and determine the tidal volume. How does this compare with normal values?
2. Develop a teaching plan that you could use in showing a client the proper use and administration of some type of inhalant therapy.
3. Develop a care plan that would promote respiratory function for a client suffering from obstructive lung disease.

36
Drugs Affecting the Reproductive Systems and Sexuality

Fertility and sexual response are affected by many factors, including the health status of the person, hormonal levels, psychosocial influences, and growth and development.

Multiple Choice Questions

For each of the following, choose the one best answer.
1. Menstrual irregularities may occur as a result of
   1. Inadequate rest
   2. Insufficient caloric intake
   3. Hormonal imbalance
   4. Rigorous sports activity
      a. All of the above
      b. 1, 2, 3
      c. 2, 3, 4
      d. 3 only
2. A diagnostic fertility workup should always include
   a. Postcoital tests
   b. Semen analysis
   c. Endometrial biopsy
   d. All of the above
3. Evaluation of the cervical mucus in fertility testing is useful in determining
   a. Obstructions in the female reproductive tract
   b. Incompatibility between sperm and mucus
   c. Microscopic fern patterns
   d. All of the above
4. Serum progesterone levels provide
   a. Predictive evidence of ovulation
   b. Evaluation of the luteal phase
   c. Information on immune reaction
   d. All of the above
5. Histories and physicals of both partners in fertility workups are necessary to
   a. Evaluate the timing of intercourse
   b. Uncover sexual infections
   c. Determine the physical status of each partner
   d. All of the above

Sequences

Arrange the following by numbering in order of occurrence during the ovarian cycle.
_____ Degenerating corpus luteum
_____ Mature corpus luteum
_____ Primary follicle
_____ Ovulation
_____ Growing follicle
_____ Mature follicle
_____ Early corpus luteum

Completion Exercises

Read each question carefully and place your answer in the space provided.
1. A female hormone that affects height in growing girls is _____. An increase in this hormone at puberty limits height through two actions, which are _____.
2. Two female sex hormones produced in the anterior lobe of the pituitary gland during the menstrual cycle are _____ and _____.
3. In the following table, describe the action and time of the highest level of each of these hormones during the menstrual cycle.

HORMONE	ACTION	TIME OF HIGHEST LEVEL
FSH		
LH		

Correct the False Statement

Indicate whether the following statements are true or false; if false, correct the underlined words or phrases.

_____ 1. In high doses, alcohol always increases sexual desire.

_____ 2. Thiazides may cause impotence.

_____ 3. β-blockers have no effect on sexual response.

Matching

Match the method of contraception in the left-hand column with the descriptive phrase in the right-hand column. Place your answer in the space provided.

_____ 1. Nonpharmacologic methods
_____ 2. Barrier methods
_____ 3. Monoclonal antibody test
_____ 4. Oral contraceptives
_____ 5. Surgical methods

a. Predictive test for ovulation
b. Absolute compliance
c. May be irreversible
d. Fertility awareness
e. Used in conjunction with spermicide

Short Answer Questions

1. Systemic illness may cause sexual problems. Name one sexual problem that can be anticipated in each of the following disorders:
   a. Diabetes mellitus: _____
   b. Cardiovascular disease: _____
   c. Kidney disease: _____
   d. Thyroid deficiency: _____

2. List at least five factors that may affect sperm production in a 25-year-old man.

3. Name at least three medications that are helpful in treating dysmenorrhea and describe their actions.

4. Identify two nonpharmacologic methods for decreasing premenstrual symptoms.

5. Osteoporosis sometimes occurs secondary to menopause. List two possible preventive measures.

6. Name the organism responsible for toxic shock syndrome and list at least four symptoms usually associated with this disease.

37
Drugs Affecting the Musculoskeletal System: Skeletal Muscle Relaxants and Antispastic Agents

Different kinds of drugs are capable of relaxing skeletal muscles and treating spasticity. Skeletal muscle relaxants are used to relieve the pain and increase the mobility of affected muscles in acute musculoskeletal disorders. Antispastic agents are used for spasticity caused by upper motor neuron disorders, such as cerebral palsy and paraplegia. There is no completely satisfactory form of therapy for alleviating skeletal muscle spasticity.

Matching

A. Match the generic names of the common skeletal muscle relaxants in the left-hand column with their trade names in the right-hand column. Place your answer in the space provided.

_____ 1. carisoprodol
_____ 2. chlorzoxazone
_____ 3. methocarbamol
_____ 4. orphenadrine
_____ 5. cyclobenzaprine
_____ 6. baclofen
_____ 7. dantrolene
_____ 8. quinine

a. Lioresal
b. Dantrium
c. Quinamm
d. Rela, Soma
e. Flexeril
f. Robaxin, Robaxisal
g. Paraflex, Parafon Forte
h. Norflex, Norgesic, Norgesic Forte

B. Match the skeletal muscle relaxant in the left-hand column with its usual adult oral dose in the right-hand column.

_____ 1. Rela, Soma
_____ 2. Paraflex
_____ 3. Robaxin
_____ 4. Norflex
_____ 5. Flexeril
_____ 6. Lioresal
_____ 7. Dantrium
_____ 8. Quinamm

a. 100 mg bid
b. 10 mg tid
c. 1 g qid
d. 5 mg tid to 80 mg qd
e. 25 mg qd to 400 mg qd
f. 260 mg qhs
g. 350 mg qid
h. 250 mg to 750 mg three or four times/day

Completion Exercises

Read the question carefully and place your answer in the space provided. Identify the extra ingredient(s) in the following compounds.
1. Soma Compound: carisoprodol and _____
2. Parafon Forte: chlorzoxazone and _____
3. Robaxisal: methocarbamol and _____
4. Norgesic: orphenadrine and _____ and _____

Short Answer Questions

1. List at least six specific conditions that cause muscle spasms intense enough to warrant medication.

2. Common side effects with all the skeletal muscle relaxants are drowsiness and dizziness. Describe what advice about side effects a nurse should give to a client who is just starting one of these medications.

3. Identify significant or unusual side effects associated with the following drugs:
   a. Parafon Forte:

   b. Paraflex:

   c. Dantrium:

   d. Robaxin:

   e. Norflex:

   f. Flexeril:

38
Drugs Affecting the Kidneys: Diuretics

The kidneys eliminate excess fluids, electrolytes, nitrogenous wastes, and toxins. The kidneys keep the body's blood chemistry properly balanced by this selective excretion of unnecessary chemicals. Diuretics increase the production of urine by inducing the body to lose fluid.

Correct the False Statement

Indicate whether the following statements are true or false; if false, correct the underlined words or phrases.

_____ 1. The force responsible for maintaining glomerular filtration is <u>an osmotic diffusion gradient</u>.

_____ 2. The glomerular filtrate is <u>more concentrated than</u> interstitial fluid.

_____ 3. Normal glomerular filtrate contains <u>little or no protein</u>.

_____ 4. The presence of red blood cells in urine is <u>abnormal</u>.

_____ 5. Diuretics are usually <u>contraindicated</u> during pregnancy.

_____ 6. Hypokalemia tends to cause <u>cramping and diarrhea</u>.

_____ 7. In digitalized persons, the effect of hypokalemia on intestinal function <u>may be opposite to</u> that in a nonmedicated person.

_____ 8. Toxic reactions to diuretics are most likely to occur in <u>cold dry</u> environments.

_____ 9. Cardiac arrest that is caused by hypokalemia is characterized by ventricular fibrillation during <u>diastole</u>.

_____ 10. To a degree, diuresis is <u>a positive feedback process (i.e., when diuresis begins, it causes further diuresis)</u>.

_____ 11. The most frequent adverse reaction to diuretic therapy is <u>dehydration</u>.

_____ 12. Furosemide is <u>highly bound</u> to plasma proteins.

_____ 13. Furosemide and ethacrynic acid are eliminated <u>only through the kidneys</u>.

_____ 14. Thiazide diuretics are most often used for the treatment of <u>acute conditions associated with edema</u>.

_____ 15. When liquid potassium supplements are administered, it is most important <u>to give them on an empty stomach</u>.

Find the Hidden Words

Hidden within the following letter grid are words and phrases from Chapter 38. They may be vertical, horizontal, or diagonal. Circle the letters as you find the hidden words.

LIST OF WORDS AND PHRASES

absorption	ethacrynic acid	mannitol
acetazolamide	fluid	nephrons
aldactone	furosemide	osmosis
amiloride	glomerulus	output
carbonic anhydrase	glycerol	reabsorption
diabetes	gout	secretion
Diamox	hydrochlorothiazide	sodium retention
diffusion	hyperkalemia	spironolactone
diuretic	hypokalemia	triamterene
Diuril	hyponatremia	tubule
Edecrin	indoline	urea
edema	intake	weight
electrolyte	Lasix	xanthine

```
c e e e r u i d o s a l i m a c e t a z o l a m i d e r i
a a l d a s i l u e c a r b l a s i n t u b u l i i d e p
a r e i u r e a b s o a a i d i a w b u t r i c n a e n o
b s c l e d i r o l i m a l a n d e n o t c a d l a s o s
d o t a a i n t a m e i b o c t r i n t a c i m a i r t o
s r r s m n t i e d r l s r h a m g i d i a m o x n e c m
m p o u o t e l e c t r o l y t e h p n o a e s a t a a s
o t l d i a a m i u r e r d d a y t y h n u r e a m b l d
s h y p o k a l e m i a p e r k a r h n k a t n i a s o b
e y t s r e a b s o r p t i o n c l i s a l a p m s o n r
c p e e a l d a o s e d i h c a g t u r l d n r u a c o a
r i p i b a i r d m a a o y h r o t m e e a o e p t a r c
e y r t s s e c i f b r n t l l d i u r i l p a i g d i e
h t e c i t e r u i d b e d o a m n e p h r y b l e l p d
y n a t r g d r m a n o c a r b o n i c a n h y d r a s e
s i s o m s o a r p e n r e o s m a n a o e c r e o s m o
e e e d e s i u e d r e a b t u b m t i r e o v r s n e p
c a r s e c r e t i o n e p h r o n s o r p p i e b a m i
a d i m d r r d e e d e d e i r i u u o n h y d i a m a n
r e i n t t e e n i e a e n a t f a l a s y h e n o t c a
b d s a n e a l t n l d m a z f t a m i l p r e a c e t a
e n b n b a b s i n t i i n i l u i d t d e l v c t r i a
t a a l a e s h o e u u a d d r b a i r e d e c r i n e p
h m l a i r t o n p g l o m e r u l u s k r e p i e e d o
a e d s a n e e y h y f c n e p l e r e a b e o m i d e n
c d d i a l d a s i n d o l i n e d e c a r b n a t n i a
r e a x a c e t o o s m o s e c r e d e c a r b e d e m o
```

Matching

A. Match each of the physiologic segments of the renal tubule in the left-hand column with all appropriate responses in the right-hand column. Place your answer(s) in the space provided.

_____ 1. Proximal tubule
_____ 2. Descending portion of the thin segment of the loop of Henle
_____ 3. Ascending portion of the thin segment of the loop of Henle
_____ 4. Diluting segment of the distal tubule
_____ 5. Late distal tubule
_____ 6. Collecting tubule

a. Reabsorption of water
b. Active secretion of hydrogen ions
c. Reabsorption of vitamins
d. Diffusion of chloride ions
e. Active transport of chloride ions
f. Reabsorption of amino acids
g. Reabsorption of urea
h. Reabsorption of sodium
i. Reabsorption of potassium
j. Responds to antidiuretic hormone
k. Responds to aldosterone
l. Secretes potassium
m. Relatively little influence

B. Match each diuretic listed in the left-hand column with its major site of action in the tubule of the kidney in the right-hand column.

_____ 1. Acetazolamide
_____ 2. Amiloride
_____ 3. Bumetamide
_____ 4. Chlorothiazide
_____ 5. Ethacrynic acid
_____ 6. Furosemide
_____ 7. Hydrochlorothiazide
_____ 8. Spironolactone
_____ 9. Triamterene
_____ 10. Xanthines
_____ 11. Indolines

a. Proximal tubule
b. Loop of Henle
c. Diluting segment
d. Distal tubule

Multiple Choice Questions

For each of the following, choose the one best answer.

1. Of the following elements, which exerts the most influence on fluid balance?
   a. Calcium
   b. Magnesium
   c. Potassium
   d. Sodium
2. The usefulness of xanthines as diuretic agents is limited by
   a. Their bronchodilating actions
   b. Their potassium-wasting effect
   c. Their stimulating effect
   d. All of the above
3. How do osmotic diuretics affect blood volume?
   a. They increase blood volume
   b. They decrease blood volume
   c. Initially they decrease blood volume and subsequently they increase it
   d. Initially they increase blood volume and subsequently they decrease it
4. Mannitol is usually administered
   a. Orally
   b. Subcutaneously
   c. Intramuscularly
   d. Intravenously
5. Glycerol is usually administered
   a. Orally
   b. Subcutaneously
   c. Intramuscularly
   d. Intravenously
6. The diuretic used most frequently to prevent acute renal failure is
   a. Furosemide
   b. Glycerol
   c. Hydrochlorothiazide
   d. Mannitol
7. A common adverse reaction to osmotic diuretics is
   a. Fluid overload
   b. Dehydration
   c. Hypokalemia
   d. Allergic reactions

8. The mechanism of action of acetazolamide is
   a. Increased hydrostatic pressure in the glomerulus
   b. Inhibition of carbonic anhydrase
   c. Inhibition of active reabsorption of sodium in the tubule
   d. Stimulation of active secretion of sodium in the tubule
9. Acetazolamide is usually administered
   a. Orally
   b. Subcutaneously
   c. Intramuscularly
   d. Intravenously
10. A frequent side effect of acetazolamide is
    a. Hyponatremia
    b. Hyperkalemia
    c. Metabolic alkalosis
    d. Metabolic acidosis
11. In addition to increasing the volume of urine, acetazolamide
    a. Increases pH of urine
    b. Decreases pH of urine
    c. Increases uric acid concentration in urine
    d. Decreases excretion of lithium
12. Clients at greatest risk for adverse reaction to acetazolamide are those predisposed to
    a. Respiratory acidosis
    b. Respiratory alkalosis
    c. Hyperkalemia
    d. Glaucoma
13. The site of action of "high-ceiling" diuretics is the
    a. Proximal tubule
    b. Loop of Henle
    c. Diluting segment
    d. Distal tubule
14. A major adverse reaction to thiazide diuretics is
    a. Hypoglycemia
    b. Metabolic acidosis
    c. Metabolic alkalosis
    d. Hypokalemia
15. The mechanism of action of spironolactone is
    a. Inhibition of aldosterone
    b. Antidiuretic hormone
    c. Carbonic anhydrase
    d. Absorption of chloride
16. A major adverse reaction to spironolactone is
    a. Hypokalemia
    b. Hyperkalemia
    c. Metabolic acidosis
    d. Metabolic alkalosis
17. Clients most vulnerable to spironolactone toxicity are those with
    a. Cardiac impairment
    b. Hepatic impairment
    c. Renal impairment
    d. Adrenal hyperfunction
18. A diuretic likely to cause feminization of male clients is
    a. Amiloride
    b. Chlorothiazide
    c. Spironolactone
    d. Triamterene
19. The most sensitive indicator of diuresis is
    a. Body weight
    b. Blood pressure
    c. Fluid intake and output
    d. Tissue turgor
20. Foods rich in potassium include
    a. Apples and raisins
    b. Bananas and oranges
    c. Cranberries and boiled vegetables
    d. Whole grain cereals
21. In persons with adequate adrenal function, what effect does stress have on potassium concentration?
    a. It increases potassium concentration in the blood
    b. It decreases potassium concentration in the blood
    c. It does not affect blood concentrations of potassium
    d. It increases potassium concentration in the intracellular fluid
    e. Both c and d
22. Hyperkalemia's effects on the gastrointestinal tract include
    a. Vasodilation and vascular congestion
    b. Atony and intestinal obstruction
    c. Increased motility and cramping pain
    d. A prolongation of intestinal transit time
23. (A) dietary component(s) that can reduce the therapeutic effect of diuretics is (are)
    a. Calorie nutrients
    b. Water and other fluids
    c. Potassium
    d. Sodium
24. When diuretic therapy is initiated, the nurse should warn clients that they will experience
    a. Some weakness
    b. Increased urination
    c. Increased number of stools
    d. All of the above

25. Therapeutic responses to diuretics should occur within
    a. 2 hours
    b. 8 hours
    c. 24 hours
    d. 48 hours

Selection of Options

For each of the following, select *all* appropriate responses. Circle correct answers.

1. Compared to glomerular filtrate, urine usually contains a
   a. Lower concentration of red blood cells
   b. Lower concentration of water
   c. Lower concentration of sodium
   d. Higher concentration of nitrogenous wastes
   e. Higher concentration of toxins
2. Mechanisms by which the kidney tubule influences the composition of urine include
   a. Filtration
   b. Passive diffusion
   c. Carrier-mediated transport
   d. Active transport mechanisms
3. Hormones that influence the function of the renal tubule include
   a. Thyroxine
   b. Aldosterone
   c. Corticosteroids
   d. Male sex hormones
   e. Vasopressin
4. When a person on restricted sodium intake is overhydrated, physiologic effects include
   a. Increased production of urine
   b. Increased loss of electrolytes in urine
   c. A tendency toward positive water balance
   d. Decreased concentration of sodium in body fluids
   e. Negative potassium balance
5. By what routes are osmotic diuretics administered?
   a. Orally
   b. Subcutaneously
   c. Intramuscularly
   d. Intravenously
6. Therapeutic uses for osmotic diuretics include
   a. Treatment of congestive heart failure with edema
   b. Prevention of acute renal failure following trauma
   c. Treatment of pulmonary edema
   d. Alleviating increased cerebrospinal fluid pressure
7. Contraindications for osmotic diuretics include
   a. Cardiac failure
   b. Hypovolemia
   c. Intracranial hemorrhage
   d. Severe dehydration
   e. Oliguria
   f. Pulmonary edema
8. Thiazide diuretics are administered
   a. Orally
   b. Subcutaneously
   c. Intramuscularly
   d. Intravenously
9. Assessment data that should be gathered regularly for clients receiving diuretics include
   a. Fluid intake and output
   b. Body weight
   c. Vital signs
   d. Tissue turgor
10. Rapid intravenous infusion of potassium can cause
    a. Phlebitis
    b. Spasm in the vein used for the infusion
    c. Prolonged systole
    d. Cardiac arrest
11. Diuretics that tend to increase gout include
    a. Acetazolamide
    b. Benzothiazides
    c. Loop diuretics
    d. Spironolactone
12. Diuretics that tend to exacerbate diabetes mellitus include
    a. Acetazolamide
    b. Benzothiazides
    c. Loop diuretics
    d. Spironolactone
13. Toxicity to various diuretics is sometimes characterized by
    a. Sodium depletion
    b. Sodium retention
    c. Potassium depletion
    d. Potassium retention
    e. Low blood volume

Short Answer Questions

1. Define the following terms:
   a. Diuretic:

   b. Edema:

2. Name three disease conditions in which diuretics are used to control edema.

3. Identify two osmotic diuretics.

4. List two therapeutic uses for carbonic anhydrase inhibitors.

5. Identify two therapeutic uses for loop diuretics.

6. Name three qualities required of a drug for osmotic diuresis.

7. Give at least two adverse reactions to loop diuretics.

8. Identify two disease conditions that tend to increase in severity when diuretics are used.

9. Name at least two fruits that are good sources of dietary potassium.

10. What class of food is a good source of dietary potassium?

11. How much will body weight decrease with a net loss of 1 liter of fluid?

UNIT TEN: DRUGS USED FOR NEOPLASTIC DISEASE

39
Theoretic Base for Chemotherapy, Alkylating Agents, and Antimetabolites

Antineoplastic drug therapy is one of three main ways of treating cancer. Seven subgroupings of alkylating agents and three subgroupings of antimetabolities include almost 20 active antineoplastic agents. A number of adverse reactions to antineoplastic drugs are very common and often complicate the care of the client receiving this therapy.

Essay Questions

Read each question carefully and write your answers on a separate sheet of paper.
1. An alkylating agent is usually used in combination with other agents to treat Hodgkin's disease in its more advanced stages. Explain the reasons for combination chemotherapy.
2. Describe five factors that affect whether or not antineoplastic drug therapy is used for a client's cancer.
3. Name the five phases of the cell cycle and identify what happens in each phase.
4. What is meant by methotrexate with "folinic acid rescue" therapy?

Matching

Match the following individual antimetabolites in the left-hand column with their subgrouping in the right-hand column. Place your answers in the space provided.

_____ 1. Thioguanine	a. Folic acid analog
_____ 2. Methotrexate	b. Pyrimidine analog
_____ 3. Floxuridine	c. Purine analog
_____ 4. Cytarabine	
_____ 5. Mercaptopurine	
_____ 6. Fluorouracil	

Short Answer Questions

1. What drugs are included in the ethylenimine and methylmelamine group of alkylating agents?

2. What alkylating agents are included in the nitrosourea grouping?

3. a. What alkylating agent causes ototoxicity?

   b. What does the term ototoxicity mean?

   c. What are its signs and symptoms?

4. Define the mechanism of action for each of the following:
   a. Folic acid analog:

   b. Pyrimidine analog:

   c. Purine analog:

5. What is topical fluorouracil used for?

6. List some interventions that would help if the client experiences anorexia, taste changes, nausea, and vomiting with antineoplastic therapy.

7. List some interventions that would help to prevent infection with the bone marrow suppression seen with antineoplastic therapy.

Completion Exercises

Read each question carefully and place your answer in the space provided.
1. Look up cyclophosphamide in the text.
    a. Adverse reactions are _____
    _____.

    b. You are caring for a client receiving this drug. Explain what you would tell her about the anticipated alopecia. _____
    _____
    _____.

2. Stomatitis is a difficult complication seen with antineoplastic therapy.
    a. The agents that might be used for general mouth care include _____
    _____.

    b. A topical anesthetic that might be used is _____.
    c. Foods that should be avoided include _____
    _____.

    d. Candidiasis would be treated with _____.
3. Dacarbazine (DTIC-Dome) has been used primarily for _____.
4. Work with the antimetabolite _____ led to the development of allopurinol.
5. An alkylating agent used in the treatment of chronic granulocytic leukemia is _____.

40
Natural Products, Hormones, and Miscellaneous Agents

Plant alkaloids, certain antibiotics, and even an enzyme have a role in antineoplastic drug therapy. The adrenocorticosteroids, estrogens, androgens, progestins, and antiestrogens are used with cancers of the reproductive system and other defined cancers.

Essay Questions
Read each question carefully and write your answers on a separate sheet of paper.
1. Describe the pulmonary adverse reaction that can occur with bleomycin.
2. Explain the difference between the two forms of cardiotoxicity that may occur when daunorubicin is used.
3. Describe the mechanism of action of asparaginase.
4. Describe the rationale for the use of estrogens and androgens in antineoplastic therapy.

Matching
A. Match the following natural products in the left-hand column with their subgrouping in the right-hand column. Place your answers in the space provided.

_____ 1. Mitomycin   a. Plant alkaloid
_____ 2. Bleomycin   b. Antibiotic
_____ 3. Vincristine   c. Enzyme
_____ 4. Plicamycin
_____ 5. Asparaginase
_____ 6. Dactinomycin
_____ 7. Vinblastine
_____ 8. Daunorubicin
_____ 9. Doxorubicin
_____ 10. Etoposide

B. Match the condition in the left-hand column with the class(es) of drugs used for treatment in the right-hand column.

_____ 1. Inoperable or recurrent endometrial cancer   a. Adrenocorticosteroids
_____ 2. Remission induction in acute lymphocytic leukemia in children   b. Estrogens
    c. Androgens
    d. Progestins
_____ 3. Advanced breast cancer to control metastatic disease   e. Antiestrogens
    f. Synthetic estrogen-antimetabolites
_____ 4. Breast cancer in postmenopausal women
_____ 5. Radiation edema
_____ 6. Prostatic cancer
_____ 7. Hypercalcemia

Short Answer Questions
1. Describe the neurotoxicities that may occur when vincristine is used.

2. How do certain antibiotics produce their antineoplastic effects?

3. Describe the renal toxicities seen with mitomycin.

4. Explain why the hypercalcemia seen with some cancers is of concern. Identify an antibiotic that may be used to treat hypercalcemia.

5. Explain why estrogen receptors are important.

Completion Exercises

Read each question carefully and place your answer in the space provided.
1. Look up etoposide in the text.
   a. Adverse reactions are _____
   _____.
   b. Some of its uses are to treat _____
   _____.
2. Hydroxyurea is used primarily to treat _____.
3. Mitotane acts on the adrenal cortex and causes _____
   _____.
4. Procarbazine does _____ so it can be used for _____.
5. Aminoglutethimide is used to treat _____.
6. The agent _____ might be used with inoperable adrenocortical cancer.
7. One unique action of plicamycin is that it _____.

UNIT ELEVEN: DRUGS AFFECTING THE IMMUNE SYSTEM

41
Drugs Used in the Treatment of Allergy

Allergic reactions may occur in persons sensitive to specific substances, including foods, fibers, environmental contaminants, and chemicals.

Completion Exercises

Read each question carefully and place your answer in the space provided.

1. The most important factor in making an accurate diagnosis of an allergy is _____ or, if a health-care professional is present when the allergy develops, _____ of symptoms.
2. Accurate reporting to the physician should include _____ and _____.
3. When possible, clinical verification should be avoided because _____.
4. Common food allergens are _____.
5. Common medication allergens are _____.
6. Environmental factors causing allergens are _____.
7. Three body areas in which atopic eczema manifests itself in children are _____, _____, and _____.
8. Treatment of allergic reactions, whenever possible, centers on _____, which requires accurate diagnosis.
9. Severe reactions may require medical intervention. One such intervention for anaphylactic shock is _____.
10. Medical intervention for bronchial asthma includes _____.
11. Corticosteroids are used for treatment of chronic asthma. Discuss the following:
    a. Clinical effectiveness (onset and maximum effect): _____.
    b. Reason for selection of this therapy: _____.
    c. Three common adverse effects: _____.
12. The regimen for discontinuing corticosteroids is _____.

13. Complete the following table of drugs that may cause a reaction.

DRUG	POSSIBLE SIDE EFFECTS OR SECONDARY EFFECTS	POSSIBLE IDIOSYNCRASY
Penicillin		
Anticonvulsants		
Chloramphenicol		
Mercurial diuretics		
Aspirin		

Multiple Choice Questions

For each of the following, choose the one best answer.

1. Symptoms of urticaria include
   1. Erythema
   2. Skin elevation that blanches with pressure
   3. Scaliness
   4. Possible pruritis
      a. All of the above
      b. 1, 2, 4
      c. 2, 3, 4
      d. only 2
2. Drug reactions may be a result of which of the following?
   1. Overdose because of synergism
   2. Overdose because of client's condition
   3. Lack of compliance
   4. Personal idiosyncrasy
   5. Side effects
      a. 1, 2, 4
      b. 3, 4, 5
      c. 1, 2, 5
      d. 2, 3, 4
      e. All of the above
3. Anaphylactic shock results most frequently from use of
   a. Chloramphenicol
   b. Thiazides
   c. Penicillin
   d. Aspirin
   e. All of the above
4. Thrombocytopenia may be associated with use of
   a. Phenothiazines
   b. Chloramphenicol
   c. Phenacetin
   d. Penicillin
   e. Aspirin

Personal Exercise: Allergies

Read each question carefully and write your answers on a separate sheet of paper.
1. Do you have any allergies? If so, in what form?
2. What medication do you take for this allergy?
3. Make up an allergy history for yourself, including such considerations as when allergies occur, possible causes, and how you treat them. (If you do not have an allergy, you may want to interview a friend or family member who has allergies.)

42
Drugs Used for Immunity

Immunization programs should take the needs of the person into account, including such factors as age, exposure to preventable disease, and possible allergies or physical conditions that might result in an adverse reaction to the immunizing agent.

Short Answer Questions

1. Immunization programs should be instituted during infancy as recommended by the Committee of Infectious Diseases of the American Academy of Pediatrics, and continued through childhood. Give the appropriate age schedules for the following:
   a. DTP:

   b. TD:

   c. OPV:

   d. MMR:

2. List contraindications to receiving measles, mumps, and rubella vaccines.

3. Explain the rationale for the following statements.
   a. Smallpox vaccinations are no longer given routinely.

   b. Tuberculin tests are given prior to or simultaneously with measles vaccine in a routine childhood immunization program.

   c. Measles vaccination should be delayed until an infant is 1 year old. If given earlier, a second dose should be given at 12 to 15 months of age.

   d. Mumps vaccine should be given to an unimmunized boy before adolescence, if possible.

   e. Anyone receiving immunization should be observed for 30 minutes following the procedure.

   f. Programs for the use of HBV for health-care workers have been instituted throughout the United States.

   g. Pregnant women should not undergo vaccination.

   h. Immunization programs should receive ongoing reevaluation.

Correct the False Statement

Indicate whether the following statements are true or false; if false, correct the underlined words or phrases.

_____ 1. <u>All</u> infants are born with some natural immunity.

_____ 2. Malnutrition is one factor <u>reducing the body's defenses against disease.</u>

_____ 3. Antibodies are supplied <u>only through the placenta, in colostrum, or by immunization with appropriate materials</u>

_____ 4. <u>Low antibody titers</u> are associated with recurrent herpes.

Completion Exercises

Read each question carefully and place your answer in the space provided.
1. _____ , an antiviral protein, is produced by the nonlymphoid cells of the body.
2. Antibodies transmitted through the _____ protect newborns against certain diseases to which their mothers have immunity.
3. Additional protection to the newborn is provided through _____ .
4. T cells produce _____ , substances that can activate other immune cells in the body.
5. The production or transfer of antibodies that results in immunity is called _____ .
6. The antibody response occurs in reaction to a _____ .
7. The best protection against pertussis in newborns is adequate immunization of _____ .
8. Theoretically, measles vaccine could activate latent _____ .
9. Measles vaccine is most effective when given at about _____ .
10. Children in kindergarten should be given priority for _____ because they are the major source of viral dissemination.
11. Immunizations are contraindicated if the child has _____ .
12. The common cold, without fever (is/is not) _____ a contraindication to immunization.
13. Failure to observe the manufacturer's storage recommendations may _____ .
14. Children should be instructed not to rub the site of an injection because _____ .

Multiple Choice Questions

For each of the following, choose the one best answer.
1. A child's defense system is usually activated between
   a. 9 and 12 months of age
   b. 6 and 15 months of age
   c. 16 and 30 months of age
   d. 3 and 15 months of age
2. Immune system disorders are affected by
   1. Congenital lack of T or B lymphocytes
   2. Body reactions to deficiencies
   3. Lack of exposure to antigens
   4. Inadequate fluid intake
   a. 2, 3   d. 1, 2
   b. 1, 4   e. All of the above
   c. 3, 4
3. In active immunization, the number of antibodies reach a peak in
   a. 4 to 8 days   c. 16 to 20 days
   b. 10 to 14 days   d. 26 to 30 days

UNIT TWELVE: NUTRITIONAL SUPPLEMENTS

43
Oral Supplements

Several therapeutic agents are administered to prevent or correct nutritional deficiencies. Although these agents are normally used in the body, when administered in high dosages they can precipitate adverse reactions. The following exercises relate to nutritional supplements that are usually administered orally.

PART 1: MINERALS AND VITAMINS

Matching

A. Match each deficiency disease in the left-hand column with the nutrient that is lacking in the right-hand column. Place your answer in the space provided.

____ 1. Beriberi		a.	Vitamin A
____ 2. Keratomalacia		b.	Vitamin B_1
____ 3. Osteomalacia		c.	Vitamin B_2
____ 4. Pellagra		d.	Vitamin B_{12}
____ 5. Pernicious anemia		e.	Niacin
____ 6. Rickets		f.	Vitamin B_6
____ 7. Scurvy		g.	Vitamin C
____ 8. Xerophthalmia		h.	Vitamin D

B. Match each vitamin in the left-hand column with its generic name in the right-hand column.

____ 1. A		a.	α-tocopherol
____ 2. B_1		b.	Ascorbic acid
____ 3. B_2		c.	Cyanocobalamin
____ 4. B_6		d.	Dihydrotachysterol
____ 5. B_{12}		e.	Pyridoxine
____ 6. C		f.	Retinol
____ 7. D		g.	Riboflavin
____ 8. E_1		h.	Thiamine

C. Match each dietary supplement in the left-hand column with the nutrient(s) it supplies in the right-hand column.

____ 1. Cod liver oil		a.	Calcium
____ 2. Dolomite		b.	Calcitriol (vitamin D)
____ 3. Kelp		c.	Fluoride
____ 4. Powdered oyster shell		d.	Iodine
		e.	Retinol (vitamin A)

Correct the False Statement

Indicate whether the following statements are true or false; if false, correct the underlined words or phrases.

____ 1. In humans, the conversion of its precursor 7-dehydrocholesterol to vitamin D requires <u>intrinsic factor</u>.

____ 2. The margin of safety of water-soluble vitamins is <u>much wider than</u> that for fat-soluble vitamins.

215

_____ 3. The cost of vitamin supplements is usually considerably higher than the cost of foods providing these nutrients.

_____ 4. To minimize vitamin loss, mineral oil should be taken with food.

_____ 5. The mineral deficiency thought to be most prevalent in the United States at present is calcium deficiency.

_____ 6. The mineral magnesium is useful in the treatment of arrhythmias resulting from hypercalcemia or digitalis toxicity.

_____ 7. A mineral used in the treatment of convulsions caused by eclampsia of pregnancy is calcium.

_____ 8. High concentrations of sodium in the intravascular fluid cause smooth muscle contraction and vasospasm.

_____ 9. Calcium deficiency in children causes osteomalacia.

_____ 10. Hard water provides more nutrients than does soft water.

Short Answer Questions

1. Define the following terms:
   a. Vitamin:

   b. Nutritional minerals:

   c. Minimum daily requirement (MDR):

   d. Recommended daily allowance:

2. Identify and define the two strengths of vitamin preparations marketed in the United States.
   a.

   b.

3. Is iron usually administered with food?

Multiple Choice Questions

For each of the following, choose the one best answer.
1. Natural vitamins differ from synthetic vitamins in
   a. Their molecular structures
   b. Their metabolic effects
   c. Their purity
   d. No way; they are identical
2. The nutritional deficiency most apt to affect corn-eating populations is
   a. Kwashiorkor
   b. Pellagra
   c. Pernicious anemia
   d. Scurvy
3. A chronic lack of vitamin C is likely to cause the deficiency disease
   a. Beriberi
   b. Kwashiorkor
   c. Pellagra
   d. Pernicious anemia
   e. Scurvy

4. How much vitamin C does Linus Pauling recommend daily for routine maintenance?
   a. 50 mg to 75 mg
   b. 100 mg to 300 mg
   c. 250 mg to 500 mg
   d. 1 g to 4 g
5. A drug helpful in the treatment of acne is derived from vitamin
   a. A
   b. B_2
   c. B_{12}
   d. C
   e. D
6. A nutrient administered as a drug to reduce blood lipids is
   a. Vitamin A
   b. Niacin
   c. Thiamine
   d. Vitamin C
   e. Vitamin D
7. The vitamin that is converted by the body to the hormone calcitriol is
   a. Vitamin A
   b. Niacin
   c. Riboflavin
   d. Thiamine
   e. Vitamin C
   f. Vitamin D
8. A vitamin useful as an antidote in warfarin toxicity is vitamin
   a. A
   b. B_1
   c. B_{12}
   d. D
   e. E
   f. K
9. A vitamin that acts as an antioxidant is vitamin
   a. A
   b. B_{12}
   c. C
   d. D
   e. E
   f. K
10. Absorption of fat-soluble vitamins is reduced by oral ingestion of
    a. Animal fats
    b. Mineral oil
    c. Starches
    d. Vegetable oils
11. Another name for the extrinsic factor required to prevent pernicious anemia is
    a. α-tocopherol
    b. Calcitriol
    c. Cyanocobalamin
    d. Thiamine
12. β-carotene is a precursor that can be converted by the body to vitamin
    a. A
    b. B_{12}
    c. C
    d. D
    e. K
13. The body can convert 7-dehydrocholesterol to vitamin
    a. A
    b. B_1
    c. B_{12}
    d. C
    e. D
    f. K
14. In the United States, the most frequent vitamin toxicity is hypervitaminosis
    a. A
    b. B complex
    c. C
    d. D
    e. E
    f. K
15. It is important that persons taking digitalis medication avoid high doses of vitamin
    a. A
    b. B complex
    c. C
    d. D
    e. E
16. Persons with liver disease may become more seriously ill if they receive treatment with certain forms of vitamin
    a. A
    b. B complex
    c. C
    d. D
    e. K
17. Vasodilation, flushing, and abdominal cramps are caused by taking large doses of
    a. Ascorbic acid
    b. α-tocopherol
    c. Calcitriol
    d. Niacin
    e. Riboflavin
18. Physical dependence can develop in persons taking large doses of vitamin
    a. A
    b. B complex
    c. C
    d. D
    e. E
    f. K
19. Growth in children may be stunted by high doses of vitamin
    a. A
    b. B complex
    c. C
    d. D
    e. E
21. People who have gastric disease or who have had gastric surgery are at increased risk for deficiency of vitamin
    a. A
    b. B_1
    c. B_2
    d. B_{12}
    e. C
    f. D
    g. K
21. Intestinal bacteria increase the supply of vitamin
    a. A
    b. B complex
    c. C
    d. D
    e. E
    f. K
22. Persons receiving L-dopa medication should
    a. Reduce dietary intake of pyridoxine
    b. Maintain a steady dietary intake of pyridoxine
    c. Decrease dietary intake of vitamin K
    d. Maintain a steady dietary intake of vitamin K
23. A regimen of gradually decreasing dosages (weaning) is desirable when persons are planning to discontinue large doses of vitamin
    a. A
    b. B complex
    c. C
    d. D
    e. E
    f. K

24. A mineral used in the treatment of psychiatric illness is
    a. Chromium   c. Magnesium
    b. Lithium   d. Iodine
25. The tissue or organ most involved in the storage of metallic elements is
    a. Bone   c. The liver
    b. Fat   d. The thyroid gland
26. The thyroid gland traps and stores the mineral
    a. Calcium   c. Magnesium
    b. Iodine   d. Sodium
27. A mineral found to be helpful in the treatment of some decubiti is
    a. Calcium   c. Iron
    b. Iodine   d. Zinc
28. The most common mineral toxicity in the United States is excess intake of
    a. Calcium   c. Potassium
    b. Iron   d. Sodium
29. Hypercalcemia tends to cause
    a. Hypertension
    b. Prolongation of cardiac systole
    c. Weak heart contraction
    d. A widening of the QRS complex on the ECG
30. The mineral most likely to precipitate allergic reaction is
    a. Calcium   d. Potassium
    b. Iodine   e. Sodium
    c. Iron
31. Osteosclerosis and mottling of tooth enamel is likely to result from chronic toxicity of
    a. Calcium   d. Iron
    b. Fluoride   e. Magnesium
    c. Iodine
32. Hyperosmotic dehydration is likely to result from toxicity caused by the mineral
    a. Calcium   d. Lithium
    b. Fluoride   e. Potassium
    c. Iron
33. For most clients with dilutional hyponatremia, the safest way to administer sodium supplements is by giving
    a. Oral salt tablets
    b. Oral table salt
    c. Intravenous infusions of 2% sodium chloride solution
    d. Intravenous infusions of normal saline solution
    e. Subcutaneous infusions of 10% sodium chloride solution
34. Whether potassium is administered orally or parenterally, it is important that
    a. The chloride salt rather than the iodide salt be used
    b. Adequate calcium is administered with it
    c. It be well diluted by fluids
    d. The client be on a cardiac monitor
35. Sodium deficit is most likely to develop in
    a. Sedentary persons in cool, dry environments
    b. Sedentary persons in hot, humid environments
    c. Physically active persons in cool, dry environments
    d. Physically active persons in hot, humid environments
36. A factor that predisposes to sodium deficit is
    a. Hypocortism
    b. Hypothyroidism
    c. Oliguria
    d. Potassium therapy
37. A factor predisposing to hypokalemia is
    a. Hypocortism
    b. Increased stress
    c. Therapy with potassium
    d. Therapy with spironolactone
38. A mineral that tends to cause constipation is
    a. Calcium   c. Magnesium
    b. Iodine   d. Sodium
39. The metal found in high concentrations in brain lesions of some persons with Alzheimer's disease is
    a. Aluminum   c. Iron
    b. Calcium   d. Magnesium
40. Lithium toxicity may be ameliorated by the administration of
    a. Calcium   c. Sodium
    b. Iron   d. Zinc
41. A mineral known to be teratogenic is
    a. Calcium   c. Lithium
    b. Iron   d. Magnesium
42. The best way to supplement dietary intake of iodine is to
    a. Take a drop of tincture of iodine diluted in water daily
    b. Supplement the diet with dolomite
    c. Increase intake of soybeans and cabbage
    d. Use iodized table salt
43. Are vitamin and mineral supplements controlled by the Food and Drug Administration?
    a. No
    b. Vitamins are, but minerals are not
    c. Minerals are, but vitamins are not
    d. Yes

Selection of Options

For each of the following, select *all* appropriate responses. Circle correct answers.

1. Vitamins that require fat and bile salts for absorption in the small intestine include vitamin(s)
   a. A
   b. B complex
   c. C
   d. D
   e. E
   f. K

2. The liver serves as a tissue storage depot for vitamin(s)
   a. A
   b. B complex
   c. C
   d. D

3. Which vitamins are teratogenic?
   a. A
   b. B complex
   c. C
   d. D
   e. E

4. Signs and symptoms of excesses of vitamins A and D include
   a. Fatigue and lethargy
   b. Abnormal bone changes
   c. Bone tenderness
   d. Headache
   e. Constipation
   f. Oliguria
   g. Soft tissue calcification

5. Intrinsic factor greatly enhances intestinal absorption of vitamin(s)
   a. A
   b. B_1
   c. B_2
   d. B_{12}
   e. C
   f. D
   g. K

6. Ingredients often used in multivitamin preparations include
   a. Citrus pulp
   b. Fish liver oils
   c. Meat extracts
   d. Vegetable oils
   e. Yeast

7. Vitamin C breakdown in food can be minimized by
   a. Pasteurization
   b. Refrigeration
   c. Reduction in pH
   d. Use of copper storage containers

8. During pregnancy, serious adverse reactions can be caused by taking megavitamin doses of vitamin(s)
   a. A
   b. B_1
   c. B_2
   d. B_{12}
   e. C
   f. K

9. Mineral elements involved in the proper physiologic function of nerves and muscles include
   a. Aluminum
   b. Calcium
   c. Magnesium
   d. Potassium
   e. Sodium

10. Substances that play important roles in the tissue distribution of calcium include
    a. Ascorbic acid
    b. Calcitonin
    c. Calcitriol
    d. Parathormone
    e. Thyroxine

11. Clients with renal failure are likely to develop high serum concentrations of
    a. Calcium
    b. Iodine
    c. Magnesium
    d. Potassium
    e. Sodium

12. Goiter (thyroid gland enlargement) is apt to develop as a result of
    a. Calcium deficiency
    b. Calcium toxicity
    c. Iodine deficiency
    d. Iodine toxicity
    e. Iron deficiency
    f. Iron toxicity

13. Substances useful in the correction of calcium deficits include
    a. Amphojel antacid
    b. Dolomite
    c. Kelp
    d. Milk
    e. Tums antacid

14. Foods rich in potassium include
    a. Bananas
    b. Cabbage
    c. Green leafy vegetables
    d. Meat
    e. Orange juice

15. To add helpful minerals to the diet, the nurse may recommend the use of cooking pots made of
    a. Aluminum
    b. Enameled steel
    c. Glass
    d. Iron
    e. Stainless steel

16. To prevent the migration of undesirable metals into food, the nurse may recommend the use of cooking utensils made of
    a. Aluminum
    b. Enameled steel
    c. Glass
    d. Iron
    e. Stainless steel

17. General measures used in the treatment of metal toxicity include
    a. Fever therapy to promote diaphoresis
    b. Administration of ion exchange resins
    c. Administration of chelating agents
    d. Diuretic therapy

18. Fruits that are good sources of potassium include
    a. Apples
    b. Bananas
    c. Cranberries
    d. Oranges

PART 2: HEMATINICS

Short Answer Questions

1. Define the term hematinic, citing two specific actions performed by hematinics.

2. Explain the roles of ferritin and transferrin.

3. Identify at least six types of individuals who would most likely have an increased need for iron.

4. List four common foods with iron content greater than 1 mg/100 g.

5. When should ferrous sulfate be administered for optimal absorption?

6. What evaluation criterion can be used to determine if the objective for the use of an iron preparation is being met?

7. What are three disadvantages of iron combination preparations?

8. Identify three instances when parenteral iron might be used instead of oral iron.

9. Which hematinic requires the presence of intrinsic factor for absorption, and where is intrinsic factor produced?

10. What is the outcome of multisystem deprivation of vitamin B_{12}?

11. List at least six situations or conditions that may result in folic acid deficiency.

12. What symptoms might a person complain of who has a decrease in available oxygen from some type of anemia? List at least eight symptoms.

Matching

Match the hematinic in the left-hand column with the human body's daily requirement for it in the right-hand column. Place your answer in the space provided.

_____ 1. Iron
_____ 2. Vitamin B$_{12}$
_____ 3. Folic acid

a. 300 IU
b. 400 mcg/d
c. 3 mcg/d
d. 10 mg (male adult)

PART 3: FEEDING FORMULAS

Correct the False Statement

Indicate whether the following statements are true or false; if false, correct the underlined words or phrases.

_____ 1. When formula feedings are ordered, the first feedings should be full strength to promote rapid correction of malnutrition.

_____ 2. Nutritional deficiencies in hospitalized persons are relatively rare because these people are under close medical supervision.

_____ 3. When preparing infant formulas, it is most important that mothers use sterile aseptic technique.

_____ 4. Physicians' prescriptions are required for the purchase of some feeding formulas.

Multiple Choice Questions

For each of the following, choose the one best answer.

1. A problem that arises frequently in clients receiving supplementary nutritional beverages is
   a. Water intoxication caused by high fluid intake
   b. Taste fatigue
   c. Glucose intolerance caused by the high carbohydrate content of these beverages
   d. Vitamin and mineral deficiencies

2. The infant feeding formula least likely to cause allergic reaction is
   a. Cow's milk formula
   b. Hydrolyzed milk formula
   c. Soybean formula
   d. Formulas low in phenylalanine

3. An adverse reaction to some feeding formulas is
   a. Dehydration
   b. An excess of fiber
   c. Hypoglycemia
   d. Water intoxication

4. In hospital settings, unused formula from opened containers may be refrigerated and reused if stored for no longer than
   a. 4 hours
   b. 12 hours
   c. 24 hours
   d. None of the above; unused formula should not be saved for reuse but should be discarded

Selection of Options

For each of the following, select *all* appropriate responses. Circle correct answers.

1. Preparations suitable for use as infant feeding formulas include
   a. Enfamil
   b. Nutramigen
   c. Condensed milk
   d. Lofenalac

2. Feeding formulas most likely to have an unpleasant odor include
   a. Enfamil
   b. Isomil
   c. Nutramigen
   d. Lofenalac

Crossword Puzzle

ACROSS

6. A hydrolyzed infant feeding formula that is low in phenylalanine
7. A powder used to make low-residue feeding formulas
8. A powder used for making foods for persons with liver disease
10. An infant feeding formula made from cows' milk
16. A life-threatening complication that can develop in persons receiving concentrated feeding formulas
17. A vegetable used as an ingredient in infant feeding formulas
18. A nutritional supplement for persons who can ingest liquids

DOWN

1. An inborn error of metabolism causing intolerance of an essential amino acid
2. A process used to reduce the allergenicity of milk formulas
3. A hydrolyzed feeding formula used for infants with multiple allergies
4. An amino acid that can cause mental retardation in children with a congenital deficiency of enzymes necessary for its complete metabolism
5. A tube feeding formula that is hypertonic
9. A liquid nutritional supplement used as a beverage
11. An infant feeding formula made from soybeans
12. A powder used to prepare feeding formulas that produce minimal pancreatic stimulus
13. An isotonic formula for tube feedings
14. A powder used to prepare a beverage for dietary supplementation that is available in most grocery stores
15. A feeding formula used for persons in renal failure

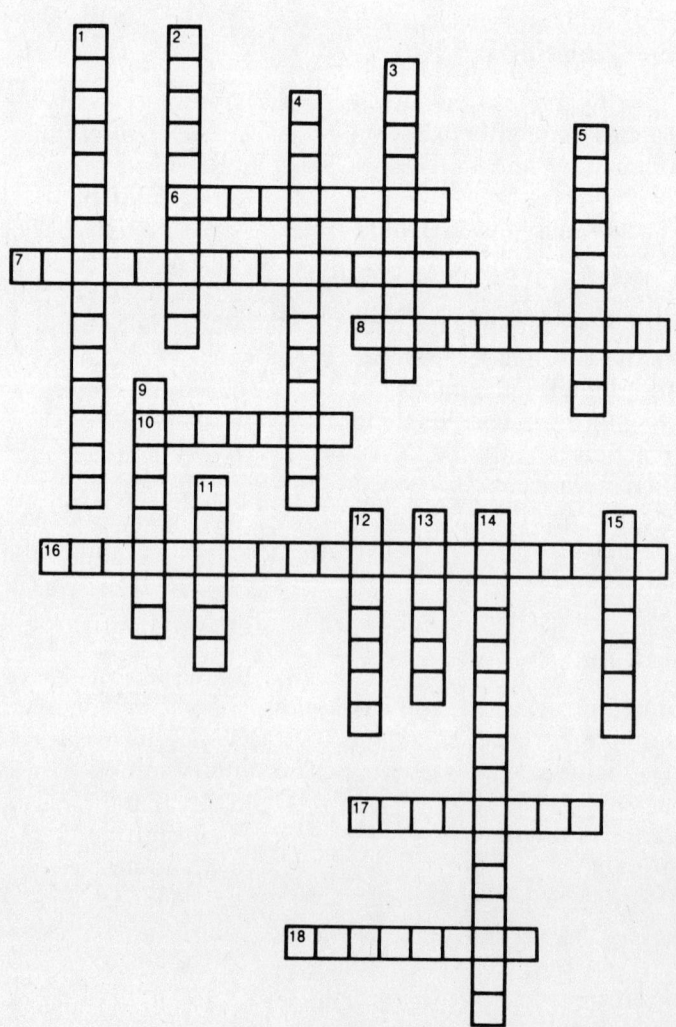

PART 4. HEALTH FOOD PRODUCTS

Correct the False Statement

Indicate whether the following statements are true or false; if false, correct the underlined words or phrases.

_____ 1. The labels on health food products <u>must adhere</u> to the standards set for over-the-counter drugs.

_____ 2. The labels on health food products <u>usually recommend</u> safe dosages.

_____ 3. Information on health food supplements is readily available from the <u>medical literature</u>.

_____ 4. Health food publications <u>are allowed</u> to accept advertisements of nutritional supplements produced by health food business.

_____ 5. Health food products <u>do not</u> exert drug efforts.

_____ 6. Linoleic acid is considered to be <u>an essential fatty acid</u>.

_____ 7. When nurses are not expert in the area of health food products, they should advise clients to <u>avoid use of all proprietary health food products</u>.

Multiple Choice Questions

For each of the following, choose the one best answer.

1. L-tryptophan is recommended by some physicians for use as a
   a. Central nervous system stimulant
   b. Hypnotic
   c. Membrane stabilizer
   d. Metabolic coenzyme
2. According to the text, recommended dosages of L-tryptophan can cause
   a. Coma   c. Mania
   b. Weight loss   d. Depression
3. To what chemical family does linoleic acid belong?
   a. Vitamin
   b. Amino acid
   c. Fatty acid
   d. Phospholipid
4. To what chemical family does lecithin belong?
   a. Amino acid
   b. Mineral
   c. Fatty acid
   d. Phospholipid
5. Kelp is a rich source of
   a. Iodine
   b. Chlorine
   c. Magnesium
   d. Calcium
6. Lecithin is most likely to prove useful as a drug for
   a. Reducing blood cholesterol level
   b. Improving the HDL/LDL ratio
   c. Aiding in weight reduction
   d. Lowering blood pressure
7. Components of garlic are under investigation for use as
   a. Anticholesterolemic agents
   b. Anti-infectives
   c. Mineral supplements
   d. Antihypertensives
8. The main ingredient in vinegar is
   a. Alcohol
   b. Ascorbic acid
   c. Citric acid
   d. Acetic acid

Selection of Options

For each of the following, select *all* appropriate responses.

1. Health food publications most often support their recommendations with
   a. Testimonials
   b. Preliminary reports from the medical literature
   c. Definitive reports from the medical literature
   d. Case histories

44
Parenteral Preparations

Parenteral nutritional supplements include clear solutions containing glucose and electrolytes, parenteral nutritional solutions containing glucose, amino acids, and fats, as well as vitamins and minerals, blood, and blood products. The following exercises relate to these treatment agents.

Matching

Match each characteristic of parenteral fluids in the left-hand column with all appropriate physiologic effects in the right-hand column.

_____ 1. Hypotonic
_____ 2. Isotonic
_____ 3. Hypertonic

a. Crenation of red blood cells
b. Lysis of red blood cells
c. Osmotic diuresis
d. Water diuresis
e. Oliguria
f. Hypervolemia with minimal disturbance of other fluid compartments

Correct the False Statement

Indicate whether the following statements are true or false; if false, correct the underlined words or phrases.

_____ 1. Clear parenteral solutions provide all nutrients required by the body.

_____ 2. Plastic tubing used for administration of intravenous lipid solutions should be free of polymers.

_____ 3. Parenteral hyperalimentation is always administered in acute care situations.

_____ 4. Tubing to be used for transfusion may be primed with dextrose solution.

Short Answer Questions

1. Name the drug administered by hypodermoclysis to facilitate absorption of clear fluids infused subcutaneously or intramuscularly.

2. What effects do dextran solutions have on coagulation?

3. Which of the substances used for parenteral hyperalimentation may be administered in a peripheral intravenous line separate from the central venous line used for the other nutrients?

4. What type of tubing is required for administration of parenteral hyperalimentation mixtures?

5. If air enters a central venous line, what should be done?

6. How long can blood be stored before being used in transfusions?

7. What is the name of the laboratory test used to determine compatibility of blood for transfusion?

8. How is whole blood stored?

9. Optimum ages for blood donation are considered to be _____ to _____.

Multiple Choice Questions

For each of the following, choose the one best answer.

1. Parenteral solutions are most rapidly absorbed and distributed when administered
   a. By hypodermoclysis
   b. Intramuscularly
   c. Intravenously
   d. Subcutaneously

2. An electrolyte likely to cause prolonged diastole, weak heart action, and cardiac arrhythmia when infused rapidly by the parenteral route is
   a. Sodium
   b. Potassium
   c. Calcium
   d. Bicarbonate

3. Maximum parenteral dosage of potassium for normal adults is
   a. 20 mEq/hour
   b. 40 mEq/hour
   c. 80 mEq/hour
   d. 100 mEq/hour

4. Parenteral hyperalimentation solutions containing multiple ingredients are usually
   a. Isotonic
   b. Slightly hypotonic
   c. Markedly hypotonic
   d. Slightly hypertonic
   e. Markedly hypertonic

5. Lipid emulsions may be administered parenterally through
   a. Filtered lines inserted into a peripheral vein
   b. Filtered lines inserted into the central vena cava
   c. Nonfiltered lines inserted into a peripheral vein
   d. Clysis tubing

6. When parenteral hyperalimentation therapy is begun, the recipient is likely to develop a transient
   a. High concentration of trace minerals
   b. Hypoglycemia
   c. Hyperglycemia
   d. Hyperphosphatemia

7. A serious adverse reaction to parenteral hyperalimentation is
   a. Glucose deficiency
   b. Infection
   c. Lysis of red blood cells
   d. Metabolic acidosis

8. The hormone administered to recipients of parenteral hyperalimentation solutions to control an adverse reaction is
   a. Insulin
   b. Glucagon
   c. Prednisone
   d. Thyroxine

9. The rate of parenteral fluid administration can be controlled most strictly by use of
   a. Hand-operated valves
   b. Alarm monitors
   c. Volume-controlled pumps

10. Clients with fluid volume deficit who respond poorly to intravenous therapy are likely to have the hormone imbalance
    a. Hypothyroidism
    b. Hypocortism
    c. Hypoinsulinism
    d. Antidiuretic hormone deficiency

11. When a central venous line is to be established, the client is placed in
    a. Fowler's position
    b. Supine position
    c. Trendelenburg position
    d. Reverse Trendelenburg position

12. Because optimum parenteral dosages for these nutrients have not yet been established, the nurse should monitor recipients for parenteral hyperalimentation closely for imbalances of
    a. Glucose
    b. Minerals
    c. Proteins
    d. Vitamins

13. A parenteral solution that must be administered through a central venous line is
    a. Hyperalimentation mixture
    b. Dextrose in water
    c. Intralipid
    d. Blood
14. At what time are infusions of fat emulsions usually begun?
    a. After early morning blood specimens for laboratory tests have been collected
    b. After the morning hygienic routine
    c. After the midday rest
    d. At bedtime
15. The parenteral fluid that contains all constituents necessary for circulatory homeostasis is
    a. Blood
    b. 5% dextrose in water
    c. Plasma
    d. Ringer's solution
16. Blood is most likely to produce the electrolyte imbalance
    a. Hypercalcemia
    b. Hyperkalemia
    c. Hyponatremia
    d. Hypoglycemia
17. Administration of multiple units of banked blood is likely to cause
    a. Hypocalcemic tetany
    b. Hypokalemic paralytic ileus
    c. Hyponatremic dehydration
    d. Iron deficiency anemia
18. The "universal recipient" is someone with blood type
    a. A
    b. B
    c. AB
    d. O
19. Incompatibility reactions are least likely to occur when the blood to be administered is
    a. Type AB, Rh+
    b. Type AB, Rh−
    c. Type O, Rh+
    d. Type O, Rh−
    e. The same ABO and Rh type as the recipient's blood
20. Someone whose religious beliefs proscribe the use of blood transfusions would be a
    a. Jehovah's Witness
    b. Hindu
    c. Mormon
    d. Seventh Day Adventist

Selection of Options

For each of the following, select *all* appropriate responses. Circle correct answers.

1. The physiologic effects of hypertonic solutions administered intravenously include
   a. Fluid shifts from the extracellular fluid compartment to the intravascular compartment
   b. A tendency toward cellular dehydration
   c. A decrease in urinary output
   d. A tendency to crenate red blood cells
2. Clear parenteral solutions are administered
   a. Subcutaneously
   b. Intramuscularly
   c. Intravenously
   d. By hypodermoclysis
   e. Intra-arterially
3. Movement of fluids through the extracellular space is inhibited by the presence of
   a. Numerous blood vessels
   b. Hyaluronic acid
   c. Intravascular hypertension
   d. Hypotensive shock
4. Rapid infusion of parenteral fluids tends to produce
   a. Circulatory overload
   b. Left ventricular failure
   c. Hypervolemia
   d. Pulmonary edema
5. Rapid infusion of clear solutions by hyperdemoclysis tends to produce
   a. Local tissue swelling
   b. Hypertension in the extracellular fluid compartments
   c. Improved local perfusion
6. Adequate hydration and renal function should be established before the following parenteral nutrients are administered:
   a. Dextrans
   b. 5% dextrose in water
   c. Normal saline solutions
   d. Potassium solutions
7. Plasma extenders include
   a. Dextrans
   b. 5% dextrose in water
   c. Hetastarch
   d. Normal saline solution

8. Nutrients administered as solutions for total parenteral hyperalimentation include
   a. Sugar
   b. Starches
   c. Amino acids
   d. Proteins
   e. Lipids
   f. Vitamins
   g. Minerals
9. Intravenous medications may be administered to clients receiving hyperalimentation solutions through the
   a. Central venous line while the hyperalimentation solution is infusing
   b. Central venous line, provided the hyperalimentation solution is not infusing at the time
   c. Peripheral line while the lipid solution is infusing
   d. Peripheral line, provided the lipid solution is not infusing at the time
10. Fat emulsions normally appear
    a. Clear
    b. Cloudy
    c. Homogeneous
    d. Layered
    e. Colored
11. Adverse effects of blood transfusions include
    a. Hyperkalemia
    b. Allergic reactions
    c. Incompatibility reactions
    d. Bloodborne infections
12. Signs and symptoms of transfusion reaction include
    a. Anxiety
    b. Back pain
    c. Bradycardia
    d. Chills and fever

UNIT THIRTEEN: MISCELLANEOUS DRUG FAMILIES

45 Diagnostic Agents

Pharmacologic agents are frequently used to carry out diagnostic procedures. Because of side effects and toxic effects, they must be conducted as carefully as any therapeutic measure to ensure that reliable diagnostic data will be obtained with the least risk to the client.

Multiple Choice Questions

For each of the following, choose the one best answer.

1. A substance administered orally and rectally to facilitate radiographic examination of the gastrointestinal tract is barium
    a. Sulfate
    b. Sulfite
    c. Sulfide
    d. Chloride
2. Screens that shield body parts from x-radiation are uncomfortable because they
    a. Feel cold to the touch
    b. Feel heavy
    c. Must be applied snugly
    d. All of the above
3. The most common side effect of barium used for radiograms is
    a. Diarrhea
    b. Constipation
    c. Nausea and vomiting
    d. Inflammation of the gastrointestinal tract
4. A contraindication for the use of barium sulfate is
    a. Abdominal pain
    b. Intestinal fistulas
    c. Peptic ulcer disease
    d. Ulcerative colitis
5. Preparation of a client for gastrointestinal x-rays using barium sulfate is likely to include administration of a(n)
    a. Laxative
    b. Sedative
    c. Analgesic
    d. Antiemetic
6. Protocols for aftercare of clients undergoing diagnostic x-rays employing barium sulfate are likely to call for administering to the client
    a. An analgesic
    b. Intravenous fluids
    c. An antidiarrheal
    d. A laxative
7. Following an upper gastrointestinal series (diagnostic x-rays using barium), clients should be monitored for
    a. Cardiac arrhythmias
    b. Allergic reaction
    c. Constipation
    d. Blood in the stool
8. Clients at high risk for complication from gastrointestinal x-ray studies are those with a history of
    a. A tendency toward diarrhea
    b. A tendency toward constipation
    c. Hypotension and frequent fainting
    d. Peptic ulcer disease
9. A serious adverse reaction to iodinated contrast media is
    a. Subclinical pulmonary embolism
    b. Inflammation of the urinary tract
    c. Anaphylaxis
    d. Intestinal obstruction
10. Iodine compounds with radiopaque properties are *not* administered to clients
    a. With hyperthyroidism
    b. Undergoing computed tomography procedures
    c. With gastrointestinal upsets
    d. With allergic hypersensitivity to iodine
11. When oral iodinated contrast media are administered in preparation for a gallbladder series, they are most likely to be given
    a. Immediately before the x-rays are taken
    b. 30 to 60 minutes before the x-rays are taken

c. Several hours before the x-rays are taken
d. Several days before the x-rays are taken

12. Following an adverse reaction to iodinated contrast media, clients should be advised to
    a. Apply iodine to the skin regularly at least once a week to minimize allergic sensitivity
    b. Avoid exposure to all halogens
    c. Avoid all radiographic diagnostic tests
    d. Wear a medical identification device

13. The most common adverse reaction(s) to radiopaque iodine are
    a. Allergic reactions
    b. Nausea, vomiting, and flushing
    c. Hypotension
    d. Persistent impairment of thyroid function

14. A nursing measure that reduces the risk of adverse reaction to barium or radiopaque iodine compounds in clients undergoing radiograms is
    a. Administration of an antihistamine prior to the test
    b. Ensuring adequate hydration prior to the test
    c. Ensuring adequate nutrition prior to the test
    d. Draping the client with a lead apron to reduce exposure of the target area to ionizing radiation

15. Most nonradioactive compounds used for volumetric diagnostic studies are administered
    a. Orally
    b. Subcutaneously
    c. Intramuscularly
    d. Intravenously

16. Clients receiving indigotindisulfonate for diagnostic testing should be reassured that
    a. The red discoloration of the stools is not harmful, and will disappear within a few days
    b. The blue discoloration of the skin is not harmful, and will subside gradually
    c. The red discoloration of the urine is not harmful, and will disappear within a few hours
    d. Green-colored stools may occur for a few days following the test, but are not harmful

17. The client at highest risk for adverse reaction to polysaccharides and dyes for volumetric testing is the person with a history of
    a. Allergic sensitivity to iodine
    b. Atopic asthma
    c. Frequent exposure to ionizing radiation
    d. Adverse reaction to barium sulfate

18. Clients who have received polysaccharides or aminohippurate for assessment of kidney function should be monitored for
    a. Hypotension
    b. Increased venous pressure
    c. Fever
    d. Hematuria

19. Dosage of radionuclides is measured in
    a. Units
    b. Micrograms or milligrams
    c. Rads
    d. Curies

20. Radioactive emissions by radionuclides cause a decline in potency of the drug. This process can be controlled by
    a. Storing the drugs in lead-lined containers
    b. Storing the drugs in opaque containers
    c. Freezing the drugs
    d. None of the above; at present, the rate of disintegration cannot be controlled by any method

21. As radioactive drugs age, the volume required for a given dose
    a. Increases
    b. Decreases
    c. Stays the same

22. Following diagnostic tests using radionuclides, what precautions are necessary to limit exposure of vulnerable persons to ionizing radiation?
    a. Urine must be diluted and dispersed by disposing it in a central sewage system
    b. Feces must be diluted and dispersed by disposing them in a central sewage system
    c. Recipients must be isolated from vulnerable persons for about 1 week
    d. All of the above
    e. None of the above

23. A physiologic antagonist of edrophonium is
    a. Atropine
    b. Muscarine
    c. Propranolol
    d. Neostigmine

24. All radionuclides should be stored in

a. Opaque containers
   b. A refrigerator
   c. A freezer
   d. Lead-lined containers
25. Autocoids used as provocative agents are usually stored in
   a. An opaque container
   b. A refrigerator
   c. A freezer
   d. A lead-lined container
26. The biologic half-life of provocative agents tends to be
   a. Very short
   b. Very long
   c. Strongly influenced by the emotions
   d. Prolonged by renal impairment
27. A serious adverse reaction to sincalide (used to assess gallbladder and pancreatic exocrine function) is
   a. Nausea and vomiting
   b. Hypoglycemia
   c. Obstruction of the hepatic bile duct
   d. Obstruction of the common bile duct
28. Which of the following adverse reactions is most likely to develop when histamine is given to someone with pheochromocytoma?
   a. Hypotensive shock
   b. Hypertensive crisis
   c. Infarction of the adrenal medulla
   d. Acute pancreatitis
29. Before clients are given edrophonium, they must be assessed for
   a. Atopic allergy
   b. Fluid and electrolyte imbalances
   c. Hormone imbalance
   d. Hyperglycemia
30. Antigenic materials that are *not* refrigerated are
   a. Antigenic extracts
   b. Concentrated solutions of antigens
   c. Materials for tine testing
   d. Skin patches
31. A contraindication for dermal reactivity indicators is
   a. Local redness and itching following a previous test
   b. Local tissue breakdown following a previous test
   c. Systemic allergic reaction following a previous test
   d. Failure to react to a previous test

Matching

Match each drug or drug class in the left-hand column with the diagnostic procedure(s) for which it may be used in the right-hand column. Place your answer in the space provided.

_____ 1. Barium sulfate
_____ 2. Iodinated contrast media
_____ 3. Indigotindisulfonate
_____ 4. Phenolphthalein
_____ 5. Polysaccharides
_____ 6. Aminohippurate
_____ 7. Sulfobromophthalein

a. Cardiac catheterization
b. X-ray of the colon
c. Test for early liver impairment
d. Volumetric assessment of kidney function
e. Arteriogram
f. CT scan of the brain
g. Location of ureteral orifices
h. Upper gastrointestinal series
i. Intravenous pyelogram

Correct the False Statement

Indicate whether the following statements are true or false; if false, correct the underlined words or phrases.

_____ 1. Toxic effects of x-rays arise from their ability to generate heat in the tissues.

_____ 2. Clients undergoing diagnostic x-rays with modern equipment are exposed to lower doses of x-rays than were clients undergoing similar studies 20 years ago.

_____ 3. A record of diagnostic x-rays and other exposure to ionizing radiation should be included as a part of an individual health history.

_____ 4. Before diagnostic gastrointestinal x-rays are to be made, clients should eat normal meals so that the barium will be diluted by the normal intestinal contents.

_____ 5. To prevent or ameliorate adverse reactions to barium, the nurse may usually recommend use of an antidiarrheal preparation following completion of the x-rays.

_____ 6. Before iodinated contrast media are administered, clients should be tested for sensitivity to these agents.

_____ 7. Following an x-ray study employing iodinated contrast media, clients should be monitored for blood pressure fluctuations.

_____ 8. Radionuclides are distributed and metabolized by the body in the same way as are similar chemicals that are nonradioactive.

_____ 9. Following use of a radionuclide, radioactivity in body tissues will decline at a slower rate than the rate of elimination of the radionuclide.

_____ 10. Adverse reactions to radioactive tracers that are likely to occur in a large number of clients include only a slight increment in lifelong exposure to ionizing radiation.

_____ 11. Allergic reactions to radionuclides are more likely to occur when the radionuclides contain iodine than when they contain other elements.

_____ 12. Workers in diagnostic centers in which radionuclides are used should wear radiation exposure detection devices.

_____ 13. Provocative agents are usually administered orally.

_____ 14. Dosages for autocoids used as provocative agents are usually quite large.

_____ 15. Because secretogogues are very selective agents, they tend to produce few side effects.

_____ 16. A serious adverse reaction common to most provocative agents is damage to rapidly growing tissue.

_____ 17. Before provocative agents are administered, a skin test for allergic sensitivity is likely to be ordered.

_____ 18. Serious reactions to provocative diagnostic tests occur frequently.

_____ 19. The time required for a reaction to dermal reactivity indicators to develop ranges from seconds to hours.

_____ 20. A positive reaction to microbial extracts used as dermal sensitivity indicators means that active infection is present.

Selection of Options

For each of the following, indicate *all* appropriate responses. Circle correct answers.

1. Precautions that should be taken when diagnostic x-rays are to be taken include
   a. Using modern equipment that is kept in good repair
   b. Filtering the x-rays by placing a thin lead apron over the area to be exposed
   c. Focusing the x-ray beam on as narrow a target area as possible
   d. Protecting radiosensitive body areas, such as the gonads, by screening them with x-ray shields

2. Contrast media used in x-ray studies often contain the elements
   a. Barium   b. Cobalt

    c. Iodine   d. Phosphorus
    e. Uranium
3. Radiopaque chemicals are administered to clients undergoing diagnostic x-rays because
    a. These chemicals make pathologic changes in bone more visible
    b. These chemicals make abnormalities in certain soft tissues more visible
    c. The presence of these chemicals in body fluids elucidates kinetic function of certain body organs
4. When x-ray study of the gastrointestinal system is undertaken, the barium can
    a. Outline the lumen of hollow structures
    b. Demonstrate kinetic movement of intestinal contents
    c. Outline the biliary ducts and gallbladder
5. Routes of administration for barium sulfate include
    a. Oral   c. Intravenous
    b. Rectal   d. Soft tissue injection
6. Clients who have taken barium sulfate for diagnostic x-rays should be told
    a. That the appearance of clay-colored stools indicates that the barium is being eliminated
    b. To avoid active exercise until after the barium has been eliminated
    c. To take measures to minimize constipation caused by the barium
7. Diagnostic uses for iodinated contrast media include
    a. Bone scans
    b. Cardiac catheterization in which moving pictures are taken
    c. X-ray study of the gallbladder
    d. Pyelograms and x-ray study of the kidney, ureters, and bladder
    e. Computed tomography (CT scans)
8. Factors that increase the risk of adverse reaction to iodinated contrast media include
    a. Poor hydration
    b. Congestive heart failure
    c. Pheochromocytoma
    d. Recent exposure to iodine-containing media
    e. Diabetic nephropathy
9. Common adverse reactions to iodinated contrast media include
    a. Nausea and vomiting
    b. Flushing and feeling of warmth
    c. Stroke
    d. Skin rash
    e. Changes in blood pressure
10. Radionuclides used for diagnostic studies commonly emit
    a. α-radiation
    b. β-radiation
    c. γ-radiation
11. Tests using radioactive tracers are avoided whenever possible for
    a. Cancer patients
    b. Growing children
    c. Women during the first week of their menstrual cycle
    d. Pregnant women
    e. Lactating women
12. Adverse reactions to accumulated exposure to low-level ionizing radiation include
    a. Tissue destruction similar to that seen in burns
    b. Increased risk of neoplastic disease, including cancer
    c. Accelerated aging of body tissues
    d. Increased risk of birth defects in progeny
    e. Infertility
13. Volumetric testing of kidney function is contraindicated for persons with
    a. Mild to moderate renal impairment
    b. Severe renal impairment
    c. Mild to moderate hepatic impairment
    d. Dehydration
14. Polysaccharides and aminohippurate are contraindicated for persons with
    a. Dehydration
    b. Pulmonary edema
    c. Hematuria
    d. Intracranial bleeding
    e. Limited cardiac reserve
15. Factors that directly influence the decline from peak concentration of residual radioactivity present in body tissues as a result of the use of radioactive tracers include
    a. Gastrointestinal absorption of the radionuclide
    b. Metabolism of the substance by the liver
    c. Elimination of the substance by excretion
    d. Number of radioactive half-lives that have elapsed
16. When radionuclides are used for diagnostic procedures, special precautions to limit exposure to ionizing radiation should be taken by

a. The client
b. The health-care staff
c. Any visitors for the client
17. Secretogogues are employed to measure production of secretions such as
    a. Bile
    b. Gastric acid
    c. Pepsin
    d. Pancreatic enzymes
18. When diagnostic tests are undertaken, the following considerations are critical for the reliability of test results:
    a. Preparation of the client
    b. Accuracy of drug dosage
    c. Timing of drug dosage
    d. Availability of antidotes
    e. Aftercare of the client
19. Dermal reactivity indicators are administered
    a. Topically to the skin
    b. Intradermally
    c. Subcutaneously
20. A negative reaction to a microbial extract used as a dermal reactivity indicator may mean that the client has
    a. Never been exposed to the pathogen
    b. Had regular, frequent exposure to the pathogen
    c. An active infection caused by the pathogen
    d. An overwhelming infection caused by the pathogen
21. Common reactions to dermal reactivity indicators include
    a. Local redness
    b. Local swelling
    c. Ulceration at the test site
    d. Necrosis of local tissue
    e. Anaphylaxis
22. Dermal reactivity indicators are used diagnostically to detect
    a. Active infectious disease
    b. Antibodies to specific allergic antigens
    c. Antibodies to infectious microorganisms

Short Answer Questions

1. What is the generally accepted safe level of exposure to ionizing radiation?

2. List at least five adverse reactions to agents used for volumetric testing.

3. Name two side effects of polysaccharides used to assess kidney function.

4. Define the following terms:
   a. radioactive:

   b. rad:

   c. rem:

   d. roentgen:

5. Identify at least two methods for measuring the relative amounts of radionuclide in body tissue.

6. How should radioactive drugs be stored?

7. Identify at least four biologic parameters that may be measured with the use of radioactive tracers.

8. List at least four parameters that should be gathered during assessment of clients scheduled for diagnostic tests using radionuclides.

9. Name three conditions that markedly increase the risk of adverse reactions to secretogogues that stimulate gastric acid secretion.

10. Identify three techniques for administering dermal reactivity indicators.

11. Why are skin tests for allergic sensitivity carried out only when emergency medical personnel or physicians are readily available?

46
Enzymes and Drugs Affecting Enzymes

Enzymes perform many functions in the body: digestion of food, metabolism of drugs, and degradation of endogenous biochemicals. As yet, the usefulness of enzyme drugs is limited because they cannot be delivered to the intracellular compartment effectively. A number have proven useful for selected purposes. The exercises that follow deal with enzymes, enzyme inhibitors, and enzyme reactivators.

Matching

Match each enzyme in the left-hand column with the substrate or substrates upon which it acts.

_____ 1. L-asparaginase
_____ 2. α-galactosidase
_____ 3. Amylase
_____ 4. Bromelain
_____ 5. Collagenase
_____ 6. Lactase
_____ 7. Papain
_____ 8. Urokinase

a. Sugar
b. Amino acid
c. Fat
d. Fibrin
e. Meat
f. Blood type B antigen
g. Insect venom
h. Pus

Correct the False Statement

Indicate whether the following statements are true or false; if false, correct the underlined words or phrases.

_____ 1. Chemically, enzymes most resemble phospholipids.

_____ 2. Enzyme systems in the body are determined primarily by environmental influences.

_____ 3. Monoamine oxidases in animals are likely to be different from those in humans.

_____ 4. Enzymes act as organic catalysts.

_____ 5. L-asparaginase is a useful antineoplastic drug because it is most toxic to actively dividing cells.

_____ 6. The drug chymopapain is measured in milligrams.

Multiple Choice Questions

For each of the following, choose the one best answer.

1. Tolerance to disulfiram
   a. Remains constant throughout therapy
   b. Tends to increase with continued therapy
   c. Tends to decrease with continued therapy
   d. Fluctuates unpredictably
2. Disulfiram is an enzyme inhibitor used to treat
   a. Insecticide poisoning
   b. Alcoholism
   c. Narcotic addiction
   d. Gout
3. The metabolism of drugs by liver microsomal enzymes is most likely to be inhibited by
   a. Drugs
   b. Enzyme inducers
   c. Protein
   d. Enzyme inhibitors
4. Lactose-intolerant individuals who eliminate milk from their diets are most likely to develop deficiency of the nutrient
   a. Calcium
   b. Essential fatty acid
   c. Vitamin A
   d. Vitamin D

5. The cause of abdominal distention and flatulence following ingestion of milk by milk-intolerant persons is
   a. Allergic reaction to lactose
   b. Inflammation of the gastrointestinal mucosa
   c. Alteration of the intestinal flora
   d. Fermentation of lactose
6. Acceleration of clysis infusions through the use of hyaluronidase is most likely to cause
   a. An acute allergic reaction
   b. Local pain and swelling
   c. A drop in blood pressure
   d. A rise in blood pressure
7. An enzyme used to decrease intraocular pressure during eye surgery is
   a. Chymopapain
   b. Hyaluronidase
   c. L-asparaginase
   d. Lactase
8. Hyaluronidase (Wydase) is used medicinally to promote
   a. Absorption of nutrients from the intestines
   b. Absorption of fluids from the intestines
   c. Absorption of fluids from subcutaneous tissues
   d. Intravenous absorption of fluids
9. Stiffness and soreness in the lumbar region following papain treatment may persist for a few
   a. Hours
   b. Days
   c. Weeks
   d. Months
10. Clients with intervertebral disk disease should avoid
    a. Walking
    b. Standing in one place
    c. Sitting
    d. Lying down
11. To detect adverse reaction, clients receiving papain should be watched for signs and symptoms of serious adverse reaction to the drug for
    a. 20 minutes
    b. 1 hour
    c. 4 hours
    d. 24 hours
12. Chymopapain treatment is carried out
    a. In the home
    b. In an outpatient clinic
    c. In a hospital medical ward
    d. In an operating room
13. The source of chymopapain is
    a. Plant tissues
    b. Animal tissues
    c. Bacterial cultures
    d. Human tissues
14. The approach most likely to reduce allergic reactions to enzyme drugs is to
    a. Desensitize the recipient before initiating treatment
    b. Use only enzymes produced from human materials
    c. Administer a glucocorticoid with each dose of enzyme drug
    d. Administer epinephrine before each dose of enzyme drug
15. How many times can papain therapy be administered to an individual?
    a. Once only
    b. Repeatedly, provided sufficient time elapses between treatments
    c. Repeatedly, provided the immune system is suppressed temporarily
    d. Repeatedly; it is not a toxic substance
16. Normal body cells can be injured by L-asparaginase because this drug
    a. Eliminates an amino acid essential to humans
    b. Blocks elimination of wastes from the cells
    c. Alters cell membranes
    d. Inhibits protein synthesis
17. Adverse reactions to enzyme drugs often take the form of
    a. Toxicity from accumulated substrates
    b. Allergic reaction to foreign proteins
    c. Reduced serum levels of therapeutic drugs taken concurrently
    d. Toxic levels of drugs taken concurrently
18. The enzyme used to treat herniated intervertebral disks is
    a. Amylase
    b. Bromelain
    c. Chymopapain
    d. Pepsin
19. Enzymes used as replacement therapy in cystic fibrosis are administered
    a. Orally
    b. Subcutaneously
    c. Intramuscularly
    d. Intravenously
    e. Intrathecally
20. At present, enzymes are available for therapeutic use in replacement of deficient enzymes in the
    a. Central nervous system

    b. Gastrointestinal tract
    c. Liver
    d. Immune system
21. Enzyme drugs manufactured from bacterial growths include
    a. Papain
    b. Amylase
    c. L-asparaginase
    d. Urokinase
22. Endogenous enzymes usually act
    a. In the intracellular compartment
    b. In the interstitial spaces
    c. In the blood
23. In comparison with most biochemicals, enzymes are present in the body in
    a. Much larger amounts
    b. Similar amounts
    c. Much smaller amounts
24. Hypertensive reactions to pralidoxime should be treated with
    a. Atropine
    b. Acetylcholine
    c. Cholinergic blockers
    d. Phentolamine
25. A drug that inhibits metabolic breakdown of many drugs is
    a. Chymopapain
    b. Disulfiram
    c. Lactase
    d. Pralidoxime

Selection of Options

For each of the following, select *all* appropriate responses.

1. In addition to alcoholic beverages, the alcoholic treated with disulfiram must avoid exposure to
    a. Medications in elixir form
    b. Medications in syrup form
    c. Wine vinegar
    d. Shaving lotion containing alcohol
2. Prior to surgery, candidates for enzyme treatment of herniated disk should be screened for allergy to
    a. Papayas
    b. Pawpaws
    c. Hard cheeses
    d. Epinephrine
    e. Meat tenderizer
    f. Monosodium glutamate

Short Answer Questions

1. How is disulfiram useful in the treatment of alcoholism?

2. How much pure alcohol is required to cause a disulfiram reaction?

3. What instructions would you give to milk-intolerant persons who would like to add milk to their diets?

4. A contraindication for the use of hyaluronidase is _____.
5. How are enzymes degraded by the body?

6. Why might children with cystic fibrosis require increasing doses of digestive enzymes after a long period of treatment?

7. Why is halothane anesthesia not recommended for surgery involving papain lysis of herniated disks?

8. The most serious adverse reaction to chymopapain is _____.
9. What precautions should be used when handling enzyme drugs? Why?

10. Can enzyme drugs cross cell membranes? The blood–brain barrier?

47
Complexes: Chelators and Ion-Exchange Compounds

Chapter 47 discusses various medications that act by exchanging ions with, or chelating chemicals that are potentially harmful to, the body so that the harmful elements are eliminated from the body. Some of these drugs (antacids and hypocholesterolemics) are discussed in detail in other chapters. The following exercises deal with material related to these medications.

Matching

A. Match each metal in the left-hand column with the drug(s) from the right-hand column used to promote its elimination.

_____ 1. Aluminum
_____ 2. Arsenic
_____ 3. Calcium
_____ 4. Chromium
_____ 5. Copper
_____ 6. Gold
_____ 7. Iron
_____ 8. Lead
_____ 9. Mercury
_____ 10. Nickel

a. Dimercaprol (BAL in oil)
b. Penicillamine (Cuprimine)
c. Edetate calcium disodium (Calcium disodium versenate)
d. Edetate disodium (Chealamide, Disotate, Endrate)
e. Deferoxamine mesylate

B. Match each biochemical in the left-hand column with the drug(s) from the right-hand column used to promote its elimination.

_____ 1. Cholesterol
_____ 2. Hydrogen ions
_____ 3. Potassium

a. Aluminum hydroxide
b. Cholestyramine
c. Magnesium hydroxide
d. Sodium polystyrene sulfonate

Correct the False Statement

Indicate whether the following statements are true or false; if false, correct the underlined words.

_____ 1. Chelating medications are used to treat <u>heavy metal poisoning</u>.

_____ 2. Chelating medications <u>are not</u> absorbed systemically.

_____ 3. When dimercaprol therapy is in progress, <u>an acid</u> urinary pH should be maintained.

_____ 4. Dialysis can be used to remove the complex <u>ferriosamine</u> which is formed by the complexing of <u>iron</u> and the chelator <u>ferriosamine</u>.

_____ 5. The use of chelators can deplete the body of <u>vitamins</u>.

_____ 6. One adverse reaction to chelator medications is <u>an increased risk of birth defects in exposed fetuses</u>.

_____ 7. Chelators are most often administered <u>orally</u>.

_____ 8. Ion exchange compounds are usually administered <u>orally</u>.

_____ 9. Ion exchange compounds are absorbed systemically and act in the blood and extracellular fluid.

_____ 10. To avoid developing allergy to ion exchange resins, the nurse should wear rubber or plastic gloves when preparing the dose.

Multiple Choice Question

For the following, choose the one best answer.
1. Clients receiving chelating drugs should be given diets rich in
   a. Protein
   b. Vitamins
   c. Potassium
   d. Trace minerals

Selection of Options

For each of the following, select *all* appropriate responses.
1. Adverse reactions to chelator drugs include
   a. Nephrotoxicity
   b. Hepatotoxicity
   c. Bone marrow depression
   d. Gastrointestinal upset
   e. Teratogenesis
2. Chelators that can be administered orally include
   a. Deferoxamine mesylate
   b. Dimercaprol
   c. Edetate preparations
   d. Penicillamine
3. Clients for whom chelation therapy is planned should be screened for
   a. Liver impairment
   b. Renal impairment
   c. Pregnancy
   d. Anemia
4. Sources of potentially poisonous metals include
   a. Paint
   b. Black ink used to print newspapers
   c. Colored inks used in magazines and colored newspapers
   d. Regular gasoline
   e. Unleaded gasoline

UNIT FOURTEEN: SPECIAL CONSIDERATIONS IN DRUG THERAPY

48
Substance Abuse

The illicit use of chemical substances has become a recognized health problem in the general population. The ability to identify and intervene in the abuse cycle will provide positive strategies for the health-care team to use in directing intervention plans. The following exercises will facilitate the development of knowledge in the area of substance abuse, and provide an understanding of the complexities of abuse cycles.

Short Answer Questions

1. Define the following terms:
   a. Abuse:

   b. Addiction:

   c. Tolerance:

   d. Dependence:

2. Describe the cycles of dependence reflected in each of the following:
   a. Pharmacologic circle:

   b. Cerebral circle:

   c. Social circle:

   d. Psychologic circle:

3. Give examples of street slang for these commonly abused drugs:
   a. Barbiturates:

   b. Heroin:

   c. Cocaine:

   d. Marijuana:

   e. Hashish:

   f. LSD:

g. Morphine:

h. Methaqualone:

i. Phencyclidine:

Completion Exercise

Read the question carefully and place your answer in the space provided. Complete the following table, which identifies several substances of abuse.

SUBSTANCE OF ABUSE	PHARMACOLOGIC EFFECTS	WITHDRAWAL SYMPTOMS	TOLERANCE–PHYSICAL DEPENDENCE
Opioid analgesic (heroin, morphine)			
Cannabis			
Alcohol			
Nicotine			
CNS depressants (Nembutal, Seconal)			
CNS stimulants (Dexedrine, cocaine)			
Psychedelics (mescaline, LSD)			

49
Drug Therapy in Maternal Care

Anything that is eaten, inhaled, injected, or used topically by a pregnant woman has the potential to harm or help the fetus. The same is true of the breast-feeding mother and her infant. Nurses must be aware of the need for maternal education to protect the fetus and infant from adverse effects of medication, as well as from pollutants found in the environment.

Labor should occur about 280 days after conception (9 calendar months, or 10 lunar months). If it starts much before the expected date of delivery, the infant may be too immature to live outside the uterus. If it occurs too long after the expected date, the fetal life may not be sustained properly *in utero* and this may result in fetal demise. In addition to the concerns about when labor will begin, nursing care centers on the safety and comfort of the mother in relation to the well-being of the fetus. Decisions have to be made regarding medications to stop labor, to help the fetal lungs mature *in utero*, and to lessen maternal pain during labor and delivery. In some instances, labor may have to be induced or made more forceful, or may take place after the baby has died *in utero*. Regardless of the circumstances, nurses attending the mother must understand the rationale and effects of any drugs that are used.

Short Answer Questions

1. Pregnancy affects the speed with which drugs pass through the placenta. Indicate in the space provided whether the reaction is slower or faster because of body changes.
   a. No increase in hepatic blood flow: _____
   b. Increased renal perfusion: _____
   c. Changes in placenta in third trimester: _____
2. Treatment of pregnancy-induced hypertension (PIH) includes dietary advice. Fill in the recommended daily allowances for the following:
   a. Protein: _____
   b. Sodium, if no edema present: _____
   c. Sodium, if edema present: _____
   d. Fluids: _____
3. Treatment also includes medication. Fill in the recommended range of doses in PIH for the following:
   a. Hydralazine PO: _____
   b. Methyldopa: _____
   c. Furosemide PO: _____
4. Discuss briefly why the following drugs are not recommended for pregnant patients with cardiac problems.
   a. Propranolol:

   b. Procainamide:

   c. Warfarin:

   d. Diuretics:

5. Name three nonpharmacologic methods of easing *breast* pain during lactation.

6. List four nonpharmacologic methods of easing *nipple* pain during nursing.

Matching

A. Match the nutrient in the left-hand column with the food in which it is found in the right-hand column. Place your answer in the space provided.

_____ 1. Iron
_____ 2. Folic acid
_____ 3. Calcium
_____ 4. Vitamin A
_____ 5. Vitamin C
_____ 6. Potassium
_____ 7. Sodium chloride
_____ 8. Fiber

a. Dairy products
b. As supplement
c. Yellow vegetables
d. Red meat
e. Citrus fruits
f. Smoked meats
g. Bran
h. Bananas

B. Match the causative agent in the left-hand column with the resulting condition in the right-hand column.

_____ 1. Maternal alcoholism
_____ 2. Anesthetic gases
_____ 3. Cigarette smoking
_____ 4. Carcinogenesis
_____ 5. Cocaine snorting

a. Small for gestational age
b. Abruptio placenta
c. Spontaneous abortion
d. FAS
e. PCB

C. Match the medication in the left-hand column with the reason for which it is given in the right-hand column.

_____ 1. Steroids
_____ 2. Erythromycin
_____ 3. Sulfa
_____ 4. Rh$_O$(D) immune globulin
_____ 5. Ampicillin with probenecid
_____ 6. Benzathine penicillin

a. Prevention of isoimmunization
b. Relief of stress during asthma
c. Treatment of *Chlamydia trachomatis* infection
d. Treatment of toxoplasmosis
e. Treatment of gonorrhea
f. Treatment of syphilis

D. Match the therapeutic drug given to a pregnant woman in the left-hand column with the fetal condition it will help in the right-hand column.

_____ 1. Digoxin
_____ 2. Rh$_O$(D) immune globulin
_____ 3. Glucocorticoids
_____ 4. Sodium levothyroxine

a. Respiratory distress syndrome
b. Hypothyroidism
c. Neonatal hydrops
d. Heart failure

Essay Question

Infants of diabetic mothers are usually large for their gestational age, and may develop hypoglycemia after birth. Explain the reasons for each of these and place your answer in the space provided.

Correct the False Statement

Indicate whether the following statements are true or false; if false, correct the underlined words or phrases and place your answer in the space provided.

_____ 1. Proper maternal weight gain during pregnancy should be <u>25 pounds or more</u> for most women.

_____ 2. Antiemetic drugs <u>taken early in the day are a safe way to control nausea and vomiting associated with pregnancy.</u>

_____ 3. Fat-soluble substances penetrate the placental barrier <u>more easily</u> than non-fat-soluble substances.

_____ 4. Overweight women should be encouraged to <u>lose weight during pregnancy.</u>

_____ 5. Immediate intervention to prevent further labor should be undertaken when <u>premature labor is diagnosed.</u>

_____ 6. Ultrasound can distinguish uterine contractions <u>producing changes in the cervix</u> from those that do not.

_____ 7. Possible maternal overhydration is a complication of <u>ritodrine combined with corticosteroids.</u>

_____ 8. Patients receiving ritodrine should be evaluated for <u>dyspnea, chest pain, pulse over 120 beats/minute, and BP below 90/60 mm Hg.</u>

_____ 9. Patients receiving ritodrine should have fluid intake limited to <u>300 ml/hour.</u>

_____ 10. <u>Drugs used for pain relief can be given at any time during labor if dose is low.</u>

Situational Exercises

What would you do in the following situations? Write your answer in the space provided.

A. Mrs. J arrives at the hospital stating that she thinks she is in labor, and that her due date is 6 weeks from now. Her physician is expected to arrive shortly, and wants certain information available at that time.

1. Provide three appropriate comments for the following procedures that have been ordered.
    a. Constant fetal monitoring:

    b. Ultrasonography:

    c. Maternal history and physical exam:

    d. Preparation for administration of ritodrine hydrochloride:

2. Nursing actions during administration of ritodrine hydrochloride for premature labor include the following:

3. Patient education following discharge with orders for taking ritodrine hydrochloride PO at home include these instructions:

B. Mrs. T has been admitted to the hospital for induction of labor because of gestational diabetes. She has completed all the necessary testing. Match each procedure in the left-hand column with its rationale in the right-hand column. Place your answer in the space provided.

_____ 1. Amniocentesis
_____ 2. Sonogram
_____ 3. PGE$_2$ given in gel
_____ 4. Oxytocic drug administration

a. Helps to ripen cervix
b. Establishes L/S ratio
c. Establishes fetal age
d. Stimulates contractions

Completion Exercises

Read each question carefully and place your answer in the space provided.
1. Following delivery of the neonate and placenta, _____ is administered to promote uterine contraction.
2. An oral drug used postpartum to contract the uterus is _____ .
3. The newborn's eyes are treated immediately after birth with _____ or _____ , because both drugs are effective against gonorrhea and *Chlamydia trachomatis*.
4. Fill in the possible side effects for the following drugs, which are frequently used for pain relief during labor.

DRUG	POSSIBLE MATERNAL SIDE EFFECTS	POSSIBLE FETAL SIDE EFFECTS
Meperidine		
Nisentil		
Hydroxyzine		
Valium		

50
Drug Therapy in Pediatric Nursing

The pediatric client is a member of a unique population in their response to pharmacologic agents. The child requires special consideration in the calculation of medication doses. Knowledge of physiology, psychology, cultural beliefs, as well as the child's age, health state, development, and genetic endowment will assist the nurse in the safe administration of therapeutic agents to this population.

Matching

A. Match the correct form of oral medication listed on the left to the appropriate age group. Assume that the child is at the normal level of physical development.

_____ 1. Capsules a. School-age children
_____ 2. Chewable tablets or liquid medications b. Infants and toddlers
 c. Preschoolers
_____ 3. Liquid medications

B. Match the appropriate site for an intramuscular injection listed on the left with the age group or groups in the column on the right.

_____ 1. Dorsogluteal a. Infants
_____ 2. Vastus lateralis b. School-age children
_____ 3. Deltoid c. Adolescents

Short Answer Questions

1. List two safety measures that would be used prior to the administration of medication to a child.

2. Discuss how knowledge of pediatric growth and development will assist the nurse in administering medication to a preschooler.

3. List two ways that play could be used to assist a school-age child prior to and following the administration of an intramuscular injection.

4. List eight factors that may influence a child's response to pharmacologic therapy.

5. List four effects an immature renal system may have on medications.

6. Give two rules or formulas for the calculation of pediatric medication doses.

Case Example

The client is a 7-year-old admitted last evening with a diagnosis of a ruptured appendix. Surgery was successfully performed, and intravenous antibiotics are ordered. Vital signs are assessed every 4 hours and are as follows: T-39.5C, P-100, R-20, BP 100.60. A nasogastric tube is in place and is connected to a low-suction machine. The child is to be ambulated this afternoon. Intramuscular analgesics are ordered.

As this is the client's first hospital admission, the parents are anxious and concerned. They are reluctant to encourage respiratory exercises or ambulation. They state that the child is fearful of needles.

Devise a care plan stating Assessment Data, Diagnosis, Goal, Intervention, and Outcome Criteria for Evaluation.

51
Drug Therapy in Gerontologic Nursing

There are many factors to consider when assessing drug use among elderly clients. Chapter 51 does not attempt to give you a "cookbook" approach to assessment, but rather attempts to facilitate your ability to view your elderly clients as people. General guidelines are presented to enable you to check for signs of developing toxicity, to assess the risk-to-benefit ratio of drugs your elderly clients are taking, and to be an advocate and teacher for an effective and safe medication regimen for your elderly clients.

Short Answer Questions

You may need to refer to other chapters for information regarding specific drugs.

1. List factors that should be included when measuring the risk-to-benefit ratio of drug use for elderly clients.

2. Name several factors that contribute to drug toxicity among elderly clients.

3. Identify some diminishing resources of the elderly that may affect their drug use.

4. Give examples of how the pharmacist may be used as a resource person.

5. What could be the adverse effects of the following drugs in an elderly client?
   a. Sedatives in a client with chronic respiratory disease:

   b. Thyroid supplements in a patient with coronary artery disease:

   c. Antihypertensive drugs in a client with arteriosclerosis or cerebrovascular insufficiency:

6. Briefly list mental symptoms that elderly clients may exhibit as a result of drug toxicity.

7. Why is it important to know the kidney function in clients taking drugs, and what are some changes you might expect in elderly clients?

Correct the False Statement

Indicate whether the following statements are true or false; if false, correct the underlined words or phrases.

_____ 1. Polypharmacy occurs among elderly clients because <u>they frequently visit their physicians with complaints of aches and pains.</u>

_____ 2. Common signs of drug toxicity among the elderly include <u>mental status changes.</u>

_____ 3. Elderly clients who have difficulty getting childproof caps off their medication bottles should be encouraged <u>to leave the caps off</u>.

_____ 4. The elderly are more prone to drug toxicity because <u>drugs are tested primarily on healthy young adults.</u>

251

_____ 5. A major problem among elderly clients is <u>compliance to their drug regimen</u>.

_____ 6. Signs and symptoms of drug toxicity in the elderly client may mimic those of <u>medical or psychiatric illness</u>.

Matching

Match the term in the left-hand column with its definition in the right-hand column. Place your answer in the space provided.

_____ 1. Toxicity
_____ 2. IM injection
_____ 3. Absorption
_____ 4. Distribution
_____ 5. Metabolism
_____ 6. Excretion
_____ 7. Calendar
_____ 8. Pharmacokinetics

a. Process affected by increased gastric pH
b. Process influenced by liver function
c. Tool that may be used to facilitate the medication regimen
d. Reaction that may first manifest as acute confusion
e. Process that may be altered by changes in body mass
f. Process influenced by kidney function
g. Procedure that should be preceded by an evaluation of muscle mass
h. Dynamic factors that influence the effectiveness of a drug in the body

Personal Exercise

Write your answers on a separate sheet of paper.
1. Go to your own or to your family's medicine cabinet and make a list of all the medicines there. Be sure to include over-the-counter drugs. Also note expiration dates, prescription dates, or both.
2. Develop various creative aids that may be used by elderly clients for the facilitation of their medication regimen.
3. Your elderly client has a history of arteriosclerosis, hypertension, emphysema, and arthritis. Her medications include digoxin, Lasix, and aspirin. You find that she also occasionally takes the following: Valium when she feels upset; multivitamins and mineral supplement; laxatives at least once a week; and an over-the-counter antihistamine when she gets a cold. This client lives with her husband, who is in good health. She frequently gets confused over how many "little white pills" to take each day. Briefly outline a teaching program you would initiate for this client.

52
Drug Therapy in Community Health Nursing

This chapter attempts to achieve two broad goals: to integrate your previous knowledge about pharmacology as it relates to various client variables, including beliefs, attitudes, and previous experiences with drugs; and to enhance your perceptions about how you view drugs, and about how those views affect your nursing ability in the home and community. Given these expected outcomes, the following questions are offered to provide you with an opportunity to test your knowledge of the chapter content, and also to assist you in applying the nursing process to at-home client situations.

Correct the False Statement

Indicate whether the following statements are true or false; if false, correct the underlined words or phrases.

_____ 1. A thorough drug history <u>at home</u> is best achieved over several visits.

_____ 2. Clients will usually comply with drugs if they understand <u>their effects and actions.</u>

_____ 3. How <u>drugs are stored in the home</u> reflects a level of safety of their use.

_____ 4. The major goal of taking a drug history is to ensure that the client takes <u>every prescribed and over-the-counter drug.</u>

Jumbled Words

For the jumble below, rearrange the three words on the left to obtain the missing letters that form the word on the right.

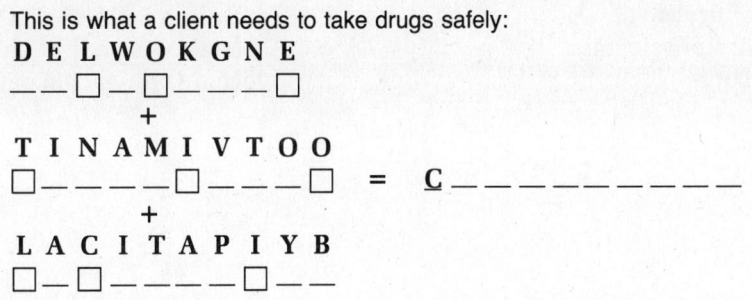

Short Answer Questions

1. List five client variables that reflect the client's knowledge of the drugs being taken.

2. Name four ways by which a prescription label is identified.

3. Explain why the following items are dangerous to the client and/or difficult for the community health nurse to assess.
   a. Multiple drug products:

   b. Sustained-release products versus tablets and capsule preparations:

4. Using knowledge acquired from other chapters in this text, name three foods that have pharmacologic effects (e.g., salt–fluid retention):

5. Identify a problem relating to drug use in the home; state the problem in measurable terms.

Situational Exercises

What would you do in the following situations?

Mr. S, a 68-year-old widower and retired prison warden, was diagnosed 10 years ago with emphysema. He recently moved to this town to live with his daughter and grandchildren. His physician has sent you a referral after diagnosing metastatic cancer to ensure that he follows his medication regimen, especially during a 6-week course of outpatient chemotherapy.

1. Before your first home visit, what further information should you obtain to prepare for a thorough drug use assessment?
   a. Past and present diagnoses
   b. Other prescribed medications
   c. His prognosis
   d. The goals of chemotherapy
   e. All of the above
2. What client variables would be of greatest importance to ascertain on the first home visit?
   1. Knowledge of drugs
   2. Names of other physicians
   3. Source of income
   4. Attitude about drugs
      a. 1 only
      b. 1, 3
      c. 2, 3
      d. 1, 4
      e. 3, 4
3. Mr. S becomes nauseated, and states that he doesn't want to continue chemotherapy. Which of the following measures would you undertake to augment his compliance?
   a. Explain how cancer cells proliferate
   b. Teach him a bland diet
   c. Ascertain his goal of chemotherapy
   d. Inform his physician of this decision

53
Drug Therapy for Pain Relief

Although pain threshold is similar for most people, pain perception varies greatly from person to person and from time to time in the same person. Because pain is a subjective experience, nurses must give credence to their clients' subjective descriptions of pain. Personal attitudes toward the use of analgesics influence their management of analgesic medication unless nurses are conscious of their biases and take measures to compensate for them.

Matching

Match each drug in the left-hand column with the dosage in the right-hand column that is equivalent in potency to the analgesic action of 650 mg aspirin. Place your answers in the space provided.

_____ 1. Sodium salicylate
_____ 2. Acetaminophen (Tylenol)
_____ 3. Codeine
_____ 4. Meperidine (Demerol)
_____ 5. Phenacetin
_____ 6. Propoxyphene (Darvon)

a. 10 mg
b. 30 mg
c. 50 mg
d. 65 mg
e. 100 mg
f. 650 mg
g. 1000 mg

Correct the False Statement

Indicate whether the following statements are true or false; if false, correct the underlined words or phrases.

_____ 1. According to the text, drugs affecting the central nervous system <u>should be considered to be dependence-producing until proven otherwise.</u>

_____ 2. Clients <u>are unlikely to develop</u> psychologic dependence on drugs that do not produce physical dependence.

_____ 3. The dosages of analgesics administered parenterally are usually <u>smaller than</u> equipotent oral dosages.

_____ 4. Overt evidence of discomfort is <u>a reliable index to level of pain perception.</u>

_____ 5. <u>The pain threshold</u> is defined as the strength of stimulus required for beginning pain perception.

_____ 6. When tested for pain threshold, people acknowledge pain sensations at <u>widely different levels</u> of stimulation.

_____ 7. In similar circumstances, individual perception of pain <u>tends to be similar</u> from person to person.

_____ 8. Pain is usually <u>less severe</u> during the hours closest to the usual hour of sleep than during the hours immediately after awakening.

_____ 9. PRN analgesics <u>should not be given</u> to clients who are pain-free.

Multiple Choice Questions

For each of the following, choose the one best answer.

1. The drugs most often ordered for treatment of severe acute pain are
   a. Anti-inflammatories
   b. Opioid analgesics
   c. Tranquilizer sedatives
   d. Hypnotics
2. According to the text, the primary goal of nursing care for clients experiencing pain should be to
   a. Alleviate severe pain
   b. Ensure that physical dependence on drugs does not develop
   c. Prevent or relieve disabling pain and discomfort
   d. Administer a minimum of pain-relieving drugs
3. To be most effective, a tentative plan for administering PRN pain medication should be projected over a period of at least
   a. The interval required between doses (e.g., 3–4 hours)
   b. An 8-hour shift
   c. A 24-hour day
   d. None of the above; the time for PRN medication cannot be anticipated
4. When is pain perception likely to be greatest?
   a. In the early morning hours, after awakening
   b. In the late afternoon and evening
   c. When the client is subject to various stimuli, whether pleasant or unpleasant
   d. None of the above; pain perception tends to be constant
5. Following common surgical procedures such as appendectomy, the use of opioid analgesics are usually limited to a period of about
   a. 24 hours
   b. 3 to 5 days
   c. 1 week to 10 days
   d. 2 weeks
6. Nonnarcotic analgesics such as aspirin are usually preferable to opioid drugs for the treatment of
   a. Incisional pain
   b. Deep visceral pain
   c. Psychogenic pain
   d. General inflammatory reaction
7. Analgesics ordered to be given as necessary (PRN) should usually be administered
   a. Before the pain begins
   b. Before the pain becomes severe
   c. When the client complains of pain
   d. When objective assessment indicates that the client is in pain
8. If a surgical client who admits to being in pain is reluctant to accept a strong analgesic, the nurse should *first*
   a. Explain the adverse effects of pain on healing
   b. Reassure the client that taking analgesics for acute pain rarely causes dependence
   c. Tell the client that the physician ordered the drug because it will aid in recovery
   d. Ask why the client prefers not to take the drug
9. Which is more difficult to treat successfully, physical or psychologic drug dependence?
   a. Physical drug dependence
   b. Psychologic drug dependence
   c. Each is equally difficult to treat
   d. Neither is difficult to treat
10. Successful treatment of physical drug dependence usually requires
    a. A few days
    b. A few weeks
    c. A few months
    d. Many months to years
11. Successful treatment of psychologic drug dependence usually requires
    a. A few days
    b. A few weeks
    c. A few months
    d. Many months to years
12. According to the text, analgesic medication should usually be used
    a. After nursing interventions have failed to relieve the pain
    b. In conjunction with nursing interventions to decrease pain
    c. Only for severe pain
    d. When time pressures limit the nursing interventions that can be carried out
13. The medications most often employed to treat non-life-threatening chronic pain are
    a. Opioid (narcotic) analgesics
    b. Nonnarcotic analgesics
    c. Nonsteroidal anti-inflammatory agents
    d. Steroids
14. Using the least potent analgesics, in minimal dosages, is conducive to

a. Decreased risk of physical drug dependence
b. Decreased risk of psychologic drug dependence
c. Optimal coping with pain
d. Development of habit of pain

15. According to the text, the approach best designed to minimize dependence on drugs is
   a. Using a minimum of all types of analgesic drugs
   b. Delaying the use of dependence-producing drugs as long as possible
   c. Avoiding the use of opioids except for severe pain
   d. Establishing early, adequate control of pain

16. Your client has been receiving 10 mg of morphine intramuscularly every 3 hours for pain. This regimen has not controlled the pain completely, and continuous intravenous infusion of morphine has been ordered. You would anticipate that the dosage of morphine ordered for this infusion would be approximately
   a. 1 mg/hr   c. 4 mg/hr
   b. 2 mg/hr   d. 6 mg/hr

17. Clients receiving continuous intravenous infusion of opioid analgesics should be monitored closely for
   a. Hypotension
   b. Tachycardia
   c. Bradypnea
   d. Pupillary constriction

18. When severe respiratory depression occurs in clients receiving long-term opioid analgesic treatment for persistent severe pain, what is the most likely treatment approach?
   a. Use of mechanical ventilation to maintain vital functions until excretion of the opioids has decreased blood concentrations below the toxic level
   b. Administration of small doses of naloxone until respirations rise to 12 or more per minute
   c. Administration of small amounts of naloxone until respirations reach 12 or more per minute and the client has regained consciousness
   d. Administration of sufficient naloxone to counteract the opioid effects

Selection of Options

For each of the following, select *all* appropriate responses. Circle correct answers.

1. Drugs used to relieve pain include
   a. Antacids
   b. Muscle relaxants
   c. Prostaglandin antagonists
   d. Opioids
   e. Acetaminophen
   f. Hypnotics

2. Overt responses to pain include
   a. An elevation of blood pressure
   b. A decrease in blood pressure
   c. An increase in activity levels
   d. A decrease in activity levels
   e. Facial grimacing
   f. Moaning or crying
   g. Stoicism

3. According to the text, advantages of early, adequate control of pain are
   a. Decreased risk of chronic pain
   b. Decreased risk of phantom pain
   c. Decreased risk of intractable pain
   d. Decreased risk of habit of pain
   e. Decreased risk of psychologic dependence on drugs
   f. An overall reduction in analgesic drug use

4. According to the text, acute pain caused by trauma or surgery
   a. May be absent immediately after injury
   b. Is most severe immediately after injury
   c. Decreases gradually and consistently with the passage of time
   d. May change in nature about 3 days following the injury

5. According to the text, repeated or prolonged pain increases the incidence of
   a. Coping behavior that tends to mask overt signs of pain
   b. Facilitation of the pain nerve pathway
   c. Development of a physiologic habit of pain
   d. Dependence on analgesics as a result of operant conditioning

6. Unrelieved pain following surgery can cause
   a. Increased risk of hemorrhage
   b. Increased risk of hypotension
   c. Increased risk of infection
   d. Delayed healing
   e. Electrolyte imbalance
   f. Chronic pain syndrome
   g. An overall increase in the total use of analgesic drugs
7. When a person experiences unusually severe or prolonged pain, contributing factors are likely to include
   a. A high level of anxiety
   b. Distracting stimuli
   c. A previously learned habit of pain
   d. Complications or a worsening of the underlying condition
   e. Acquired tolerance to the analgesic in use
8. Caution should be exercised when administering opioid drugs to clients who
   a. Greatly fear becoming dependent on opioids
   b. Have an illness that has not been diagnosed definitively
   c. May have a brain injury
   d. Have a history of opioid dependence
9. Psychologic mechanisms most likely to influence the development of dependence on drugs include
   a. Classic stimulus-response conditioning
   b. Generalization of response to similar stimuli
   c. Extinction of learning
10. Drugs used for analgesia by continuous parenteral infusion include
    a. Opioids
    b. Tranquilizer sedatives
    c. Local anesthetics
11. Analgesic drugs that relieve pain by interacting with opioid receptors on nerve cell membranes include
    a. Morphine
    b. Phenacetin
    c. Propoxyphen (Darvon)
    d. Pentazocine (Talwin)
12. Advantages of intravenous infusion of analgesics include
    a. A more constant blood concentration of analgesic
    b. Good pain relief with nonsteroidal anti-inflammatories
    c. Improved pain relief for refractory pain
    d. Ease in titrating dosage
13. Routes used for continuous parenteral infusion of analgesics include
    a. Subcutaneous (SC)
    b. Intramuscular (IM)
    c. Intravenous (IV)
    d. Local
    e. Epidural
    f. Intrathecal

Short Answer Questions

1. Name two drugs or classes of drugs that act as nonnarcotic analgesics.

2. Define the following terms:
   a. Analgesic:

   b. Physical dependence:

   c. Psychologic dependence:

   d. Tolerance:

   e. Withdrawal:

   f. Physiologic habit of pain:

3. List two characteristics of physical dependence on drugs.

4. In terminal illness characterized by pain, the client may be given considerable control over analgesic drug therapy. Name at least four advantages and one disadvantage of this approach.

5. List the types of drugs usually found in Brompton's mixture.

6. Identify at least one disadvantage of continuous parenteral infusion of analgesic drugs.

7. What is the oral dose of meperidine (Demerol) that is equipotent to 75 mg administered parenterally?

8. List at least four assessment parameters useful to the nurse who is considering the administration of a PRN analgesic.

Sequences

Arrange the following goals in order of the relative priorities that should be assigned in situations of terminal illness characterized by pain, according to the philosophy expressed in the text, by numbering each in sequence.
_____ Prevention of drug dependence
_____ Minimization of tolerance to drugs
_____ Relief of pain and promotion of comfort
_____ Avoidance of excessive sedation

Situational Exercises

Write your answers to the following questions in the spaces provided.
  Your client's pain has not been well controlled on a regimen of 60 mg of morphine PO q4h. Continuous intravenous infusion of morphine has been ordered.
1. What is the IM morphine dose equipotent to 60 mg PO?

2. What is the dosage of morphine administered by continuous IV infusion that is equipotent to 60 mg PO q4h?

3. Would you anticipate that the continuous IV dosage of morphine ordered for your client would be the same as your answer to 2 above, less than that dosage, or greater than that dosage?

Personal Exercise

What are your personal biases concerning the use of dependence-producing analgesics for the relief of pain? What life experiences led to their development? What effect are these biases likely to have on your nursing judgment in situations involving medication for clients in pain? What do you do to minimize their influence? Write your answer on a separate sheet of paper.

54
Self-Medication with Over-the-Counter Drugs

A wide range of drugs are marketed without prescription. These medications are readily available to the consumer in drugstores, grocery stores, restrooms, and vending machines, and their use is promoted through extensive advertisement in the media. The practice of self-medication has greatly increased recently. As professionals in the health-care system, nurses are in a position to minimize hazards associated with self-medication.

Personal Exercise: Drug History

Review the personal list of drugs developed in the workbook material for Chapter 1. Identify drugs on this list that are sold without a prescription. How does their number compare with the number of prescription drugs? Evaluate each nonprescription drug on the list considering the following factors: safety as you habitually use them; efficacy; and risks for adverse reactions. Identify and list drugs that you feel should be eliminated or replaced by other preparations. Are there other nonprescription drugs that you feel might be useful to you? Identify these, and the health problem for which you might find them useful. List measures that you would take to enhance the safety and efficacy of self-medication with over-the-counter drugs. Write your answer on a separate sheet of paper.

Completion Exercise

Complete the following table, which compares prescription and nonprescription drugs, by listing both advantages and disadvantages of their use.

TYPE OF DRUG USE	ADVANTAGES	DISADVANTAGES
Prescription		
Nonprescription		

Correct the False Statement

Indicate whether the following statements are true or false; if false, correct the underlined words or phrases.

_____ 1. Federal regulations require that specific warnings be included on the labels of certain drugs.

_____ 2. Many nonprescription drugs contain more than one active ingredient.

_____ 3. The number of drugs available for prescription is about twice the number of drugs allowed in over-the-counter preparations.

_____ 4. The ingredients and formulations of some nonprescription drugs are identical to those prescribed by physicians for similar medicinal purposes.

_____ 5. Use of nonprescription drugs could be eliminated without serious disruption of health-care delivery in the United States.

_____ 6. All "health products" sold over the counter at pharmacies have been found to be safe and effective by the Food and Drug Administration.

_____ 7. Nonprescription drugs contain substances of low potency and rarely cause significant adverse reactions.

Multiple Choice Questions

For each of the following, choose the one best
1. In recent years, what trends have characterized the use of prescription and nonprescription drugs?
   a. Use of both prescription and nonprescription drugs has declined
   b. Use of both prescription and nonprescription drugs has increased
   c. Use of prescription drugs has increased while use of nonprescription drugs had decreased
   d. Use of prescription drugs has decreased while use of nonprescription drugs has increased
2. When was the first legislation enacted in the United States to control the manufacture and sale of drugs?
   a. 1866   c. 1938
   b. 1906   d. 1970
3. The federal law(s) on which current regulation of nonprescription drugs in the United States is based is (are) the
   a. Food and Drug Act of 1938
   b. Durham–Humphrey Amendment of 1952
   c. Kefauver–Harris Act of 1962
   d. All of the above
4. The legal terms "legend" and "over-the-counter drugs" were first established by the
   a. Food and Drug Act of 1938
   b. Durham–Humphrey Amendment of 1952
   c. Kefauver–Harris Act of 1962
   d. Controlled Substance Act of 1970
5. The federal agency responsible for enforcement of most drug regulations is the
   a. Food and Drug Administration
   b. Department of Health and Social Services
   c. Public Health Department
   d. Treasury Department
6. The federal government is concerned with
   a. Safety of nonprescription drugs
   b. Efficacy of nonprescription drugs
   c. Truth in labeling of nonprescription drugs
   d. All of the above
7. A dietary aid recently classified as a drug and removed from the market because of unproven safety and efficacy is
   a. Hexachlorophene
   b. Aspartame
   c. Saccharin
   d. Starch blockers
8. Preparations that are *not* classified as drugs and are *not* controlled by federal regulations are most likely to have a label
   a. That contains no guidelines for use
   b. Stating that the preparation is not a drug
   c. Warning that it has not undergone FDA testing
   d. All of the above
9. Childproof caps are designed to
   a. Preclude access to medication by children
   b. Delay access to medication by children
   c. Facilitate access to medication by persons with impaired manual dexterity
   d. Protect the drug from being tampered with
   e. All of the above
10. If the seal on a package of nonprescription drugs is not intact at the time of purchase, the consumer should
    a. Return the package to the pharmacy for exchange or refund
    b. Return the package to the pharmaceutical house that manufactured the drug
    c. Turn the package over to the local police
    d. Keep the package and notify the Food and Drug Administration

Selection of Options

For each of the following, select *all* appropriate responses. Circle correct answers.

1. Disadvantages of multiple drug preparations include
   a. Fixed dosage combinations
   b. Excessive medication by inappropriate drugs
   c. Increased risk of allergic reaction
2. Nonprescription drugs advertised for the relief of both premenstrual tension and dysmenorrhea are likely to
   a. Contain different medicines for treating each condition
   b. Be ineffective against one of the two conditions
   c. Medicate the client excessively, because premenstrual tension and dysmenorrhea do not occur concurrently
3. Most over-the-counter preparations for the relief of colds and sinus conditions contain a combination of
   a. Antihistamines
   b. Aspirin or acetaminophen
   c. Anti-inflammatory drugs (nonsteroidals)
   d. Decongestants
   e. Hypnotics
   f. Laxatives
   g. Sympathomimetics
   h. Scopolamine
   i. Sedatives
4. Federal regulations require that the label on nonprescription drugs
   a. Identify all active ingredients
   b. Use terminology readily understood by laypeople
   c. List all adverse reactions caused by the drugs
5. Factors influencing the trend toward self-medication include
   a. The high cost of medical care and prescription drugs
   b. Sales promotion by intensive advertising
   c. The trend toward increased personal autonomy in health care
6. Criteria for discontinuing a nonprescription drug and seeking professional health care or advice include
   a. Failure to improve or increased severity of the illness
   b. A need to take nonprescription drugs longer than 3 days
   c. A need for increased dosage for continued effectiveness
   d. Development of adverse reactions
7. Characteristics of nonprescription drugs include
   a. Selection of drugs from a limited number of approved substances
   b. Use of a single drug per remedy
   c. Exploitation of physiologic actions normally considered (in prescription drugs) to be side effects
   d. Aggressive marketing through intensive advertising

Short Answer Questions

1. List at least four criteria for safe use of nonprescription medications.

2. Give three examples of warnings required by federal regulations on the labels of certain nonprescription drugs.

3. Identify at least three ingredients used in nonprescription drugs that are harmful to certain people; for each of these, identify the client(s) at risk.

4. Name one reference dealing with nonprescription drugs that you could recommend to a client wishing to learn more about over-the-counter remedies.

ANSWER SECTION

1
Orientation to Pharmacology: Historical Overview

Sequences

___2___ Ebers Medical Papyrus (Egypt)
___5___ Use of foxglove by William Withering
___1___ Codification of mixtures for medicine (China)
___4___ Sophisticated Arabian pharmacology
___6___ Injection techniques
___7___ Drug production as a major technical industry
___3___ Roman Materia Medica

Checklist

1, 3, 4, 6, 7

Short Answer Questions

Large drug industry with advanced technology; large numbers of medicinal drugs; growing problems of drug abuse; growing problems of chemical pollution; renewed interest in herbal and traditional medicines; increased concern about overuse of chemicals

Matching

1. a 2. a 3. b 4. a 5. a 6. b 7. a 8. a

Completion Exercises

1. Prunes
2. Coffee, tea, chocolate, peyote, pituri, fly agaric, caapi, kavi
3. 19th
4. Markedly diluted preparations
5. Avoided harmful heroic measures

Personal Exercise: History of Pharmacologically Active Substances

The following are examples of entries that may be included:

DRUG NAME	RESPONSE	DESIRABLE	UNDESIRABLE
		(Check one)	
Prescription Drugs			
Penicillin	Decrease in pain and soreness of throat (tonsilitis)	x	
	Itchy skin rash		x
Erythromycin	Decrease in pain and soreness of throat	x	
Patent Medicines			
Hydrocortisone ointment	Relief of skin itching	x	
Tylenol	Lowering of fever	x	

265

DRUG NAME	RESPONSE	DESIRABLE	UNDESIRABLE
			(Check one)
Folk Remedies			
Tea (applied to skin for relief of itching)	None		
Herbs			
Chamomile tea	Relaxation	x	
Mint tea	Relaxation	x	
Foods			
Prunes	Relief of constipation	x	
Social Drugs			
Nicotine (cigarettes)	Elevated mood	x	
	Relaxation	x	
	Stimulation	x	
	Cough		x
	Bad breath		x
	Stained teeth and fingers		x
Alcohol	Relaxation	x	
	Silliness	Undecided	
	Irritability		x
Poisons			
HCl (spilled in lab)	Pain in burned area		x
Pollutants			
Exhaust fumes (e.g., in underpass in traffic jam)	Headache		x

2
Standards and Controls

Matching

A. 1. a, b, c, d 2. c, d (possibly b in some areas) 3. a, b, c, d 4. a, c, d
   5. None of the above 6. a, b
   7. a, b, c, d

B. 1. d 2. a 3. a 4. e 5. d 6. b 7. b
   8. b 9. a 10. c

Correct the False Statement

1. F; Drug Enforcement Agency of the Department of Justice
2. F; more severe
3. T
4. F; the United States Pharmacopeia and the National Formulary
5. F; was never enforced in relation to drug efficacy
6. F; the Harrison Narcotic Act of 1914
7. T
8. T
9. F; nonprescription or over-the-counter
10. F; any health-care practitioner

Multiple Choice

1. a 2. c 3. d

Completion Exercises

1. Thalidomide
2. Salk polio vaccine
3. Effective
4. Kefauver–Harris Amendment of 1962
5. Personal choice

Short Answer Questions

1. Unlike the drug-dependent person, the drug addict either endangers the public or has lost the power to control the addiction.
2. Among the possible answers are the following: prohibition of alcohol in the 1920s and severe penalties for the use of marijuana in the mid-20th century. In both cases there was widespread noncompliance with the law.
3. a. Potency
   b. Safety margin (or safety)
   c. Efficacy
   d. Purity
   e. Bioavailability
4. It is used to test substances for mutagenicity, a property believed to reflect carcinogenicity.
5. Examples of some family practices and attitudes (from our experience) include the following: religious beliefs that the use of alcohol is sinful (leading to pressure toward total abstinence); cultural patterns regarding the use of wine as a table beverage, even for children; permissiveness in relation to the use of marijuana; either strictures against or permissiveness toward the use of tobacco; avoidance of local anesthetics because (1) the numbing of gums is believed to promote careless drilling on the part of the dentist, or (2) the drugs are totally ineffective in some family members; avoidance of drugs to which many family members develop allergies (e.g., aspirin, penicillin); avoidance of drugs to which many family members develop unpleasant side effects (e.g., depression following the use of diazepam); reliance on the use of Antiphlogistine (a patent medicine used to prepare topical poultices); a tendency to discontinue dosing with a prescription drug as soon as the symptoms subside because the use of drugs is feared and distrusted; persistence in seeking medical help from different physicians until a drug is prescribed because of belief that medication is required to treat most illnesses.

3
Nursing Process in the Management of Drug-Related Problems

Personal Exercise: Nursing Care Plan

The personal nursing care plan is a learning experience that can influence the student's self-care practices. Even when substances not commonly considered to be true "drugs" such as nutritional supplements (vitamins and minerals) or aspirin are involved, the student will find that the use of the substance involves some risk, the effects of the medicine may be enhanced by nondrug measures, and the properties of the chemicals involved must be considered if optimal health care is to result.

Correct the False Statement

1. F; involves many independent as well as dependent nursing functions
2. T
3. F; clients in the community; treatment of acute or chronic health problems
4. F; use judgment in deciding whether to encourage or discourage drug use by individual clients
5. F; each time goals are established or revised

Short Answer Questions

1. Promotion of optimal response to drugs; decreasing the risk of adverse reactions to drugs; assisting clients to achieve optimal health through proper use of drugs
2. Assessment; diagnosis; planning; intervention; evaluation
3. Drugs prescribed by physicians; self-prescribed medicines; nonmedicinal drugs used; chemical exposure in the recent past
4. Minimization of side effects; prevention of drug dependence; prompt detection of adverse reactions; withdrawal from a dependency-producing chemical; reduction (or promotion) of drug use
5. Therapeutic response; adverse reactions; unusual reactions; allergic reactions; tolerance; dependence
6. Because unusual reactions are often associated with inherited (genetic) factors that may be shared by the client
7. The quality of the desired change; the magnitude of the change desired; a method for measuring the magnitude of change; a time limit for achieving the desired change

Multiple Choice Questions

1. a 2. b 3. d 4. a 5. d 6. b 7. c

Selection of Options

1. a, b 2. c, d 3. a, b, c, d

4
Development of a Knowledge Base in Pharmacology

Personal Exercise: Drug File

1. ASPIRIN

1. Acetylsalicylic acid
2. Analgesic, anti-inflammatory, antipyretic
3. Headache, arthritis, excessive fever
4. 6
5. 1
6. 5
7. 3
8. No
9. 2
10. 4
11. 4 (rectal suppositories)
12. It is hydrolyzed by tissue esterases, principally in the liver, and excreted by the kidneys
13. 2
14. 1

2. REGULAR INSULIN

1. Hormone, protein
2. When it occupies insulin receptors on the surfaces of body cells, it facilitates the movement of glucose into the cells.
3. It accelerates the storage and metabolism of glucose. In clients suffering from diabetes mellitus, it corrects the distorted nutrient metabolism and tends to lower blood glucose levels toward normal.
4. 1
5. 3
6. 1; hypoglycemia, which occurs more frequently than allergy, is a toxic effect.
7. 2
8. 2
9. a, c, d
10. Oral carbohydrates, glucose infusions, or glucagon injections
11. 4
12. 4
13. Unopened bottles should be refrigerated. The bottle in use should be kept at room temperature.
14. 3
15. 3

3. MEPERIDINE

1. 2
2. a. T
   b. F; a central nervous system depressant
   c. F; drowsiness
   d. T
   e. T
3. It occupies opioid receptors on body cells, producing the same effects as the autacoid endorphins and enkephalins and as opiates such as morphine.
4. 4
5. 4
6. 2
7. 1

Matching

1. b 2. c 3. d 4. c 5. b 6. d 7. a

Short Answer Question

The pharmacist (or pharmacy) who dispensed the drug

5
Toxicology

Short Answer Questions

1. a. Antidote: an agent that counteracts the action of a poison
   b. Toxicology: the study of the effects of chemicals on biologic systems that focuses on the harmful effects of the substance
   c. FEP: free erythrocyte protoporphyrin, an essential element in the composition of hemoglobin
   d. Chelate: to combine an element at the receptor site of a metal in a weakly dissociated complex, allowing the metal to be excreted from the body

2.
TOXIN ROUTE	EXAMPLE
Percutaneous	DDT, hexachlorophene
Gastrointestinal	Lead, drugs
Inhalational	Carbon monoxide
Parenteral	Medications

3. a. With gag reflex present, and in a conscious victim, give milk or water to dilute the poison. Induce emesis if not contraindicated.
   b. Remove victim to fresh air
   c. Flood the skin with water for 2 to 3 minutes. Remove affected apparel when patient is under the stream of water; after flooding the skin, gently wash with soap and water.
   d. Irrigate the eyes copiously with lukewarm water for 15 minutes. Do not use eye drops.

4. Skin decontamination; emesis; lavage; charcoal; cathartic

5. Forced diuresis; peritoneal dialysis; hemodialysis; exchange transfusions; hemoperfusion

6. a. Two successive venous Pb levels ≥ 70 µg/dl, with or without symptoms
   b. FEP ≥ 250 µg/dl and venous Pb level of 50 µg/dl, with or without symptoms
   c. FEP > 109 µg/dl and elevated venous Pb level of ≥ 30 µg/dl with symptoms
   d. Venous Pb level > 49 µg/dl with symptoms and evidence of toxicity, such as abnormal FEP and positive results from provocative chelation

6
Approaches to Drug Therapy

Matching

1. b   2. a   3. c   4. c   5. b

Completion Exercise

The following are examples of answers that might be given:

SUBSTANCE USED	WHO PRESCRIBED	REASON FOR USE	TYPE OF APPROACH REPRESENTED
Aspirin	Self	Headache	Empiric–rational
Tetracycline	Physician	Acne	Rational
Saline gargle	Self	Sore throat	Empiric

Short Answer Questions

1. a. Hippocrates lived around 460 to 370 BC. He was recognized in Greek medicine for his role in the evolution of rational thinking in the field of medical science.
   b. Galen was a Greek physician who lived from about AD 129 to 200 in Rome. He was the most influential medical writer of his times and was unchallenged until the 16th century. He was noted for large-scale use of medicinal plants and prepared his own prescriptions using the theory of "humors." He was also recognized as a renowned anatomy teacher and illustrator.
   c. Pliny (AD 23–79) wrote the Historia Naturalis. His writings reflect early attempts at experimentation in the use of medicines. He is credited with finding the medicinal value of certain remedies.
   d. Magendie (AD 1783–1855) outlined specific problems confronting the scientist in the use of the rational approach to pharmacology.
   e. Thales (about 460–370 BC) was known as the "Father of Science." He sought to differentiate between magical and natural causes of phenomena.
2. a. The dose–effect relationship of a drug
   b. Time and chemical factors involved in absorption, distribution, chemical transformation, and removal of a drug into and out of living material
   c. Localization of the site of action of a drug
   d. Scientific mechanism of action of a drug
   e. Relationship between the chemical constitution of a drug and its biologic activity

Multiple Choice Questions

1. b   2. b   3. c

7
Pharmacodynamics and Pharmacokinetics

Matching

A. 1. b 2. a 3. a 4. c 5. a 6. b 7. c
   8. c
B. 1. b 2. d 3. a 4. c

C. 1. b 2. a 3. a 4. d 5. c 6. a
   7. b, c, d 8. a

Computation

1. 20,000   2. 1.875   3. 10

Checklist

2, 5, 6, 7, 9

Correct the False Statement

1. F; a decrease
2. T
3. F; wider
4. F; higher
5. F; very narrow to nonexistent (because it is as likely to kill as to produce a therapeutic effect)
6. F; lipid-soluble
7. T
8. F; for both local and systemic effects
9. T
10. F; acidic
11. F; retards and may reduce
12. F; acidic
13. F; duodenum or small intestine
14. F; gradual absorption
15. F; lesser
16. T
17. F; decrease
18. F; only when a prompt therapeutic response to a drug is critical
19. T
20. F; liver
21. T
22. F; is sometimes
23. T

Completion Exercises

1. Intra-arterial infusion; extracorporeal perfusion; topical application for local effect; injection for local effect (e.g., regional anesthesia, joint injections)
2. Hyaluronidase (Wydase)
3. Epinephrine (Adrenalin)
4. Less than 100
5. Liver by way of the biliary tract
6. Constant rate intravenous infusion

*Draw a Drug Map**

1. penicillin G procaine

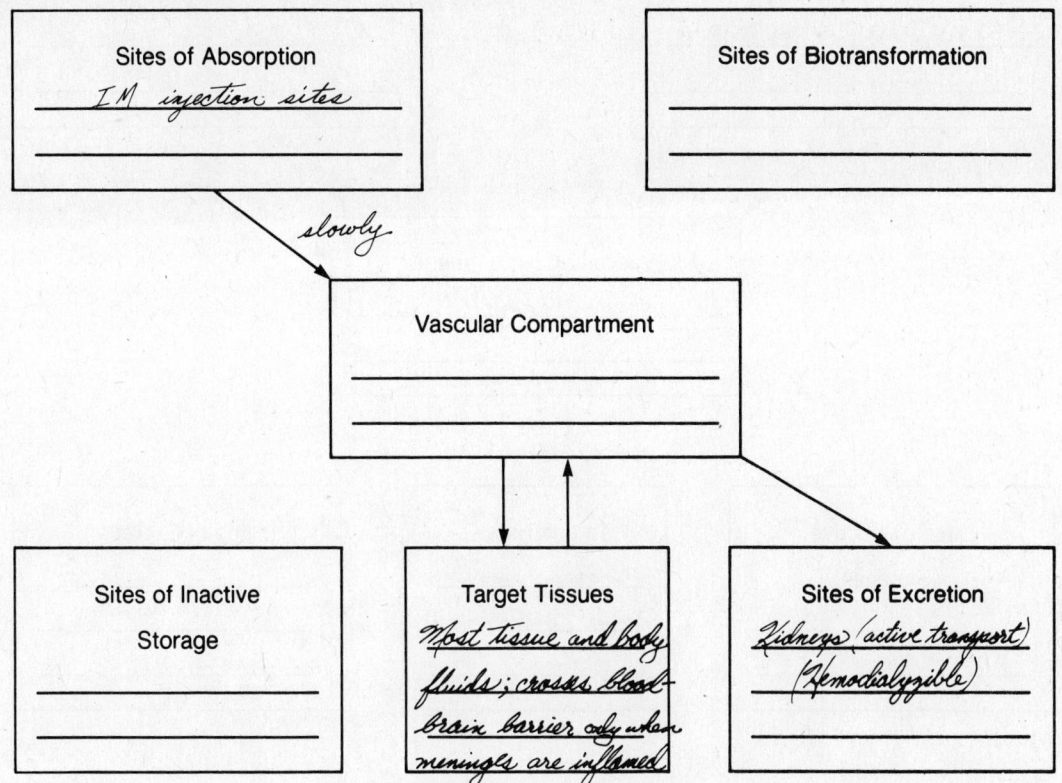

* All information in this section has been taken from the American Society of Hospital Pharmacists: American Hospital Formulary Service, Sections 8:12.16, 68:04, 68:20.08, 56:12, 28:08, and 10:00. Bethesda, American Society of Hospital Pharmacists, 1983.

2. prednisone

Sites of Absorption: GI mucosa; IV or IM injection sites

Sites of Biotransformation: Most tissues, but especially the liver

Vascular Compartment: Binds to transcortin

Sites of Inactive Storage: ___

Target Tissues: Muscles, liver, skin, intestines, kidneys

Sites of Excretion: Kidneys; Appears in milk

3. Insulin

Sites of Absorption: SC, IM, or IV injection sites; some preparations are treated to delay absorption

Sites of Biotransformation: Liver (primarily by enzyme glutathione insulin dehydrogenase); some by kidney and muscle

Vascular Compartment: ___

2% unchanged
98% metabolite

Sites of Inactive Storage: Binding to insulin antibodies

Target Tissues: Throughout ECF

Sites of Excretion: Kidneys

4. milk of magnesia

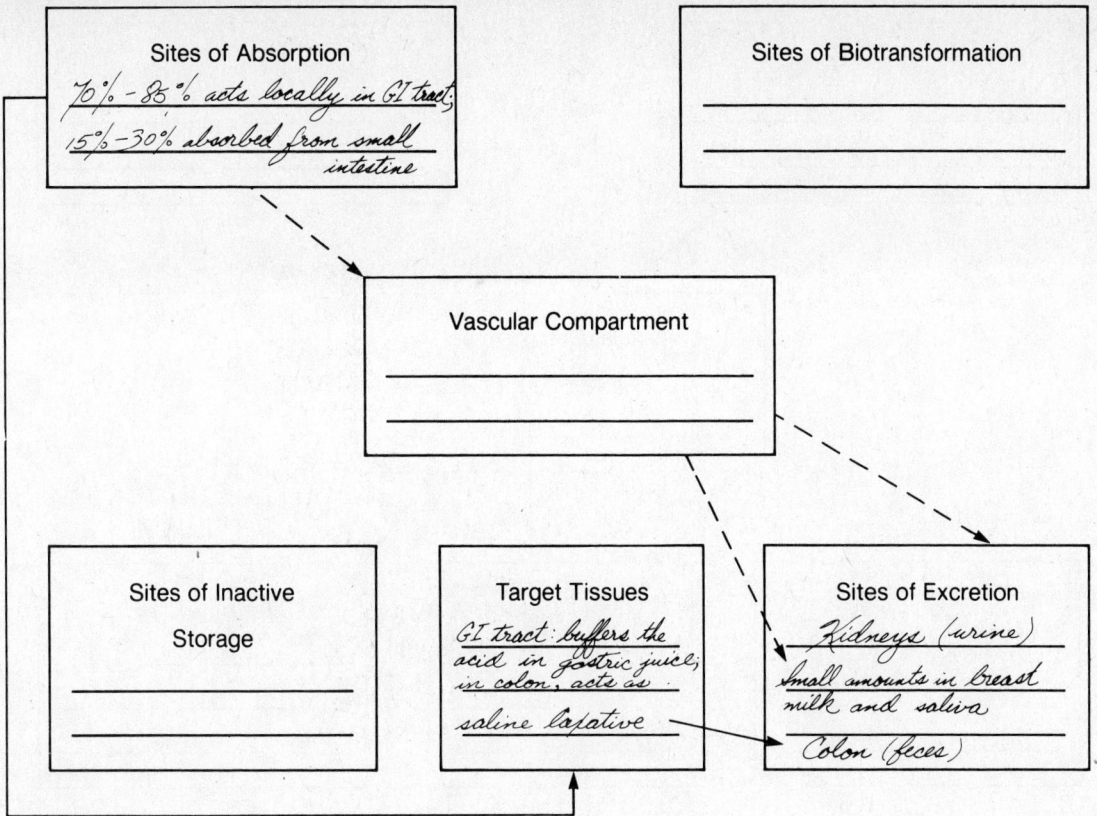

5. morphine sulfate

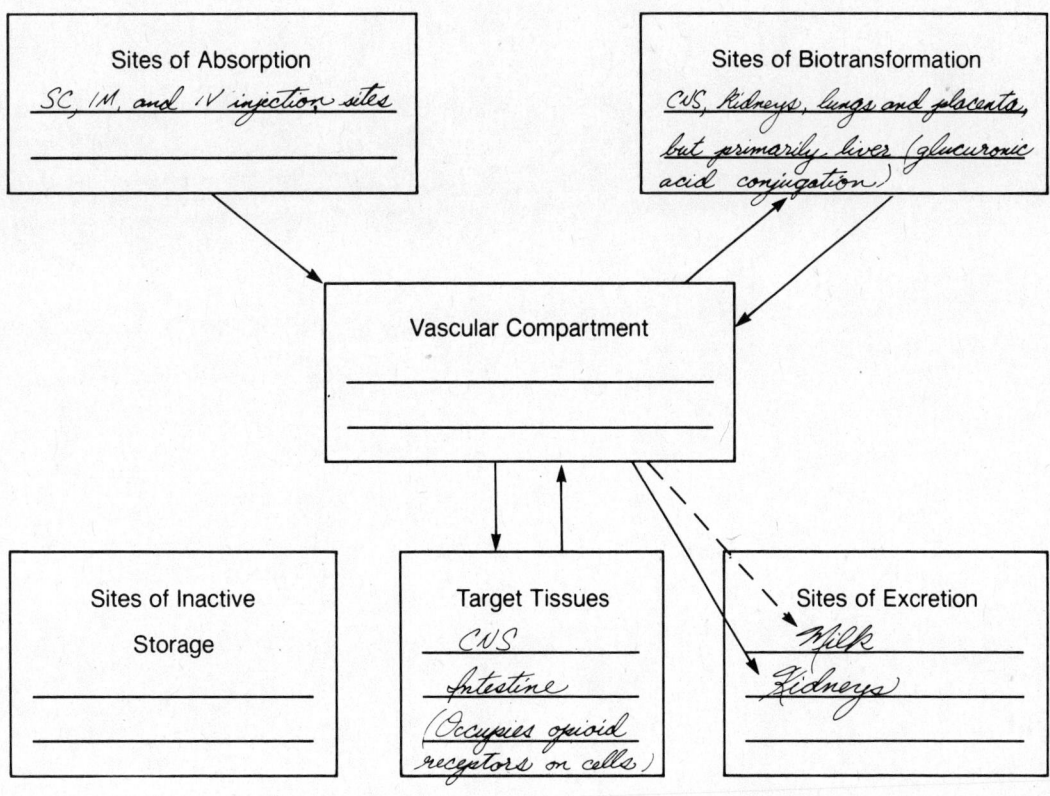

6. methotrexate sodium

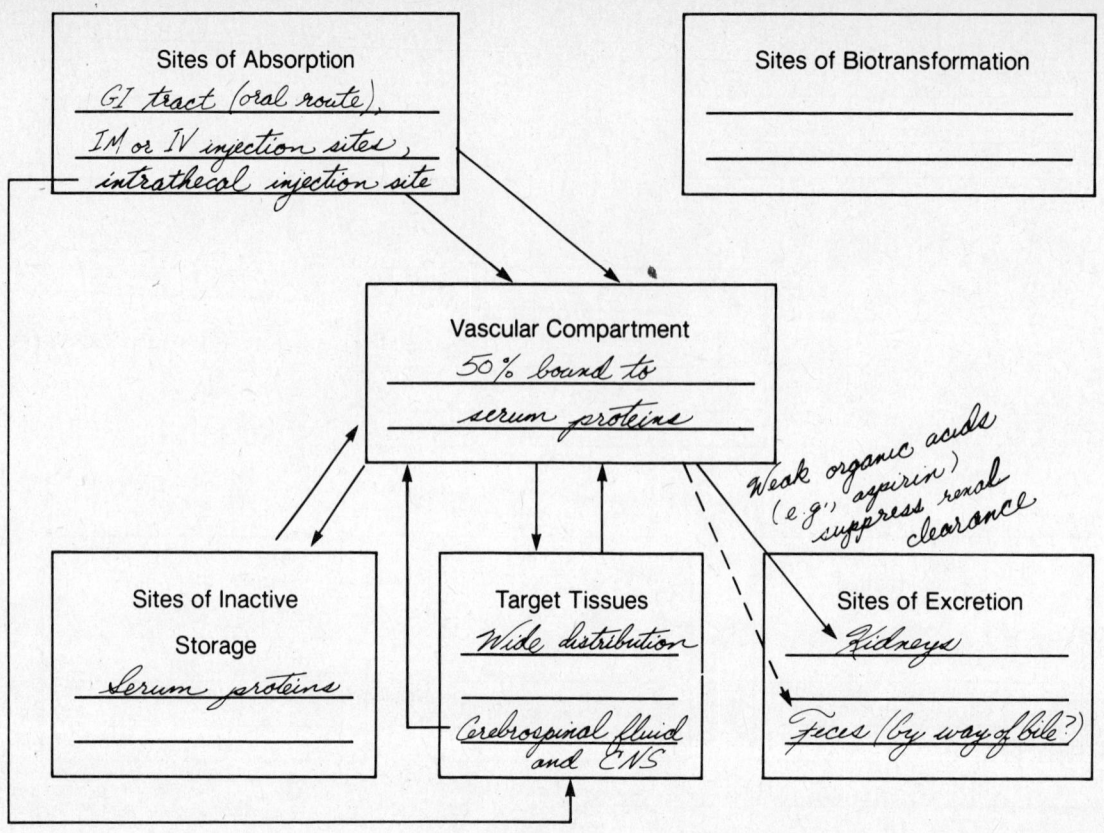

8
Drug Preparations

Matching

1. e, f, h   2. d, f   3. b   4. a, g   5. c   6. d, f
7. d, f   8. c   9. g   10. a   11. e   12. b   13. d

Correct the False Statement

1. F; trade, brand, or proprietary
2. T
3. T
4. T
5. F; are
6. F; prevent them from sticking to the machines used to press the tablets
7. F; volatile
8. F; an emulsion

Multiple Choice Questions

1. c   2. c   3. b   4. b   5. a   6. b   7. d   8. d   9. d   10. b   11. a   12. a   13. c

Selection of Options

1. b, d, e   2. b, c, d, e   3. c, d, e   4. d only

Rank-Order Question

c, f, e, d, a, b

Short Answer Questions

1. Emulsions
2. Tablets
3. Suppositories
4. Liniments
5. Aromatic waters
6. Fluidextracts
7. Elixirs
8. Alkaloids

9
Drug Reactions and Interactions

Short Answer Questions

1. a. Iatrogenic: arising from or caused by medical treatment
   b. Adverse reaction: any of several undesirable reactions that can occur when a drug is taken
   c. Side effect: any physiologic effect other than that for which a given drug is administered
   d. Allergic reaction: an adverse response to a chemical caused by the presence in an organism of immune bodies whose production was stimulated by previous exposure to that chemical
   e. Idiosyncratic reaction: an abnormal response to a drug that may take the form of extreme sensitivity to low doses, extreme insensitivity to high doses, or a response that is qualitatively different from the usual response
   f. Chain reaction: a response that occurs when the use of one drug necessitates the use of multiple additional drugs to control side effects of the first drug
   g. Cumulative reaction: toxicity caused by the accumulation of a drug in the body that occurs when the dosage exceeds the amount the body can degrade through metabolism or excretion.
   h. Tolerance: a condition of decreased responsiveness that is acquired after a single or repeated exposure to a given drug or to one closely allied in pharmacologic activity
   i. Dependence: a condition in which the user of a drug has a compelling desire to continue taking the drug, either to experience its effects or to avoid the discomfort of its absence
   j. Detrimental drug interaction: a drug interaction that is hazardous or deleterious to the client
2. a. Nausea, vomiting, epigastric discomfort, skin rashes, diarrhea, vertigo, insomnia, euphoria, nervousness, hematuria, blurred vision, retention of sodium and chloride, reduction in urine volume, increase in plasma volume
   b. Anti-inflammatory agents, oral anticoagulants, warfarin, oral hypoglycemics, sulfonamides, thyroid hormone
3. a. Skin rash is the most common adverse reaction to penicillin. Generalized rashes often take the form of urticaria. Local reactions to injections are characterized by erythema and itching. Skin problems often precede more serious allergic reactions.
   b. Anaphylaxis is the most serious allergic reaction to penicillin. In this life-threatening condition, swelling of tissues of the respiratory tract, bronchospasm, and generalized vasospasm cause cardiorespiratory collapse.
4. DRUG WITH
   DECREASED

ABSORPTION	INTERACTANT DRUG
tetracycline	aluminum and magnesium antacids and laxatives; milk products; ferrous sulfate
aspirin	cholestyramine
digoxin	kaolin-pectin suspension (e.g., Kaopectate)
rifampin	p-aminosalicylic acid
isoniazid	aluminum hydroxide gel
griseofulvin	phenobarbital

5. Do not give the drugs simultaneously. For example, give digoxin 2 hours before Kaopectate; give the antacid 3 hours after tetracycline.
6. a. Phenylbutazone and warfarin
   b. Valproic acid and phenytoin
   c. Methotrexate and acetylsalicylic acid
7. a. Drug inhibitor: a drug that reduces the metabolism of others, such as allopurinol, cimetidine, or phenylbutazone
   b. Drug inducer: a drug that can induce the synthesis of hepatic drug-metabolizing enzymes, such as glutethimide, griseofulvin, or nicotine
8. Phenylbutazone, phenytoin
9. Uric acid is formed by xanthine oxidase-catalyzed oxidation of hypoxanthine and xanthine. Allopurinol inhibits the xanthine oxidase. This inhibition reduces plasma concentration and urinary excretion of uric acid and increases plasma concentration and renal excretion of uric acid precursors.
10. When tyramine is not oxidized it is freely absorbed and can reach the adrenergic nerve endings through the circulating blood. Here there is an accumulation of noradrenaline as a result of the preceding effect of the MAO inhibitor. Tyramine causes the release of this surplus noradrenaline, resulting in an accentuated hypertensive effect. Fatal cerebral hemorrhages have occurred.

11. The acceleration of metabolism caused by smoking can result in a reduction of blood levels and reduction of therapeutic effects of the interactant drug.
12. Kidney, hepatobiliary route, lung, skin, saliva, milk, sweat
13. By alkalinizing the urine through the use of antacids in large doses

Matching

A. 1. b 2. a 3. d 4. c 5. a 6. b 7. c
   8. d 9. b 10. d 11. c 12. a
B. 1. d 2. c 3. a 4. a 5. b 6. d 7. c
   8. a
C. 1. d 2. f 3. c

Completion Exercises

1.
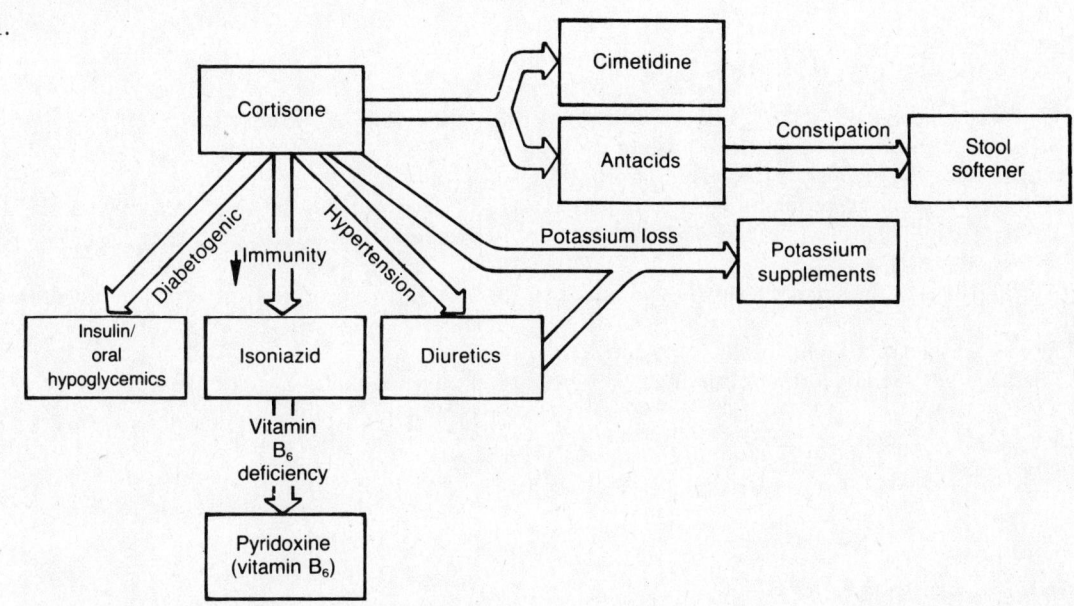

2. Weak acids are excreted <u>more</u> rapidly in <u>alkaline</u> urine. Weak <u>bases</u> are excreted more <u>rapidly</u> in <u>acidic</u> urine.

Short Answer Questions

1. Client is under treatment by two or more physicians at the same time; client has other temporary or permanent medical or dental problems, client uses over-the-counter preparations; client's diet includes components that will conflict with medications that are to be prescribed
2. a. Eliminate noxious stimuli; advise the client to remain still or move slowly; serve frequent small feedings; offer food favored by the client; present food attractively; administer antiemetics, when ordered, prior to meal time; consult with the physician about a change in medication order.
   b. Advise client to change position slowly, especially when arising from a lying position; promote ample fluid intake to maintain hydration and blood volume; assist client with ambulation; consult with physician about a change in medication.
   c. Consult physician promptly about a change in medication; keep client comfortably cool; apply cold compresses to affected areas; teach client to exert pressure on affected area rather than scratching; encourage engrossing activities.
   d. Encourage foods and fluids to replace intestinal losses of fluid and salts; advise client to avoid laxative or irritating foods (prunes, pears, rhubarb, raisins, coffee, saccharin, sucaryl, and other individual foods that increase the client's discomfort); suggest moderate use of tea.
   e. Encourage client to consume laxative foods (prunes, pears, rhubarb, raisins); teach client to avoid large intake of berries or tea; encourage ample fluids; encourage exercise; promote a regular habit of defecation (recommend allotting time after breakfast for attempts to defecate); consult with physician about a change in medication.

10
Interactions between Food and Medications

Matching

A. 1. e 2. a 3. f 4. g 5. a 6. d 7. b
    8. g 9. c
B. 10. f 11. j 12. b 13. c

C. 14. e 15. a, b, h 16. a, h 17. h 18. h
    19. g 20. d 21. f

Correct the False Statement

1. F; may be used as foods if the toxins are present in low concentrations (or if the toxins are removed from the food prior to consumption)
2. F; the concentration of toxins is so low that the body can metabolize them as fast as they are absorbed
3. F; helps alleviate the symptoms of the common cold
4. F; do not alter blood lipids because the active oils have been removed by processing
5. T
6. F; only those foods to which he or she reacts adversely
7. T
8. F; is not necessarily safe to use
9. F; harmless yellow pigmentation of the skin
10. T
11. F; need not list the specific names of all ingredients and additives
12. T
13. F; reduce absorption of drugs by adsorbing them
14. T
15. F; liquids that will not raise stomach pH
16. F; vitamin D and calcium

Multiple Choice Questions

1. d 2. c 3. c 4. d 5. d 6. d 7. b 8. b
9. a 10. b 11. b 12. a 13. d 14. a
15. b 16. b 17. d 18. b 19. b 20. d
21. c 22. d 23. d 24. b 25. d 26. c
27. b 28. d 29. d 30. d 31. b

Selection of Options

1. b, c 2. a, f, h, i 3. b, c, e, f 4. c, e, f
5. b, e 6. a, e 7. c, e 8. b only 9. c, d, e
10. b, d 11. a, b, c, d, e 12. d, e 13. a, d
14. d, e

Short Answer Questions

1. Lack of fiber in the diet, dehydration, inactivity, stress, hypokalemia, excessive intake of tea
2. Preservatives (anti-oxidants), conditioners, emulsifiers, moisturizers, dyes, flavoring agents, stabilizers, thickeners, nutrients
3. Amylases, ascorbic acid (vitamin C), beta-carotene, calcium salts, caramel, casein, carbon dioxide, gelatin, lecithin, proteases (meat tenderizer), vanillin (vanilla)
4. Aged (or hard) cheeses, chocolate, beer, yeast, Chianti wines, cold cuts, sausages, chicken liver
5. Poverty, pre-existing malnutrition, long-term dietary restriction, anorexia, pregnancy, lactation, rapid growth, chronic disease (thyrotoxicosis, diabetes mellitus, maldigestion, bowel disease), prolonged or severe stress, chronic dialysis, use of oral contraceptives, long-term medication regimens

11
Psychological Aspects of Drug Therapy

Short Answer Questions

1. a. Enhancement: the drug is more effective than expected
   b. Negation: the drug is not, or is only minimally, effective
   c. Adverse reaction: an allergic or undesirable effect that is unwanted is experienced
2. Feelings of dependency, anger, hostility, resentment; feelings of security and well-being; anxiety
3. Alleviating pain and anxiety; inducing sleep; decreasing or minimizing allergic reactions
4. Refusing to take the medication; taking enough of the medication to feel better without having to give up the sick role; taking the medication but developing other symptoms
5. Taking a larger dosage than prescribed; taking the drug more often than indicated; taking the drug longer than indicated; taking several drugs concurrently in spite of drug–drug interactions

Matching

1. c 2. d 3. a 4. f 5. e 6. b

Multiple Choice Questions

1. a 2. b 3. b 4. b 5. d 6. a

12
Cultural Aspects of Drug Therapy

Short Answer Questions

1. a. Ethnomedicine: holistic approach to illness that takes into consideration folk beliefs and psychosocial, cultural, physiologic, and spiritual forces
   b. Medicinal plant: any plant containing substances that can be used for therapeutic purposes
   c. Ethnopharmacology: the observation, description, and experimental study of indigenous drugs and their biologic activities
   d. Doctrine of signatures: belief in the principle that "like cures like"; selection of a particular plant may depend on such factors as its color, odor, shape, and its relationship to the illness, (e.g., red plant may be used for blood-related problems; "milk" from dandelion stem may be used to stimulate lactation)
   e. Decoction: the use of roots, stem, or bark of a vegetable drug to form a medicinal liquid by soaking the parts in cold water and bringing to a boil
   f. Tisane: most common way to use dried plants for medicinal purposes; recipe for a tisane requires the basic remedy, adjuvant, complement, and correctors
   g. Maceration: method used to prepare a tisane when the active ingredients of the medicinal plant are found in the mucilage; it is an aqueous extraction of the product that has soaked in cold water for 2 to 12 hours
   h. Infusion: form of tisane used when the active ingredient is found in the flower, seeds, or leaves of the plant; boiling water is poured over the plant parts

2. a. Black Americans: health denotes harmony with nature and the body, mind, spirit; restoring harmony restores sense of self
   b. Hispanic Americans: God is responsible for allowing health or illness; fatalism is dominant; maintaining a balance between hot and cold forces promotes wellness
   c. Native Americans: human body is one with the universe; respect for the body; belief that the body and universe are interdependent; belief in cause and effect; illness is purposeful and is related to past or future events
   d. Asian Americans: universal balance is dependent on harmony between elemental forces of fire, water, wood, earth, and metal

3. Degree of cross-cultural influences; socioeconomic status; language facility; strength and significance of kinship ties; degree of acceptance of dominant culture's values

4. Part of plant collected; amount of processing required to render the plant useful; time of day harvested; life cycle of plant at the time of harvest; season of the harvest

Completion Exercises

1.
GROUP	COMMON ILLNESS	REMEDY
Black Americans	Cold	Hot toddie, hot lemon water, honey tea
	Fever	Herbal tea
	Boils	Raw eggshell skin applied to the boil
Hispanic Americans	Stomachache	Tea made from rue, sweet basil, wormwood
	Pneumonia	Tea made from mint, mallow
Native Americans	Cough	Tea made from wild cherry bark
	Stomachache	Tea made from milkweed, birch, mountain ash
European Americans	Sore throats	Salt water gargle
	Burns	Tannic acid (tea bags)

2.
CHEMICAL COMPONENT	EFFECT ON THE BODY
Vitamins	Vital nutrients for overall body health
Alkaloids	Nitrogenous organic compounds that affect the vascular and central nervous systems

CHEMICAL COMPONENT	EFFECT ON THE BODY
Antibiotics	Attack microorganisms
Heterosides	Interact with body elements to produce various effects on body systems, such as diuretics, irritants, antispasmodics, laxatives

3.

MEDICINAL PLANT	ACTIVE INGREDIENT(S)	MEDICINAL USE
Purple foxglove	Digitalin, gitoxin, digitoxin	Cardiotonic, used in treatment of heart failure
Rauwolfia	Reserpine	Hypotensive, sedative
American mandrake	Alkaloids scopolamine and hyoscyamine	Sedative, diuretic, purgative; treatment for condyloma acuminatum
Periwinkle	Alkaloids vinblastine and vincristine	Treatment of malignancies
Cocaine	Alkaloid cocaine	Reduce pain, local anesthesia
Opium poppy	Alkaloids morphine and narcotine	Pain relief, sedation

Checklist

1. a 2. b 3. d 4. c

13
Basic Principles of Medication

Matching

A. 1. a, c, f
   2. b (provided that the cart is completely stacked before medications are begun); d, e (provided that the cart is locked each time the nurse leaves it); g, h

B. 1. a, b, c 2. c 3. a, b 4. c 5. a, b, c

Correct the False Statement

1. F; the physician should be consulted to determine the route desired
2. F; physicians, nurses, and respiratory therapists
3. F; refuse to carry out drug orders that are likely to cause harm to the client (other answers, such as questioning inappropriate order, would also be correct)
4. T

Multiple Choice Questions

1. a. A remaining half-tablet should be given the next time the drug is administered to even out any discrepancy of dose as soon as possible
2. d. For most drugs, accuracy within 10% of the dose ordered is acceptable. The physician is responsible for informing the client, initially, about the benefits and risks of the treatment.
3. b. In community and hospital settings nurses need to consult with physicians, but the degree of influence exercised by nurses over drug regimens is usually less than in skilled nursing facilities in which physicians rely on nurses to manage most aspects of care of the chronically or terminally ill. In most states, nurses in independent practice cannot diagnose illness or prescribe medication, although they are allowed to counsel clients regarding the use of over-the-counter preparations and measures to optimize response to prescription drugs.
4. a. In institutional settings vocational–technical nurses practice under the supervision of professional nurses.
5. a. Enteric-coated tablets should not be broken, because the drug would be released prematurely in the stomach. Solutions made from tablets are usually unpalatable.

Selection of Options

1. a, d. Only in selected situations would b or c be appropriate.
2. d. Most medicine glasses do not have scales containing markings for 18 ml or its factors. Whereas 4 drams would be approximately equal to 18 ml (1 dram is 4 to 5 ml), a syringe would be more accurate. Fill the 6-ml syringe three times and eject the drug into a medicine glass.
3. b, c. The nurse would also be responsible if the client were harmed by the drug.
4. a, b, c. Although a large dose might alert the nurse to an increased risk of toxicity, individual responses to a given dose of drug vary greatly, and absolute level of dosage does not predict client response.

Sequences

__3__	Notify the physician of the client's failure to improve.	__1__	Interview the client to determine whether the oral antibiotic has been retained.
__2__	Check the chart to see how many doses of antibiotic the client has received.		

Short Answer Questions

1. (In any order) the right drug, the right client (patient), the right dose, the right route, the right time
2. 7. Drug levels decline as follows: after 1 half-life, 50%; after 2, 25%; after 3, $12\frac{1}{2}$%; after 4, $6\frac{1}{4}$%; after 5, $3\frac{1}{8}$%; after 6, $1\frac{9}{16}$%; after 7, $\frac{25}{32}$%.
3. 7 half-lives, or 7 full days

Completion Exercises

1. Dispensing 2. Prescribing 3. Compounding

Situational Exercises

1. In this situation, drawn from the author's experience, administration of the drug would violate one of the rules of dosage preparation, namely that unscored tablets should not be divided. In this case, the need of the client for medication outweighs the risk of breaking an unscored tablet—that is, the risk of inaccurate dosage. However, it is critical that the tablet be divided as accurately as possible, especially in this client, whose ability to eliminate the drug is limited.

In the real situation, controversy arose among the members of the nursing staff regarding whether or not the drug should be administered. The situation was resolved when the team leader used a sharp knife to carve a line in the middle of the tablet, which subsequently was broken into two beautifully even halves. The pharmacist was consulted to determine whether the glazed coating had any protective function that would be lost by administering the broken tablet. It did not, and the medication was administered successfully.

2. When the nurse asked the physician to spell the name of the drug, it was recognized as Evacugen (Ē-văć-ū-jĕn'), a common laxative preparation.

3. Determine whether or not food interferes with the absorption of the drug. In this case it does not. Remove the drug and store it in a secure place until tray time, when you would again offer it to the client. It would be wise to change the time assigned for administration of the drug so that in the future it will be given at mealtime. If the drug had been ordered more than once a day (bid or tid), the times for subsequent administration on this day would need adjusting to prevent dosage at too-short intervals.

Personal Exercise: Drug History

Of particular importance in this situation would be foods or other chemicals that might be toxic and therefore be the cause of the pain. Also of concern would be exposure to antibiotics, because use of such drugs could alter the intestinal flora, resulting in superinfection or in predisposition to antibiotic-resistant infections (and, in this situation, surgery might be required). All chemicals to which you have been exposed within the last 14 days should be listed, as should all drugs that produce an adverse reaction in you.

14
Special Skills Related to Drug Administration

Matching

1. g   2. c   3. a, d   4. f   5. b   6. h

Correct the False Statement

1. F; until the first dose is drawn from it, after which it is stored at room temperature
2. F; to place the container in a pocket near the body until the container no longer feels cool to the touch
3. F; in a locked cabinet in a cool, dry room
4. T
5. F; a stock bottle
6. F; the physician must be consulted to determine the route to be used
7. F; the nurse should not administer the dose unless he or she no longer considers the dose likely to harm the client
8. T
9. T
10. F; water

Multiple Choice Questions

1. b   2. c   3. b   4. a

Selection of Options

1. c, e, f, h   2. b, c, e

Short Answer Questions

1. Intravenous
2. Right eye
3. Once a day
4. Before meals
5. At bedtime
6. One drop
7. One ounce
8. Milligram
9. Gram
10. Milliliter
11. Once when necessary
12. When necessasry
13. After meals
14. Once a day
15. Once an hour
16. Immediately
17. Intramuscular
18. Hypodermic
19. Five
20. One-half
21. Saturated solution of potassium permanganate
22. Soap suds enema
23. Morphine sulfate
24. Milk of magnesia
25. Mineral oil
26. Tap water enema
27. Gram
28. Microgram
29. Kilogram
30. Cubic centimeter
31. Liter
32. Aspirin

Completion Exercises

1. Standing orders accompanied by criteria for their use
2. Superscription, inscription, and subscription
3. Household, apothecary, and metric
4. Metric

Computation: Review of Mathematics

1. a. 20
    b. 11
    c. 4
    d. 2
    e. 24
    f. 15
    g. $7\frac{1}{2}$
    h. 32
    i. 60
    j. $1\frac{1}{2}$
    k. 9
    l. 42
    m. 154
    n. 65
    o. 2000
    p. 95

2. a. ii
    b. x
    c. vi
    d. xiv
    e. xxix
    f. xcvi
    g. cxliv
    h. lxiii
    i. xxxix
    j. lxxxvi
    k. xvii
    l. mcmlxxxiv
    m. viiss

3. a. $2\frac{1}{2}$
    b. $5\frac{1}{3}$
    c. $6\frac{1}{4}$
    d. $1\frac{3}{12}$, which reduces down to $1\frac{1}{4}$
    e. $2\frac{2}{7}$
    f. $4\frac{3}{10}$
    g. $6\frac{2}{9}$
    h. $\frac{90}{11} = 8\frac{2}{11}$
       $5 + 8\frac{2}{11} = 13\frac{2}{11}$

4. a. $\frac{5}{10}$, or $\frac{1}{2}$
    b. $\frac{3}{100}$
    c. $\frac{305}{1000}$, or $\frac{61}{200}$
    d. $\frac{11}{1000}$
    e. $\frac{13}{100}$
    f. $\frac{25}{10,000}$, or $\frac{1}{400}$
    g. $\frac{125}{1000}$, or $\frac{1}{8}$
    h. $\frac{875}{10,000}$, or $\frac{7}{80}$
    i. $\frac{326}{1000}$, or $\frac{163}{500}$
    j. $\frac{4004}{10,000}$, or $\frac{1001}{2,500}$
    k. $\frac{7}{100,000}$

5. a. 0.75
    b. 0.666666 or 0.67
    c. 0.125 or 0.13
    d. 0.3
    e. 0.875 or 0.88
    f. 0.1666666 or 0.17
    g. 1.5
    h. 3.375 or 3.38
    i. 10.777 or 10.78
    j. 3.3125 or 3.31

6. a. About 4 or 5 ml
    b. About 15 ml
    c. About 30 ml
    d. 4–5 g
    e. 60, 64, 65, or $66\frac{2}{3}$ mg
    f. $\frac{1}{16} - \frac{1}{15}$ ml
    g. 4–5 ml
    h. 480, or 500 ml
    i. 960, or 1000 ml

7. a. $\frac{2}{5}$
    b. $\frac{3}{4}$
    c. $\frac{2}{3}$
    d. 5
    e. $\frac{1}{2}$
    f. $\frac{8}{13}$
    g. $\frac{3}{4}$
    h. $\frac{16}{39}$
    i. $\frac{2}{5}$
    j. $\frac{3}{4}$
    k. $\frac{9}{16}$
    l. $\frac{3}{7}$
    m. $\frac{39}{53}$
    n. $\frac{1}{2}$

8. a. $1\frac{1}{2}$
    b. $1\frac{1}{4}$
    c. $2\frac{1}{2}$
    d. $1\frac{2}{3}$
    e. 2
    f. $2\frac{2}{3}$
    g. $4\frac{2}{5}$
    h. $9\frac{1}{2}$
    i. $1\frac{1}{2}$
    j. $1\frac{3}{5}$
    k. $1\frac{1}{5}$
    l. 2
    m. $1\frac{1}{2}$
    n. $2\frac{2}{3}$

9. a. $\frac{1}{3}$
    b. $\frac{2}{7}$
    c. $\frac{2}{3}$
    d. $\frac{1}{150}$
    e. $\frac{1}{200}$
    f. $\frac{1}{16}$
    g. $\frac{3}{50}$
    h. $\frac{3}{500}$
    i. $\frac{1}{1000}$
    j. $\frac{1}{75}$
    k. $\frac{1}{150}$

10. a. 0.4
    b. 0.4666, or 0.47
    c. 0.625
    d. 1.75
    e. 2.6
    f. 1.6666, or 1.67
    g. 0.5
    h. 2.08333, or 2.08
    i. 2.0

j. 1.5
k. 1.25
l. 1.666, or 1.67
m. 0.777, or 0.78
n. 0.5

11. a. $\frac{7}{10}$
b. $1\frac{7}{20}$
c. $\frac{7}{8}$
d. $\frac{2}{5}$
e. $\frac{89}{100}$
f. $\frac{3}{4}$
g. $\frac{3}{8}$
h. $1\frac{67}{100}$
i. $7\frac{3}{10}$
j. $3\frac{13}{80}$
k. $5\frac{33}{50}$
l. $8\frac{1}{8}$
m. $\frac{11}{100}$
n. $6\frac{1}{3}$

12. a. $\frac{4}{7}$
b. $\frac{17}{30}$
c. $\frac{5}{6}$
d. $\frac{11}{12}$
e. $\frac{5}{7}$
f. $\frac{1}{2}$
g. $3\frac{5}{6}$
h. $4\frac{8}{9}$
i. $12\frac{5}{18}$

13. a. $\frac{1}{2}$
b. $\frac{1}{6}$
c. $\frac{1}{18}$
d. $\frac{1}{12}$
e. $\frac{1}{6}$
f. $\frac{13}{36}$
g. $\frac{29}{60}$
h. $4\frac{11}{18}$
i. $28\frac{20}{39}$
j. $\frac{19}{22}$

14. a. $\frac{1}{6}$
b. $\frac{3}{20}$
c. $\frac{1}{4}$
d. $\frac{3}{10}$
e. $\frac{5}{16}$
f. 50
g. 20
h. 12
i. $18\frac{3}{4}$
j. 1
k. $487\frac{1}{2}$

15. a. $1\frac{1}{2}$
b. $\frac{3}{4}$
c. $1\frac{1}{6}$
d. $\frac{1}{300}$
e. $\frac{3}{5}$
f. $\frac{3}{4}$
g. 1
h. $\frac{1}{4}$

16. a. $\frac{9}{2}$
b. $\frac{169}{10}$
c. $\frac{43}{4}$
d. $\frac{107}{8}$

e. $\frac{287}{11}$
f. $\frac{161}{12}$

17. a. 0.55
b. 0.99
c. 2.25
d. 0.375
e. 1.25
f. 6.191

18. a. 15.32
b. 2.25
c. 3.2
d. 1.8
e. 6.17

19. a. 1.25
b. 50
c. 7,500
d. 100
e. 7.14
f. 12.06
g. 0.625, or $\frac{5}{8}$
h. 0.125, or $\frac{1}{8}$
i. 0.45, or $\frac{9}{20}$

20. a. 0.30
b. 0.025
c. 5,000
d. 2
e. $\frac{1}{8}$, or 0.125
f. 0.55
g. 0.0001
h. 0.0875
i. 0.0003

21. a. 25%
b. 60%
c. $37\frac{1}{2}$%
d. $16\frac{2}{3}$%
e. 60%
f. 7%
g. 0.1%
h. 0.9%
i. 6%
j. 350%
k. 10%
l. 0.02%
m. 0.5%

22. a. 0.0009
b. 0.5
c. 0.03
d. 0.75

23. a. $\frac{1}{10}$
b. $\frac{3}{8}$
c. $\frac{2}{3}$
d. $\frac{1}{11}$
e. $\frac{1}{4}$
f. $\frac{3}{5}$
g. $\frac{7}{8}$
h. $\frac{1}{6}$

24. a. 125
b. 9
c. 4.5
d. 120
e. 0.025

f. 0.002
g. 50%
h. 20%
i. 9%
j. 5%
k. 2000%
l. $33\frac{1}{3}$%

25. a. 3:4
b. 1:2
c. 7:8
d. 13:20
e. 65:83
f. 10:30 or 1:3
g. 22:30 or 11:15
h. 3:100
i. 10:1
j. 8:1
k. 75:100 or 3:4
l. $33\frac{1}{3}$:100 or 1:3
m. $\frac{1}{4}$:10 or 1:40
n. $\frac{1}{10}$:100 or 1:1000

26. a. $x = 2$
b. $x = 2$
c. $x = 2$ tab
d. $x = \frac{2}{3}$ ml or 10 minims
e. $x = 25$ mg
f. $x = \frac{8}{9}$
g. $x = 2.8$
h. $x = 2$
i. $x = \frac{18}{63}$, or $\frac{2}{7}$, or 0.285, or 0.29
j. $x = 5$
k. $x = 1$
l. $x = 2$
m. Terms within the equation must match. Therefore mg must be changed to μg (or vice versa). $\frac{0.4 \text{ mg}}{1 \text{ mg}} = \frac{x}{1}$ ml, or $x = 0.4$ ml.
n. $x = \frac{2}{3}$

27. a. 1
b. 1000
c. 1
d. 3,000
e. 5,300
f. 0.5 or $\frac{1}{2}$
g. 1,900
h. 0.35
i. 4,030

28. a. 1,480 ml, or 1.480 liters
b. 3,270 ml, or 3.27 liters

29. a. 2,000 mg
b. 500 mg
c. 0.00025 g
d. 0.6 g
e. 0.1 mg

f. 0.03 mg
g. 400 μg
h. 0.001 g
i. 3 mg
j. 0.000005 g

30. a. 1:20, 5%
b. 7:10, 70%
c. (gr xxx = 2 g) 1:100, 1%

31. a. $\frac{2}{5}$, or 0.4 ml
b. $1\frac{1}{2}$, or 1.5 ml
c. $\frac{7}{10}$, or 0.7 ml
d. $\frac{3}{4}$ ml or 0.75 ml, or 12 min
e. $\frac{3}{8}$, or 0.38 ml
f. 400 ml. 1000 ml of 1:5000 solution must contain $\frac{1}{5}$ g or 200 mg of pure Zephiran chloride. Each ml of 1:2000 stock solution contains $\frac{1}{2}$ mg or 0.0005 g of pure Zephiran chloride.

32. a. gr x = 600 mg (or 625 mg or 650 mg or 667 mg)
b. 150 mg = gr iiss (60 mg/gr i)
c. 400 μg = 0.4 mg
d. 0.5 g = gr viiss (gr xv = 1 g)
e. gr iss = 100 mg ($66\frac{2}{3}$ mg = gr i)
f. gr $\frac{1}{300}$ = 0.2 mg or 200 μg (60 mg = gr i)
g. 200 mg = gr iii ($66\frac{2}{3}$ mg = gr i)
h. 3 oz = 90 ml; 8 oz = 240 ml (30 ml = ℥ i)
i. $\frac{3}{4}$ ml = 12 minims (16 minims = 1 ml)
   $\frac{1}{3}$ ml = 5 minims (15 minims = 1 ml)

33. a. 2 tablets
b. 2 tablets
c. 4 tablets
d. $\frac{1}{2}$ tablet
e. 2 tablets
f. 2 tablets
g. $\frac{1}{2}$ tablet
h. 2 tablets
i. 4 tablets

34. a. 4 ml
b. 6 ml
c. 1.2 ml (60 mg = gr i)
d. $\frac{1}{4}$ fl oz, or ℥ ii
e. $\frac{1}{3}$ ml, or 5 minims, or 0.33 ml
f. $1\frac{1}{2}$ or 1.5 ml
g. 3 fl oz (60 mg = gr i)
h. 60 mg% = 60 mg drug in 100 ml solution; gr $\frac{1}{100}$ = 0.6 mg; use 1 ml solution
i. 2 fl oz, or 60 ml
j. (gr i = 60 mg); $1\frac{1}{5}$ ml or 1.2 ml

35. a. $\frac{12}{10,000}$ g, or 1.2 mg or gr $\frac{1}{50}$
b. $\frac{3}{10}$ g, or 0.3 g, or 300 mg
c. 5 g

Sequences

1. $\frac{3}{4}, \frac{2}{3}, \frac{1}{2}, \frac{5}{12}, \frac{1}{4}$
2. $\frac{5}{6}, \frac{3}{4}, \frac{1}{2}, \frac{3}{8}, \frac{1}{12}$
3. $\frac{5}{6}, \frac{1}{3}, \frac{2}{7}, \frac{3}{13}, \frac{1}{6}$

4. 125.1, 60.001, 4.48, 3.00125, 0.219
5. 10.038, 4.0680, 0.902, 0.32158, 0.000976
6. 134.6, 29.10, 3.209, 1.999, 0.832

Completion Exercise

DRUG	RATIO	%	FRACTION	DECIMAL
Normal saline solution	9:1000	0.9	$\frac{9}{1000}$	0.009
Epinephrine	1:1000	0.1	$\frac{1}{1000}$	0.001
Disinfectant alcohol	7:10	70	$\frac{7}{10}$	0.7
Rubbing alcohol	5:10 or 1:2	50	$\frac{5}{10}$ or $\frac{1}{2}$	0.5
Neo-Synephrine nose drops	1:400	$\frac{1}{4}$	$\frac{1}{400}$	0.0025
D_5W	5:100 or 1:20	5	$\frac{5}{100}$ or $\frac{1}{20}$	0.05

Situational Exercises

A. 1. a. 0.6 ml
   b. 0.5 ml
   c. 0.25 ml, or 4 minims
2. a. One 40-mg tablet and two 5-mg tablets
   b. One 20-mg tablet and three 5-mg tablets
   c. One 20-mg tablet and two and one-half 5-mg tablets
   d. One 20-mg tablet and one 5-mg tablet
   e. Three and one-half 5-mg tablets
3. a. $\frac{2}{3}$ ml or 10 min of 6 mg/ml solution; 0.266 or 0.27 ml of 15-mg/ml solution
   b. $1\frac{2}{3}$ ml or 1.7 ml or 25 min of 6 mg/ml solution; $\frac{2}{3}$ ml or 0.67 ml or 10 minims of 15 mg/ml solution
   c. $1\frac{1}{3}$ ml or 1.3 ml or 20 min of 6 mg/ml solution; $\frac{8}{15}$ or 8 min or 0.53 ml of 15 mg/ml solution
   d. This is an unusually large dose of morphine, and should be questioned. Unless there are special circumstances (e.g., an unusually large client, a client with some tolerance for the drug, a need for deep sedation, under close observation), this drug dose is likely to be harmful to a client. 5 ml of 6 mg/ml solution would be required (too large a volume to give); 2 ml of 15 mg/ml solution could be used.
   e. 1 ml of 6 mg/ml solution; $\frac{6}{15}$ or 6 min or 0.4 ml of 15 mg/ml solution
   f. 2 ml of 6 mg/ml solution; $\frac{12}{15}$ or 12 min or 0.8 ml of 15 mg/ml solution
4. a. 0.6 ml of 1 mg/ml solution; 1 ml of 0.6 mg/ml solution; $1\frac{1}{2}$ or 1.5 ml of 0.4 mg/ml solution
   b. 0.3 ml of 1 mg/ml solution; $\frac{1}{2}$ or 0.5 ml of 0.6 mg/ml solution; $\frac{3}{4}$ or .75 ml or 12 minims of 0.4 mg/ml solution
   c. 400 µg = 0.4 mg
   0.4 ml of 1.0 mg/ml solution; $\frac{2}{3}$ ml or 10 minims or 0.67 ml of 0.6 mg/ml solution; 1 ml of 0.4 mg/ml solution
   d. 200 µg = 0.2 mg
   0.2 ml of 1.0 mg/ml solution; $\frac{1}{3}$ ml or 5 min or 0.33 ml of 0.6 mg/ml solution; $\frac{1}{2}$ or 0.5 ml of 0.4 mg/ml solution
   e. gr $\frac{1}{100}$ = 0.6 mg (60 mg/gr)
   0.6 ml of 1.0 mg/ml solution; 1 ml of 0.6 mg/ml solution; $1\frac{1}{2}$ or 1.5 ml of 0.4 mg/ml solution
   f. gr 1/150 = 0.4 mg (60 mg/gr)
   0.4 ml of 1.0 mg/ml solution; $\frac{2}{3}$ ml or 10 min or 0.67 ml of 0.6 mg/ml solution; 1 ml of 0.4 mg/ml solution
5. a. Four tablets containing 0.0125 g each or two tablets containing 0.025 g each
   b. Three tablets containing 0.0125 g each or one and one-half tablets containing 0.025 g each (the latter can be given only if the tablets are scored). The dose administered would equal $37\frac{1}{2}$ mg, which is within 10% of the ordered dose, 40 mg.
   c. The 100-mg or 1000-mg tablets could be used. Administer five tablets containing 100 mg, or one-half tablet of the 1000-mg size per dose. A total of 30 tablets containing 100 mg each or three tablets containing 1,000 mg each would be needed to complete the dosage regimen. Because ten tablets of the 50-mg size would be needed per dose (60 tablets total), it would not be as advantageous to use this size, although to do so would not be an error in medication.

B. 1. For an adult, up to 1000 ml may be needed for an enema. Normal saline solution is 0.9% sodium chloride, so 9 g of salt will be needed. Because scales are rarely available in clinical settings, a volumetric quantity is needed. Salts have a specific gravity very close to that of water, so 9 ml of sodium chloride (℥ ii) are approximately equal to 9 g.

Procedure: Measure ℥ ii of sodium chloride in a medicine cup. Obtain a plastic enema bag. Clamp the tubing. Pour up to 1 pint of lukewarm water into the bag (to prevent dry salt from entering the tubing). Add the measured salt. Mix solution thoroughly. Add enough additional lukewarm water to make 1000 ml of solution. Hang the bag from a hook. Elevate the end of the tubing above the level of solution in the bag and unclamp the tubing. As solution fills the tubing, lower the tip of the tubing to the level of the solution. Clamp the tubing tightly. Verify that the temperature of the solution is lukewarm. The enema is now ready to be administered.

2. Except for the amount of solution needed, the first paragraph of B1 (above) applies. About 100 ml of solution will suffice for a mouthwash. Therefore, about 1 g (0.9 g) or 1 ml of salt is needed. Because 1 tsp, 1 dram, and 4 ml are approximately equivalent, $\frac{1}{4}$ tsp of salt will be needed.

Procedure: Place $\frac{1}{4}$ tsp of salt in a graduated cup, such as a new urine specimen container. Add water of the desired temperature to the 100-ml mark. Mix thoroughly.

3. About 1000 ml are required for a douche. 5% Na_2Co_3 = 5 g drug/100 ml solution; therefore 50 g or 50 ml Na_2Co_3 will be needed to make 1000 ml solution.

Procedure: Measure 50 ml of soda bicarbonate (using a medicine cup). Pour about 1 pint of lukewarm water into a douche bag. Add the soda bicarbonate. Mix thoroughly. Add enough additional lukewarm water to make 1000 ml solution. Expel air from the tubing (as above). Verify that the temperature of the solution is lukewarm.

4. 1 g is equivalent to 1000 mg.
Procedure: Give two tablets, 3 times daily.

5. Gr iv is equivalent to 240 mg to 267 mg (using equivalents ranging from 60 mg = gr i to $66\frac{2}{3}$ mg = gr i). The 324-mg tablet is too much to give, even if the 10% "margin for error" is considered. (10% of 267 = 26.7; added to 267, this means that 293.7 mg is the maximum allowable dose.) Because enteric-coated tablets cannot be divided, a different dose form or a different dose ordered is required.

Procedure: Call the pharmacy to determine whether or not another dose form containing the proper amount is available. If it is not, inform the physician (who may then alter the dosage ordered or request a liquid preparation that can be measured more precisely).

6. This is an incomplete order, because the route is not specified. (30 mg is the usual adult *oral* dose of Thorazine.)

Procedure: Call the physician to clarify the order. If 30 mg is to be given IM, administer 0.6 ml.

7. Verify that Lanoxin and digoxin are the same drug. (They are.) Five 0.25-mg tablets will be needed. This is a large (digitalizing) dose and should be verified by the physician.

8. Measure 33 ml of hydrogen peroxide stock (3%) solution into a graduated cup such as a new urine specimen container. Add water to make 100 ml of solution.

9. A sterile solution is required. Because sterile graduated flasks are seldom available in clinical situations, a flask containing 1000 ml of sterile water may be used. If the dry drug is added to the sterile water, the resulting solution may not be exactly 1000 ml but the difference will be less than 10%.

Procedure: Warm a 1000-ml flask of sterile water. Aseptically, "pour" five tablets of potassium permanganate into the flask. Cover and agitate to dissolve the tablets completely. Cool the solution to lukewarm. Verify the temperature of the solution by pouring a small amount on your wrist. (If a sterile thermometer is available, use it to verify the temperature of the solution.) Use with a sterile foot basin to soak the foot.

10. Measure 10 minims ($\frac{2}{3}$ ml) to administer.

11. Because no more than two drugs should be mixed together for parenteral administration, and because the volume of the three drugs would be too large, at least two injections will be needed. Meperidine hydrochloride (Demerol) and atropine sulfate are salts with cation components of active drug and so are likely to be compatible. If possible, verify their compatibility with a chart or with a pharmacist. (The two drugs can be mixed.) If the atropine is drawn up without mixing any other drug with it, the remainder of the vial can be used for subsequent medications as a stock drug.

Procedure: Verify that the Tubex contains exactly 1 ml of Demerol; eject all air and any excess drug from the Tubex syringe. Using a new 2-ml or 3-ml syringe, inject 0.4 ml of air into the vial containing the atropine. Cap the empty syringe and save for measuring the Vistaril. Holding the atropine vial upside down, insert the tip of the needle on the Tubex syringe into the vial and allow 0.4 ml of atropine solution to flow down into the Demerol solution. Do not allow air to enter the Tubex syringe and do not push any solution from the Tubex into the atropine vial. When a total of 1.4 ml of solution is in the syringe, withdraw from the vial and cap the needle. Using the syringe previously reserved, measure 1 ml of Vistaril. Administer the contents of both syringes to the client. (*Note:* If these medications are prepared ahead of time, be sure to attach an adhesive label denoting their contents to both syringes.)

12. Obtain a medicine cup, a graduated cup that will measure 100 ml, and a spoon or straw. Take these and the packet of K-Lyte to the bedside. Place the K-Lyte powder in the bottom of the larger cup. Add water to make 100 ml of solution. Stir with a spoon or straw until completely dissolved. Pour out 40 ml into the medicine cup and discard. Administer the remaining 60 ml of solution ($\frac{3}{5}$ of the packet).

13. There is a rule stating that unscored tablets cannot be broken for fractional doses. The purpose of this rule is to ensure optimum accuracy of dosage. The nurse cannot simply omit the medication, however, because this drug is critical to the prevention of stress ulcers. The nurse with a sound rationale knows when it is necessary to break the rule, and how to minimize the risk when doing so.

    Procedure: Call the pharmacist to determine whether there is another dosage form that will allow accurate measurement of the dose. If there is not, ascertain whether or not the hard coating serves a critical purpose that will be defeated by breaking the tablet. (In this case, it does not.) Using a sharp knife, score a line in the middle of the tablet. Break the tablet. Administer one-half tablet, reserving the remaining half for the next dose.

14. $11\frac{2}{3}$ ml are required but cannot be measured precisely.

    Procedure: Administer 12 ml, which is within the 10% margin of safety. Flush the tubing with 30 ml of water or with some other clear liquid after injecting the medication.

15. Administer 12 ml. Flush the tubing as described in B14 (above).

16. 15 ml of pure alcohol is needed to make 1 oz (30 ml) of rubbing alcohol solution. The amount of 70% alcohol containing that amount of pure alcohol is approximately 21.4 ml. (Use the ratio 70:100::15:x.)

    Procedure: Place 20 ml of 70% alcohol in a medicine cup and add water to make 30 ml of solution.

15
Major Antimicrobial Drugs

Personal Exercise: Antimicrobials

Most students will probably have received antimicrobial drugs in the fairly recent past. Evaluating this experience will promote a sensitivity to the needs of clients who are placed on anti-infective therapy.

Short Answer Questions

1. a. Effectiveness
   b. Broadness of spectrum
   c. Inability to induce resistance in microbial populations
   d. Retention of potency in presence of tissue materials and other drugs
   e. Penetration to all tissues and fluids in therapeutic concentrations
   f. Lack of toxicity to host cells and organs
2. Cell wall; cell wall synthesis; protein synthesis; metabolism; nucleic acid synthesis.
3. Selected reproduction; transduction; transformation; conjunction
4. The spectrum of an anti-infective is the number and type of organisms vulnerable to its action
5. Ample hydration, cleansing of the perineum from front to back, application and removal of perineal pads from front to back, avoidance of the use of bath salts or bubble bath solution
6. Adrenalin or epinephrine
7. First-generation cephalosporins exert good action against gram + organisms, but only moderate action against gram − organisms

   Second-generation cephalosporins are more effective against gram − organisms than are first-generation cephalosporins

   Third-generation cephalosporins are most effective of all against gram − organisms but have less activity against gram + organisms than do first-generation cephalosporins

Multiple Choice Questions

1. b 2. a 3. d 4. d 5. a 6. b 7. a 8. c
9. b 10. b 11. d 12. c 13. c 14. b
15. b 16. d

Selection of Options

1. a, c, d, e 2. a, b 3. a, c 4. a, b, c
5. c only 6. b, c, d

Crossword Puzzle

Crossword Puzzle

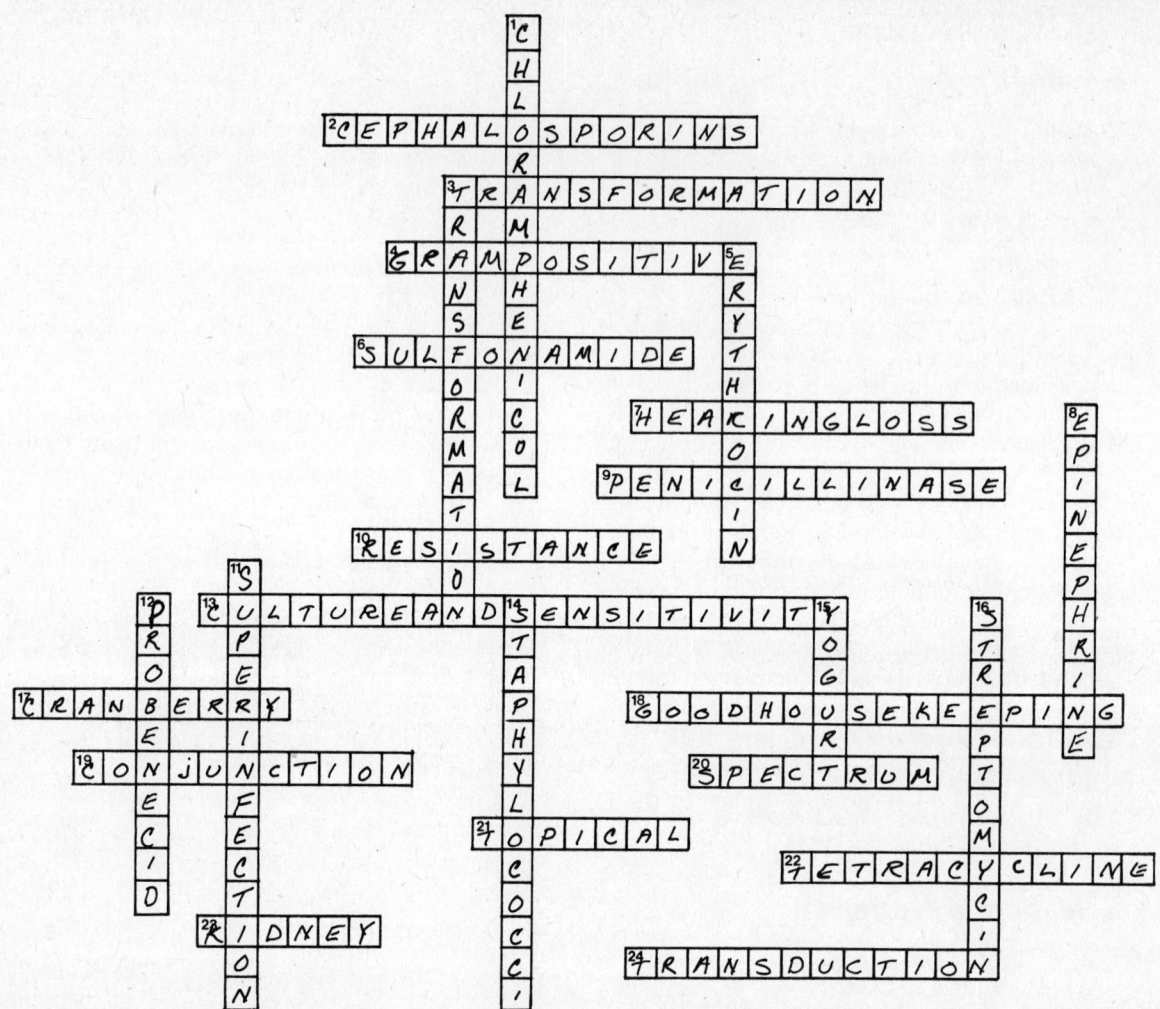

16
Antimycobacterial Agents, Miscellaneous Antimicrobials, and Urinary Tract Antiseptics

Crossword Puzzle

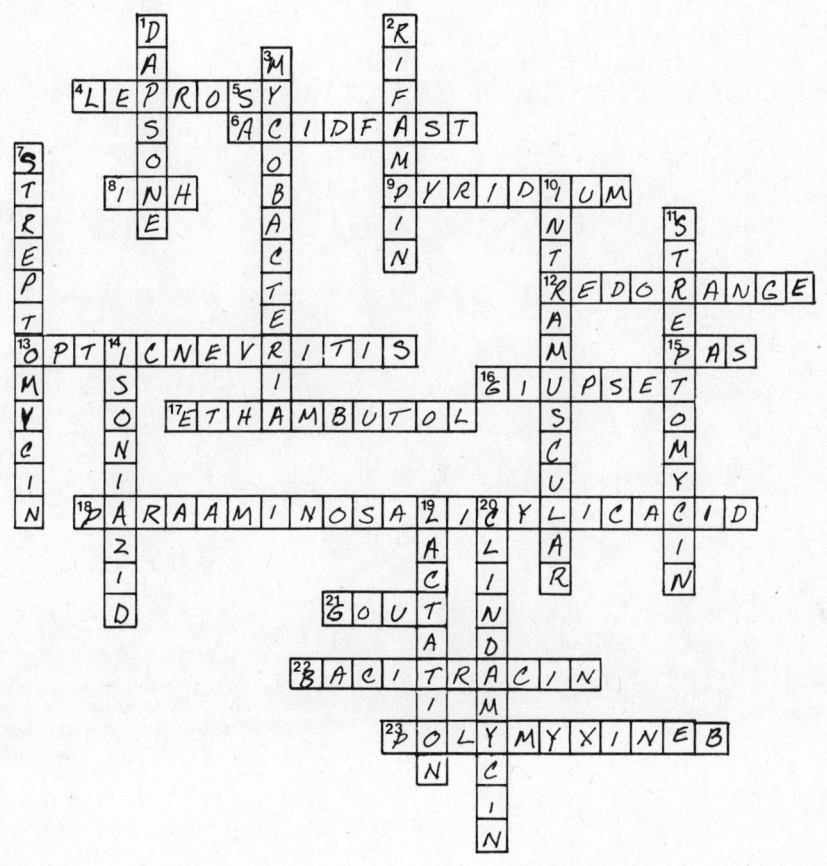

Matching

A. 1. e, f, g 2. d 3. a, c, d, f, h 4. b, c, d, f
   5. a, c, h 6. f, h 7. d, f, g
B. 1. b 2. c 3. d, e 4. a, c

Multiple Choice Questions

1. a 2. d 3. b 4. d 5. c 6. b 7. f 8. b
9. c 10. b 11. d 12. d

Selection of Options

1. a only 2. c only 3. a, c, d, f 4. a, c, g
5. b, c, e, f 6. d, f 7. a, d, f 8. a, c, d, e
9. d, e

Short Answer Questions

1. Tuberculosis and leprosy
2. Streptomycin
3. Ethambutol, isoniazid, rifampin
4. a. Rifampin
   b. Sweat, urine, feces, saliva, tears and cerebrospinal fluid tend to become orange-red in color
5. Increase fluid intake, perineal cleanliness from urinary meatus outward, applying and removing perineal pads from front to back, decreasing use of bath salts or bubble baths, decrease fecal contamination of perineum (bowel training programs, prompt cleaning after fecal incontinence), eliminate use of urinary catheters (bladder training)
6. To prevent activation of the drug by stomach acids

17
Drugs Used to Treat Infections Caused by Viruses and Fungi

Personal Experience: Antiviral and Antifungal Drugs

Drugs discussed in Chapter 17 that are most likely to have been used are fungicides (to treat athlete's foot or ringworm), vitamin C, and viral vaccines. You may find that you were not well informed in the past, either about methods for preventing nonbacterial infectious diseases or about the risks of such drugs.

Matching

A. 1. d 2. d 3. c 4. a 5. e 6. b 7. a
B. 1. b 2. a 3. e 4. g 5. a, d 6. c, g
   7. b 8. a

Short Answer Questions

1. a. Rubeola
   b. Acute infectious parotitis
   c. Rubella
   d. Varicella
   e. Poliomyelitis
   f. Variola
   g. Pertussis
2. The ability to reproduce
3. The property of forming crystals
4. Paralysis (anterior motor horn damage from defective Salk vaccine, Guillame Barre syndrome from swine flu vaccine), fever, malaise
5. Ringworm, athlete's foot, "jock itch," thrush, some types of diaper rash
6. Alcohol, witch hazel, tannic acid, zinc salts, aluminum salts
7. Promoting ventilation of superficial tissues by using absorbent porous clothing (e.g., leather shoes, cotton underwear); avoiding the use of oily application to the feet; avoiding the use of broad-spectrum antibiotics; boiling socks between wearings; alternating shoes to allow for thorough drying between wearings

Completion Exercises

1.

ANTIVIRAL COMPOUND	a. TRADE NAME(S)	b. THERAPEUTIC USES	c. ADVERSE REACTION(S)
Vidarabine	Vira-A	Treatment of herpes simplex keratitis, herpes simplex keratoconjunctivitis, herpes simplex encephalitis	Local inflammation
Idoxuridine*	Herplex Stoxil	Treatment of herpes simplex keratitis, genital herpes	Local inflammation; severe tissue inflammation when combined with boric acid
Azidothymidine	AZT	Palliative treatment of acquired immune deficiency syndrome (AIDS)	Bone marrow suppression
Acyclovir	Zovirax	Treatment of viral infections in immunosuppressed persons, genital herpes	Local inflammation

* Use of this drug remains experimental.

ANTIVIRAL COMPOUND	a. TRADE NAME(S)	b. THERAPEUTIC USES	c. ADVERSE REACTION(S)
Ribavirin	Virazole	Treatment of lower respiratory infections caused by viruses	Impaired respiratory and cardiac function

2. ANTIFUNGAL	a. ROUTE(S)	b. MODE(S) OF ACTION	c. ADVERSE REACTION(S)
Amphotericin B	Intravenous	Systemic (local when injected intrathecally or intra-articularly)	Chills and fever; GI upset
Clotrimazole	Topical; oral; intravenous	Local; systemic	Local tissue inflammation; GI upset
Griseofulvin	Oral	Systemic	Abnormal white cell counts; skin rash; photosensitivity; nephrotoxicity; elevated porphyrins
Ketoconazole	Oral	Systemic	GI upset; hepatotoxicity
Micanazole	Topical; oral; intravenous	Local; systemic	Local tissue inflammation; GI upset; skin rash

Correct the False Statement

1. F; preventing contact between virus and host and use of vaccines to stimulate active resistance
2. T
3. F; intravenously, orally, or topically
4. T
5. T
6. F; for reasons of safety; acute care settings

Multiple Choice Questions

1. c 2. a 3. d 4. c 5. b 6. c 7. d 8. c
9. a 10. c 11. d

Selection of Options

1. a, b, d   2. b, c, d   3. a, b   4. a, d, e, g
5. b, c, e   6. b, c, d, e   7. a, b, c   8. a, b

18
Drugs Used to Treat Rickettsiae, Protozoa, Helminths, and Ectoparasites

Matching

1. e   2. d   3. f   4. g   5. d   6. a   7. c
8. a, c   9. c   10. e

Short Answer Questions

1. a. Use insecticides as a last resort after employing all possible nonchemical control measures.
   b. Use as sparingly as possible to avoid environmental contamination.
   c. Follow directions regarding use carefully to minimize the risk of poisoning or of environmental contamination.
   d. Use protective clothing and procedures to minimize personal risk.
   e. Remove people, pets, and plants from areas in which spray, fog, mist, or "bomb" insecticides are to be used.
   f. Seek assistance of experts in the field of pest control for reliable instruction on the use of insecticides.
2. a. Use poisons as a last resort after employing all possible nonchemical control measures.
   b. Use as bait a substance (e.g., grain) that is not a usual food for children.
   c. Place the bait in places that are not accessible to children or pets.
3. a. Louse
   b. Scabies mite

Correct the False Statement

1. F; insecticides that are polychlorinated hydrocarbons
2. T
3. F; the addition of chloroquine to table salt
4. F; whites of Mediterranean origin and blacks
5. F; vegetative forms of the organism and abscesses caused by the protozoa, but not amebic cysts
6. T
7. F; reduction of the population of parasites and prevention of reinfection (severely affected persons cannot tolerate the vigorous treatment required for elimination of the parasite)
8. F; ova
9. T
10. T
11. T
12. F; should not be used; because the residues of the drugs are likely to contaminate the food
13. T
14. F; vinegar, laundry bleach

Multiple Choice Questions

1. d   9. d   17. b
2. a   10. c   18. b
3. d   11. c   19. b
4. a   12. b   20. a
5. d   13. d   21. c
6. c   14. e   22. b
7. c   15. d   23. c
8. b   16. a   24. b

Selection of Options

1. a, b, c   2. a, c   3. b, c   4. b, c   5. a, b, c
6. a, b, c, d   7. a, b, c

19
Antipyretics

Find the Hidden Words

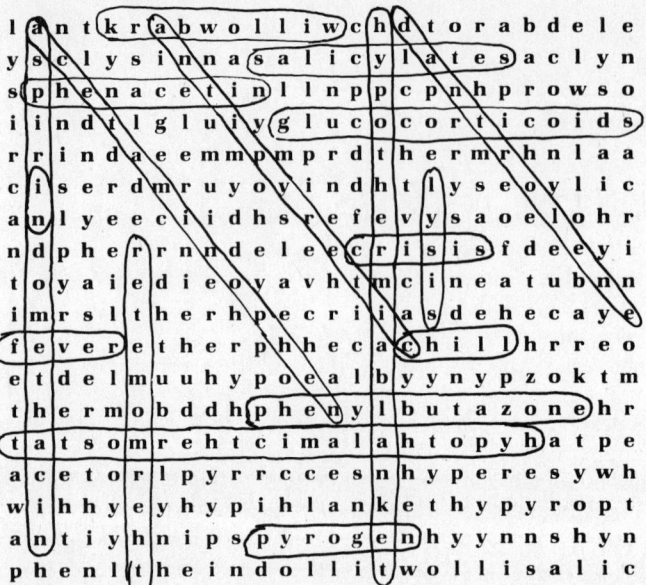

Matching

1. b, c, d   2. e   3. e   4. b   5. a

Multiple Choice Questions

1. b   2. b   3. a   4. c   5. b   6. d   7. c   8. f

Selection of Options

1. a, b, c   2. a, c

Short Answer Questions

1. A decrease in endogenous pyrogens that stimulate receptors on the hypothalamic cells controlling body temperature; resetting of the thermostat to a lower level; vasodilation, muscular relaxation, and sweating; a rapid lowering of body temperature.
2. Dehydration; nutritional depletion; stress on the heart; breakdown of enzyme systems; tissue damage (including brain damage)
3. Factors that vary directly with temperature are muscular activity, progesterone levels, and emotional excitement and infectious illness; a factor inversely related to temperature is age; time of day is also a factor, with temperatures highest about 10 to 14 hours after arising from sleep.
4. Take several successive temperatures under controlled conditions, preferably before arising from bed in the morning; average the data.
5. a. Immersion in tepid water
   b. Wrapping in hypothermia blankets

20
Agents Used in Debridement of Wounds

Matching

1. c 2. b

Correct the False Statement

1. F; a stinging sensation
2. F; 3%
3. T

Multiple Choice Questions

1. b 2. d 3. d 4. c 5. d 6. e

Crossword Puzzle

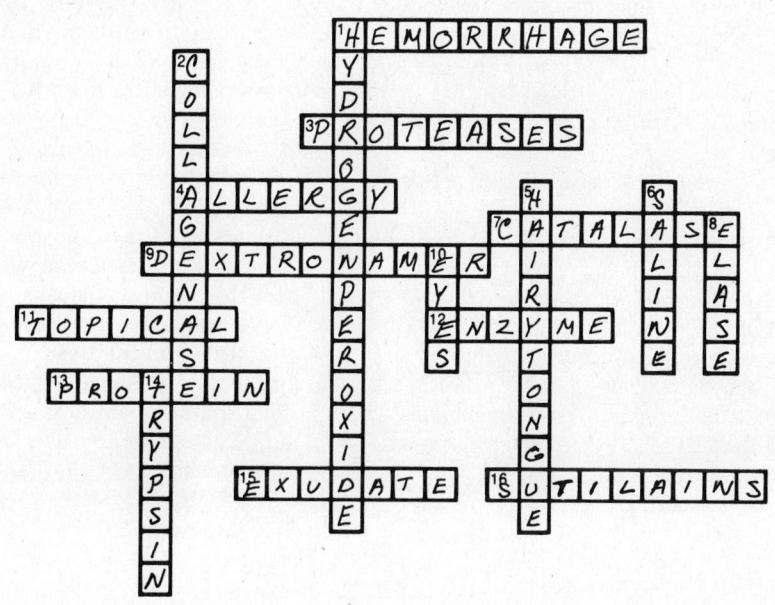

21
Anti-inflammatory and Related Agents

Matching

1. b 2. g 3. k 4. j 5. e 6. c

Short Answer Questions

1. Prostaglandins exist in increased concentrations in inflammatory exudates. The inflammatory process damages cell membranes and arachidonic acid is released. Arachidonic acid is a precursor of prostaglandins, and prostaglandin synthetase or cyclooxygenase catalyzes the conversion of arachidonic acid to intermediary substances. Certain prostaglandins promote the inflammatory process.
2. Many drugs inhibit the release of prostaglandin synthetase; thus, prostaglandin production will be decreased and, hence, pain will be decreased.
3. a. Anti-inflammatory property: acetylsalicylic acid's ability to inhibit prostaglandin synthetase
   b. Analgesic property: acetylsalicylic acid's ability to relieve pain
   c. Uricosuric property: acetylsalicylic acid's ability to increase the urinary excretion of uric acid, thereby reducing the concentration of uric acid in the blood
   d. Antipyretic property: acetylsalicylic acid's ability to reduce fever
4. a. Headache, neuralgia, myalgia, dysmenorrhea, arthralgia
   b. Rheumatic fever
   c. Rheumatoid arthritis
   d. Bartter's syndrome
5. Salicylism is mild salicylate intoxication, and usually occurs after repeated administration of large doses. This syndrome is characterized by headache, dizziness, tinnitus, decreased auditory acuity, dimness of vision, mental confusion, lassitude, drowsiness, sweating, thirst, hyperventilation, nausea, vomiting, and (occasionally) diarrhea.
6. Acetylsalicylic acid prevents the formation by the platelets of thromboxane A_2, a potent aggregating agent, through the acetylation of platelet cyclooxygenase. Platelets cannot regenerate the cyclooxygenase enzyme, apparently because they do not have the capacity for protein biosynthesis. A dose of acetylsalicylic acid inhibits the cyclooxygenase for the life of the platelet (8 to 11 days). Consequently, a single dose of acetylsalicylic acid approximately doubles the bleeding time of normal persons, for 4 to 7 days.
7. a. With meals or during meals
   b. With milk
   c. With antacids
8. Acetylsalicylic acid; warfarin; tolbutamide
9. Frontal headache
10. Para-aminophenol derivatives (phenacetin and acetaminophen) have the analgesic and antipyretic properties but not the anti-inflammatory or uricosuric properties of aspirin.
11. In this nephropathy papillary necrosis seems to be the primary lesion, with secondary chronic interstitial nephritis. The nephropathy is usually insidious in onset, but may progress to irreversible renal insufficiency. People at risk for this nephropathy are those who have taken large doses of analgesics over a period of years. It is believed that the nephrotoxic substance is phenacetin, which is available in over-the-counter analgesic mixtures.
12. Acetaminophen normally is detoxified by glutathione in the liver. Toxic doses of acetaminophen exhaust glutathione stores, allowing a toxic acetaminophen metabolite to accumulate and damage liver cells; acetylcysteine (Mucomyst)
13. 6 to 8 weeks
14. Skin lesions range from erythema to exfoliative dermatitis. The most common response is a rash with pruritus. Mucous membrane lesions include stomatitis, gingivitis, glossitis, pharyngitis, tracheitis, gastritis, colitis, and vaginitis. Some people have a metallic taste in their mouths or itching of the oral mucosa before stomatitis develops. A gray to blue pigmentation may occur in skin and mucous membranes, especially in areas exposed to light.
15. Agranulocytosis and aplastic anemia
16. Primary gout represents a group of inborn metabolic disorders causing hyperuricemia and deposition of sodium urate crystals in joints. Secondary gout occurs in certain diseases in which there is an increased breakdown of nucleic acids, producing hyperuricemia, or in patients who have an interference with renal excretion.

17. Its mechanism of action appears to involve the inhibition of the migration of leukocytes into the inflammed area. The net result is to decrease the inflammatory response, thus reducing the pain.
18. a. Prevention of hyperuricemia secondary to chemotherapy for neoplasms
    b. Treatment of drug-induced hyperuricemia (e.g., by diuretics)
19. Uric acid is formed by the xanthine oxidase-catalyzed oxidation of hypoxanthine and xanthine. Allopurinol inhibits the xanthine oxidase. This inhibition reduces plasma concentration and urinary excretion of uric acid and increases plasma concentration and renal excretion of uric acid precursors.
20. If penicillin and probenecid were given simultaneously, the effect of the probenecid would be to decrease the excretion of penicillin by inhibition of its tubular secretion. If the two drugs are given together, there are higher (double) concentrations and more prolonged concentrations of the penicillin in the plasma than when the penicillin is given alone.
21. There is the possibility of precipitating renal calculi because of the mobilization of urates. Uric acid tends to crystallize out of an acidic urine. Therefore alkalinization is recommended, and may be accomplished through the use of 3 g to 7.5 g of sodium bicarbonate daily or 7.5 g of potassium citrate daily.

22
Autonomic Drugs

Matching

A. 1. b 2. d 3. b 4. b 5. a 6. b 7. c
B. 1. b 2. b 3. a 4. b 5. a 6. b 7. a
   8. a

C. 1. b,e,i,k 2. c,j 3. a,l 4. d,g 5. b,f
   6. b,k 7. b,h

Find the Hidden Words

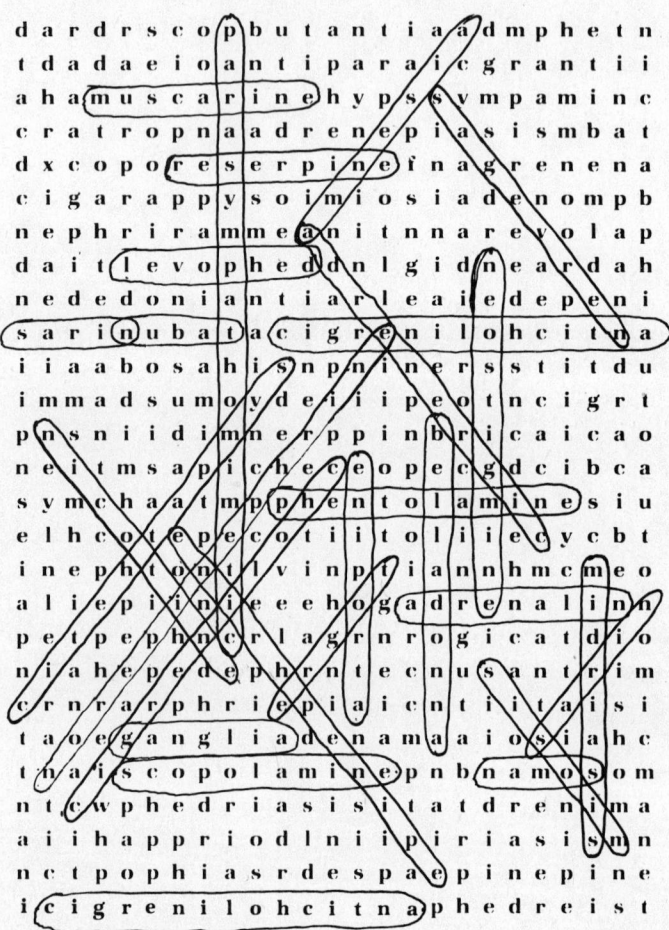

Correct the False Statement

1. F; longer
2. T
3. F; is not dependent on
4. T
5. F; discontinued 2 to 3 weeks prior to the surgery
6. F; anticholinesterases
7. T
8. F; muscarinic
9. T
10. T
11. F; gently compress the tear duct to reduce drainage of drug through this passageway

Completion Exercise

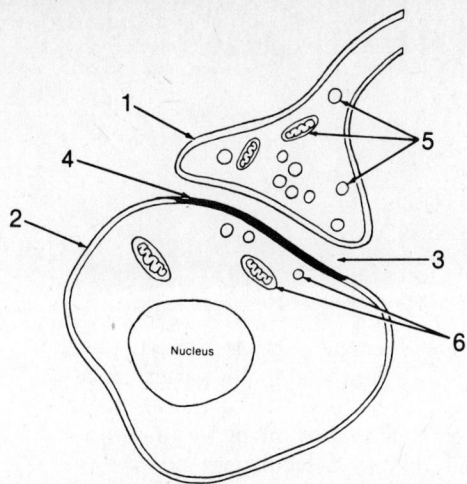

Multiple Choice Questions

1. b 2. d 3. c 4. d 5. a 6. b 7. c 8. c
9. d 10. c 11. c 12. b 13. b 14. c
15. a 16. b 17. a 18. b 19. e 20. e
21. d 22. a 23. c 24. a 25. d 26. d
27. c 28. b 29. c 30. b 31. a 32. d
33. c 34. b 35. b

Selection of Options

1. b, c 2. a, b, c, e 3. b, c 4. a, b, d, e
5. b, c 6. b, c 7. b, d, e 8. d only 9. b, c
10. a, b, d 11. a, b, c 12. a, b 13. a, c, d
14. b, c 15. a, b, c 16. b, c, d 17. a, c, e
18. a, c, d 19. a, c 20. b, c 21. a, b, d
22. a, b

Short Answer Questions

1. Brain; spinal cord
2. Cortex; brain stem
3. Respiratory; cardiac; vasomotor; appetite; vomiting
4. α_1-receptors, α_2-receptors, β_1-receptors, β_2-receptors
5. Nicotinic receptors; muscarinic receptors
6. Sympathomimetic (adrenergic); parasympathomimetic (cholinergic); sympatholytic (antiadrenergic, sympathetic blocking agents); parasympatholytic (anticholinergic)
7. Treatment of myasthenia gravis, glaucoma (as a miotic), intestinal atony, atony of the urinary bladder
8. The cranial nerves are part of the parasympathetic system.
9. Duration of effect in the person; mealtime; sleep–wake cycle (drugs are best taken before meals and before and after sleeping, but must be scheduled frequently enough to prevent respiratory arrest)
10. Nausea, salivation, abdominal pain, dizziness, change in hearing, change in vision, confusion, weakness, respiratory arrest, cardiovascular collapse, convulsions.
11. Cancer; peptic ulcer; obstructive airway disease; vascular degeneration; (in women) placental inadequacy, low-birth-weight babies
12. Failure to respond to a drug that develops rapidly on repeated administration of the drug

23
Central Nervous System Stimulants

Matching

A. 1. d 2. c 3. a

Short Answer Questions

1. Theophylline
2. Reduce stimuli; use cool colors (blue, green); keep client warm; give sedative massage
3. Nervousness, irritability, restlessness, agitation, tremor, insomnia
4. Wave the broken ampule before the client's face; administer only whiffs
5. Nausea, vomiting, weight loss, nasal septum perforation
6. Topical
7. A temporary return of signs and symptoms of drug effects although drug use has been discontinued
8. Decrease stimuli; therapeutic communication ("talking down")
9. Increased mental alertness; increased capacity for work; improved motor performance (particularly of skills that have been mastered); euphoria; stimulation of respirations, heart function, and metabolism
10. Tremor, restlessness, insomnia, impaired motor performance, hypertension, exhaustion
11. Treatment of narcolepsy; treatment of hyperkinesis, learning disabilities, and behavioral problems stemming from minimal brain dysfunction in children; treatment of catalepsy; initiation of weight reduction regimens

Find the Hidden Words

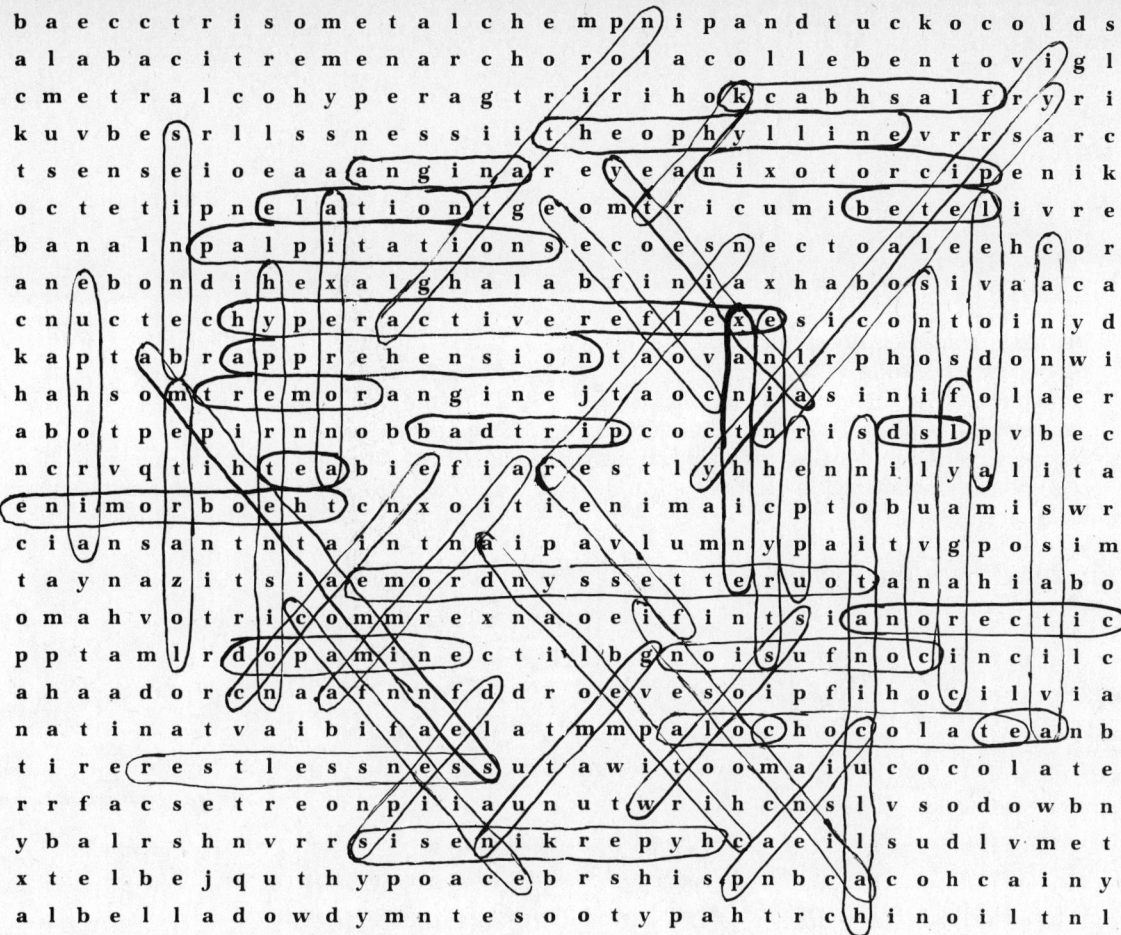

Correct the False Statement

1. F; stimulating release of endogenous neurotransmitters in the nervous system
2. T
3. T
4. F; impair
5. F; from an inactive substance to an active drug
6. F; it cannot cross the blood–brain barrier
7. F; a relatively high dose of levodopa to maintain brain tissue concentrations
8. F; 6 to 8 weeks
9. T
10. F; stimulants; depressants
11. F; agonists
12. F; descending
13. T
14. F; sometimes; do not always abolish
15. F; includes tissues perfused by endarteries, such as fingers, toes, ears, nose, or penis
16. T

Multiple Choice Questions

1. a 2. d 3. d 4. c 5. b 6. d 7. b 8. d
9. c 10. b 11. d 12. d 13. b 14. a
15. b 16. a 17. b 18. b 19. b 20. d
21. b 22. b 23. c 24. a 25. d 26. c
27. d 28. b 29. d

Selection of Options

1. a, b, d   2. a, c, e, f   3. a, b, d, e   4. b, c
5. a, b, c, d   6. b, c, d   7. c, d   8. a, b, c, d

24
Central Nervous System Depressants

Matching

A. 1. b 2. a 3. a 4. b 5. a 6. b 7. a
B. 1. c 2. b 3. a 4. a 5. d 6. b

Short Answer Questions

1. Lethargy, coma, cardiovascular collapse, respiratory arrest, death
2. Hypnotics the night before surgery; narcotic analgesics, tranquilizers, and anticholinergics preoperatively; rapid-acting induction agent; one or more inhalant anesthetics; oxygen; skeletal muscle relaxants
3. Gradual resumption of independence; halfway houses; self-help groups
4. Schedule IV
5. Yes, in some people
6. Eliminate stimuli; promote muscle relaxation; alleviate stress and anxiety; promote comfort; follow the client's personal bedtime ritual.

Find the Hidden Words

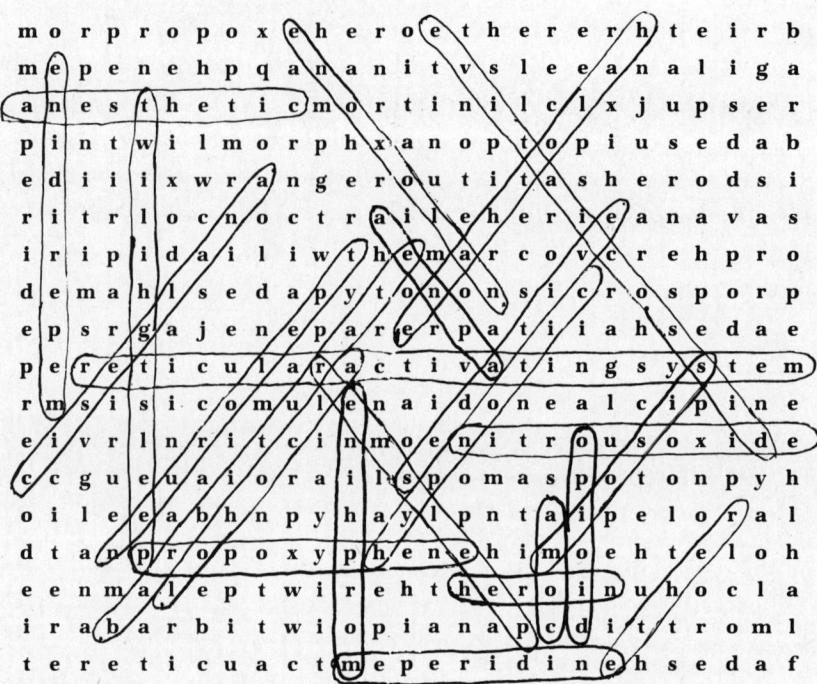

Correct the False Statement

1. T
2. F; only fractional parts
3. T
4. F; hyperthyroidism
5. T
6. F; double-locked cabinets
7. F; benzodiazepines
8. F; active metabolites
9. F; quiet activities
10. F; outside the bedroom or in the care of another person
11. F; central nervous system depressants
12. T
13. T
14. F; is neither more dangerous nor more difficult
15. F; central nervous system depressant
16. T
17. T
18. F; drying or astringent agent
19. T
20. F; disulfiramlike

308

Multiple Choice Questions

1. a 2. a 3. d 4. b 5. b 6. d 7. c 8. b
9. b 10. d 11. b 12. d 13. a 14. d
15. d 16. d 17. d 18. a 19. b 20. b
21. c 22. b 23. c 24. c 25. c 26. c
27. d 28. c 29. b 30. d 31. c 32. d
33. d 34. b 35. a 36. c 37. c 38. d
39. a 40. b 41. c 42. b 43. a 44. c
45. b 46. d 47. d 48. a 49. b

Selection of Options

1. a, b 2. c only 3. b, d 4. a, b, d
5. a, b, c 6. a, c, d 7. b, c, d 8. a, c, d
9. a, c 10. a, d, e, f 11. a, b, c, d 12. a, c
13. a, b, d 14. b, c 15. c only 16. a, b, c
17. a, c, d 18. b, c, d, e, f 19. a, b, d
20. a, c, d 21. a, b, c, e
22. a, b, c, d, e, f, g, h, i, j 23. a, b, d, e
24. a, b 25. a, b, d 26. a, d

25
Anticonvulsants

Correct the False Statement

1. F; occipital lobe
2. F; is not influenced when
3. F; whether or not
4. T
5. F; central nervous system depressants
6. T
7. T
8. F; phenobarbital and phenytoin
9. F; ethosuximide
10. T
11. F; impair
12. F; other weak acids
13. F; slow; 12 to 15 hours
14. T
15. F; binds highly
16. F; more
17. T
18. F; still carries a stigma

Short Answer Questions

1. Epilepsy is the name of a syndrome characterized by seizure disorder.
2. Seizure threshold is the relative level of excitation at which seizure activity is initiated in the brain.
3. Level of the basal seizure threshold; presence of foci that initiate abnormal stimuli; irritation of nerve cells as a result of biochemical changes in the body.
4. Eating regular meals; limiting salt intake; getting adequate rest and sleep; engaging in physical exercise; avoiding exhaustion; practicing good mental hygiene; avoiding alcoholic beverages; avoiding stimulant drugs; prevention or early treatment of infections
5. Shaving, bleaching the hair; electrolysis of hair follicles

Matching

1. a, b, c, f, g, h, i, j, n, o, p   2. c, e, i, j, k, l, m
3. a, i, n, q   4. c, d, h, i, r   5. c, e, h, i
6. e, h, k, s

Multiple Choice

1. d   2. c   3. b   4. b   5. c   6. a   7. b   8. d
9. d   10. a   11. b   12. c   13. a   14. d
15. d   16. b   17. a   18. c   19. c   20. b
21. b   22. c   23. c   24. d   25. d   26. d
27. c   28. b   29. a   30. b   31. d   32. a
33. d   34. b   35. d   36. e

Selection of Options

1. a, b, c, e   2. a, d   3. a, c, d   4. a, b, d, e
5. a, c   6. a, c, d   7. c, d   8. a, b, d   9. b, c

26 The Psychoactive Drugs

Multiple Choice Questions

1. a 2. d 3. d 4. a 5. a 6. b 7. d 8. f
9. b 10. a 11. c 12. a 13. d 14. a
15. c 16. a 17. d 18. a 19. a 20. c
21. d 22. c

Matching

A. 1. c 2. a 3. b 4. d
B. 1. d 2. a 3. e 4. b 5. c
C. 1. d 2. e 3. a 4. b 5. c
D. 1. b 2. c 3. d 4. a

Completion Exercises

1. Subcortical
2. Hypothalamus, limbic, reticular activating
3. Dopamine, acetylcholine, serotonin, norepinephrine
4. Antipsychotic, antianxiety, antidepressant–mood stabilizers
5. Endogenous, reactive, neurotic
6. Tricyclic and heterocyclic compounds, MAO inhibitors, antimanic drugs, psychomotor stimulants
7. Should not

Correct the False Statement

1. F; depression
2. T
3. F; may
4. F; voluntary

Short Answer Questions

1. a. Hypothalamus
   b. Reticular activating system
   c. Limbic system
2. Neurotic anxiety; neurotic or reactive depression; muscle spasticity; preoperative sedation; nonepileptic convulsions; status epilepticus; acute alcohol intoxication
3. Aged cheeses; red wines; chicken livers; beer; bananas; avocados
4. a. Lithium alters sodium transport in nerve and muscle cells, making it necessary to maintain an adequate salt and water intake.
   b. MAO inhibitors and tyramine interact to increase norepinephrine levels in the blood.

27
Cardiac Drugs

PART 1: CARDIOTONIC GLYCOSIDES

Correct the False Statement

1. T
2. T
3. F; enhancing tissue perfusion in the kidney
4. F; digitoxin
5. F; will not
6. F; congestive heart failure
7. F; palliative
8. F; a relative
9. T

Crossword Puzzle

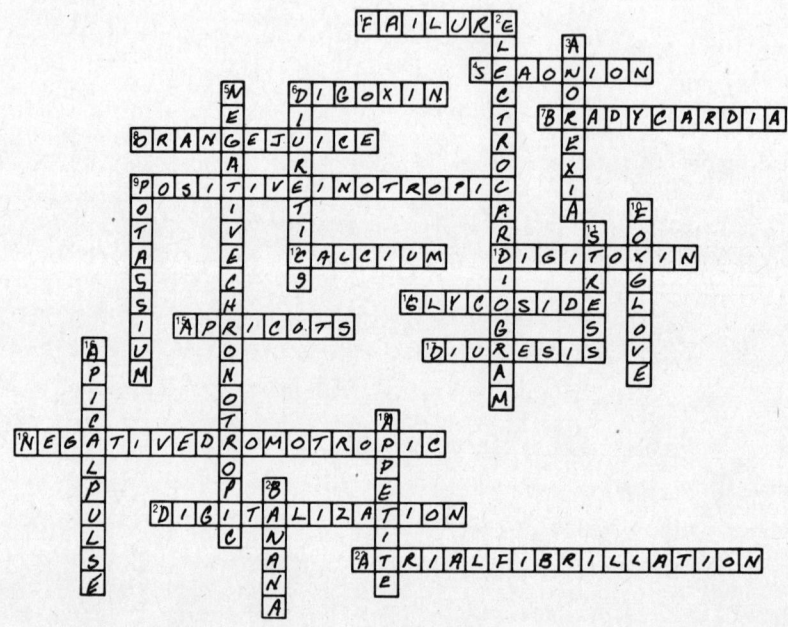

Multiple Choice Questions

1. c 2. a 3. d 4. b 5. b 6. b 7. d 8. a
9. d 10. b 11. c 12. b 13. c 14. b
15. b

Matching

A. 1. c 2. a 3. d
B. 1. a 2. c 3. e 4. d 5. f

Selection of Options

1. b, c, d, e 2. a, c 3. a, b, c 4. a, c, d, e, f
5. a, b, c 6. a, b, d 7. a, b 8. a, b, d, f, g
9. a, c, d 10. a, b, c, d, e 11. a, c, e 12. a, c
13. a, b, c, e, f, g

312

PART 2: ANTIARRHYTHMIC DRUGS

Correct the False Statement

1. T
2. F; adrenergic blocking agents
3. T
4. F; arterial embolism
5. T
6. F; hypoglycemia
7. F; brown
8. F; prolongation of repolarization

Multiple Choice Questions

1. a 2. d 3. b 4. a 5. d 6. d 7. c 8. a
9. d 10. c

Crossword Puzzle

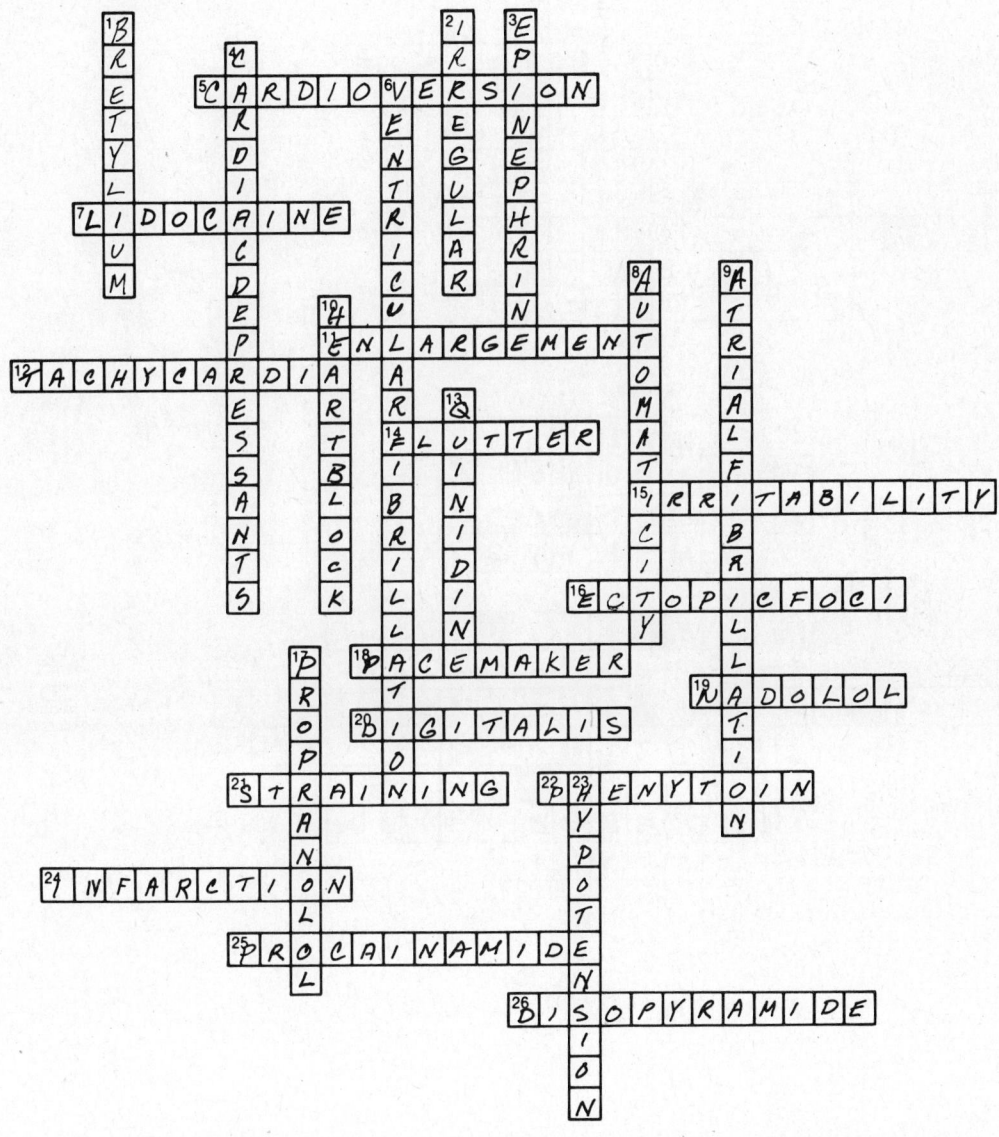

Selection of Options

1. a, b, c, d   2. a, b, c, d, e, f, g   3. a, d
4. a, b, d   5. b, d

28
Vascular Drugs

Anagram–Scrabble

1.
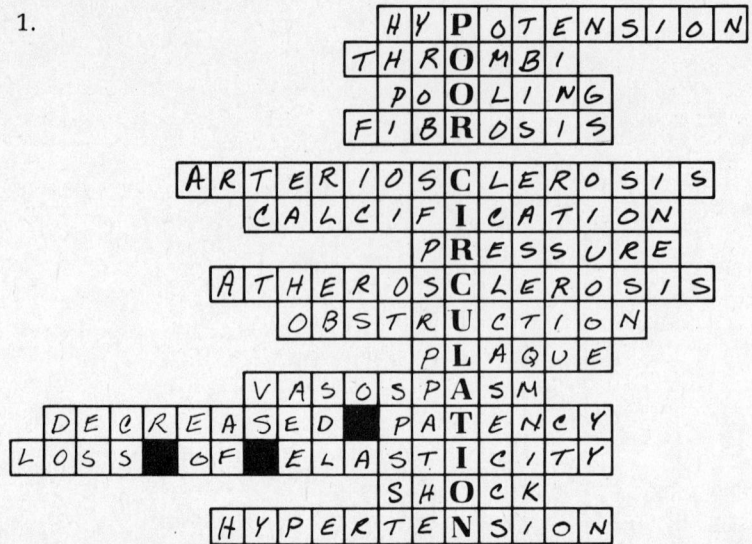

2.
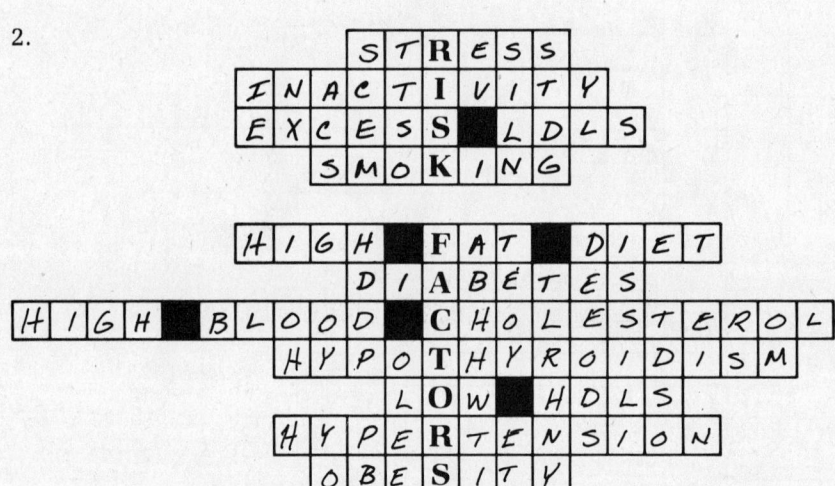

PART 1: ANTILIPEMIC DRUGS

Multiple Choice Questions

1. b 2. b 3. c 4. d 5. b 6. b 7. b 8. c
9. d 10. d 11. d 12. b 13. a 14. c
15. d

Correct the False Statement

1. T
2. F; renal impairment
3. F; does
4. F; are not; locally in the gastrointestinal tract
5. T
6. T
7. F; must be well diluted in fluids prior to ingestion
8. F; with food
9. F; do not indicate
10. F; do not indicate
11. F; cutaneous flushing and pruritus
12. F; dextrothyroxine
13. F; is highly bound
14. T

Selection of Options

1. b, d 2. a, b, c, d, e 3. a, b, d, e 4. a, b
5. a, b, d, e, f 6. a, b, d, e 7. b, c 8. a, c
9. a, b 10. b, d, f 11. a, c, d, e 12. b, c, d
13. a, b, c, d, e

Short Answer Questions

1. PO
2. In urine and feces
3. They are used only when older, more conventional methods of treatment are unsuccessful
4. Avoid inhaling the powder; mix the powder with ample fluids; do not administer with other drugs; advise an increased intake of fluid and fiber

PART 2: VASODILATORS

Find the Hidden Words

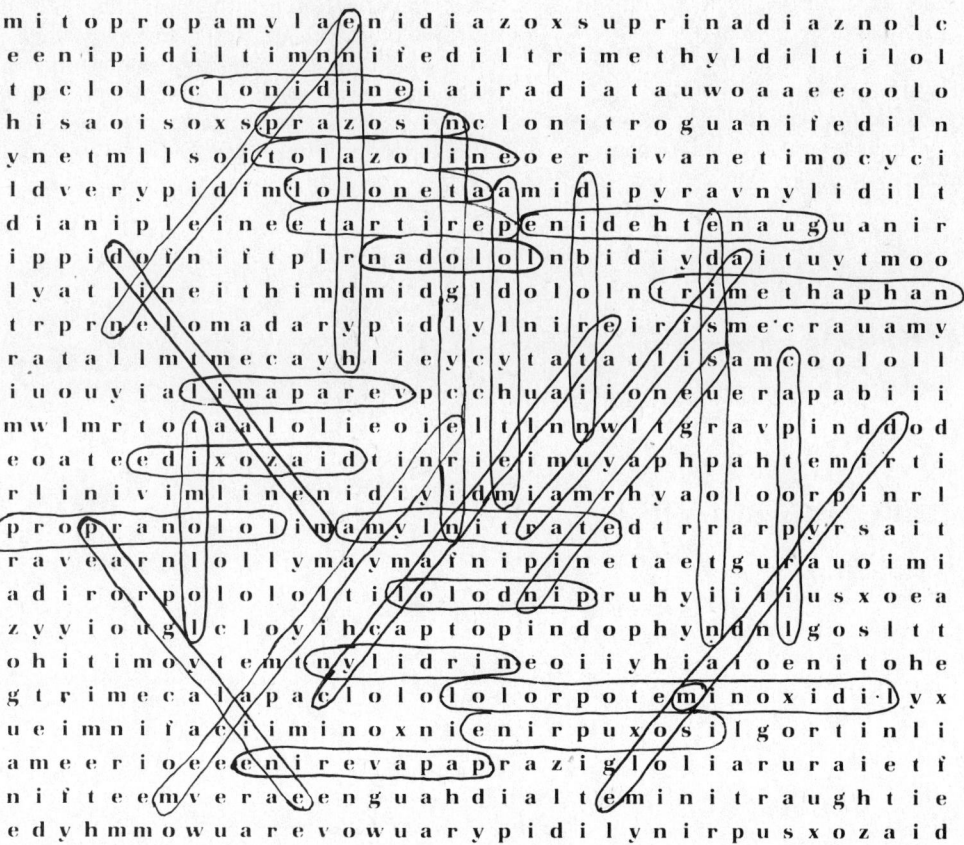

Multiple Choice Questions

1. c 2. c 3. b 4. d 5. d 6. a 7. b 8. b
9. b 10. d 11. c 12. a 13. b 14. c
15. d 16. b 17. c 18. c 19. d 20. b
21. b

Correct the False Statement

1. F; 140 mm Hg; 90 mm Hg
2. F; should be applied to the affected part (e.g., hands) because a local effect is desired
3. F; palliative
4. F; where they will be readily available, but away from body heat
5. T
6. F; do not cross the blood–brain barrier in significant amounts
7. T
8. T
9. T
10. F; several times a day
11. F; maintain hydration to decrease the risk of kidney damage

Selection of Options

1. a, b, d, e, g, h 2. a, b 3. a, c, d 4. a, d
5. d only 6. b, c 7. c, d 8. a, c 9. a, b, d
10. a, b, c, d, e 11. c, d, e 12. a, c, d, e

Short Answer Questions

1. Epinephrine, norepinephrine, angiotensin, vasopressin, prostaglandins (possibly)
2. Once daily
3. Three months after unsealing the bottle
4. Congestive heart failure, heart block; asthma, bradycardia, diarrhea, peptic ulcer, hypoglycemia, impotency
5. Place the client on a cardiac monitor; use an infusion pump or regulator; monitor vital signs; cover fluid reservoir in the intravenous infusion with opaque material; monitor drug solution for color changes; use intravenous line for no drugs except nitroprusside

PART 3: VASOCONSTRICTORS

Selection of Options

1. a, c, d 2. b only 3. c, d 4. a, b, c
5. b only

PART 4: SCLEROSING AGENTS

Multiple Choice Questions

1. d 2. d 3. b 4. a 5. a 6. a

Selection of Options

1. a, b, c, d, e, g, i 2. b, c 3. a, c 4. a, c

Short Answer Question

1. Doing active exercises; avoiding prolonged sitting or standing; avoiding use of constricting bands on the legs; avoiding obesity; limiting the number of pregnancies; using supportive hose

29
Drugs Affecting Coagulation

PART 1: HEMOSTATICS

Correct the False Statement

1. F; fresh whole uncitrated blood
2. F; calcium
3. T
4. F; through tubing containing a filter to remove solid particles
5. F; a continued tendency toward hemorrhage
6. T
7. F; fibrinolytic kinases
8. F; renal impairment
9. F; blood or blood plasma
10. T
11. F; acute hypotension

Multiple Choice Questions

1. b 2. d 3. b 4. c 5. b 6. a 7. d 8. c
9. b 10. c 11. c 12. a 13. b 14. d
15. a 16. a 17. c 18. b 19. b 20. b
21. b 22. a

Selection of Options

1. a, b, d 2. a, b, c 3. a, b 4. a, c, d, e
5. b, c 6. a, b, c 7. a, b, c 8. d only
9. a, d 10. a, b, c, d, f 11. b, c, d 12. a, d
13. c, d

Short Answer Questions

1. Damaged platelets release an enzyme that activates thromboplastin; thromboplastin catalyzes the conversion of prothrombin to thrombin; thrombin catalyzes the formation of fibrin from fibrinogen. Approximately twelve different biochemicals are involved in the process
2. Protamine sulfate molecules combine with heparin molecules so that the active sites of both drugs are buried within the molecule of the complex, rendering both physiologically inactive
3. Hypercoagulability, because intravascular thrombi disrupt circulation and perfusion promptly and disastrously
4. It is in limited supply; it requires intravenous infusion through filtered tubing; the drug is relatively unstable and requires careful handling and storage; it is a blood product and may (rarely) carry infectious organisms

PART 2: ANTICOAGULANTS

Correct the False Statement

1. F; but will not dissolve clots already formed in the blood vessels
2. F; improperly cured clover hay
3. F; two to three times
4. F; an inhibitor of platelet aggregation
5. T
6. F; decrease the therapeutic effect of the anticoagulant
7. F; delayed healing and dehiscence
8. F; heparin
9. F; citrate
10. F; heparin
11. F; coumarin

Multiple Choice Questions

1. b 2. c 3. b 4. c

Selection of Options

1. a, b, d   2. a, b, d, e, f, g   3. a, c   4. a, b, d
5. a, b, c, e, f   6. a, c, d

Short Answer Questions

1. No, it is destroyed by digestive enzymes
2. It results in large ecchymoses
3. No, they increase the risk of hemorrhage in the infant
4. Heparin
5. Aspiration is omitted; massage is omitted; an abdominal site is used
6. No, but intake should be kept stable
7. Yes, but dosages of coumarin may have to be adjusted when dosages of the other drugs are changed

Completion Exercise

	COUMARIN	HEPARIN
Mechanism of action	Inhibits prothrombin production by the liver by competing with vitamin K	Inhibits enzymes involved in several steps of coagulation
Route(s) of administration	PO	SC or IV
Unit of measurement of doses	mg	Units (bioassay)
Frequency of dosage	Once daily	Several times a day to continuous infusion
Onset of action	Days	Depending on route, immediate to less than an hour
Antidote(s)	Vitamin K, whole blood, or plasma	Protamine sulfate
Laboratory test for monitoring response	Prothrombin time (PT)	Partial thromboplastin time (PTT)
Toxic reaction	Hemorrhage	Hemorrhage
Other adverse reaction(s)	Allergy	Allergy

PART 3: FIBRINOLYTICS

Matching

1. a   2. a, c   3. b   4. a

Correct the False Statement

1. F; enzymes with protein structures
2. F; 6 hours for tAPT; 12–14 hours for SK and UK
3. F; intra-arterially or into the coronary artery

Multiple Choice Questions

1. d   2. b   3. b   4. b   5. b

Selection of Options

1. a, b, c, d   2. a, b, c, e   3. a, c   4. a, b

Short Answer Question

1. Store at temperatures less than 70°F; do not freeze; do not agitate when adding diluent; use solutions before they become outdated

PART 4: DRUGS THAT ENHANCE PERIPHERAL CIRCULATION

Selection of Options
1. a, d

PART 5: EXERCISES RELATING TO THE ENTIRE CHAPTER

Multiple Choice Questions
1. a   2. b   3. a   4. c

Short Answer Questions
1. Encourage client and family to express their concerns, acknowledge them and take appropriate action; perform procedures competently and efficiently; express a warm personal concern for the client and family; acknowledge the gravity of the situation but do not destroy hope.
2. Eliminate noxious stimuli (noise, glare, odors, pain); establish a trusting relationship with the client and offer realistic reassurance; anticipate the client's needs and take action to satisfy them; respond quickly to the client's requests for help; listen to the client's concerns; teach the client one or more techniques for stress management

30
Agents Affecting the Upper Gastrointestinal Tract

Matching

A. 1. a, b 2. a, b, d, e 3. a, b, c
B. 1. a, c, g 2. b, e, f 3. a, e, f 4. b, d, f

Crossword Puzzle

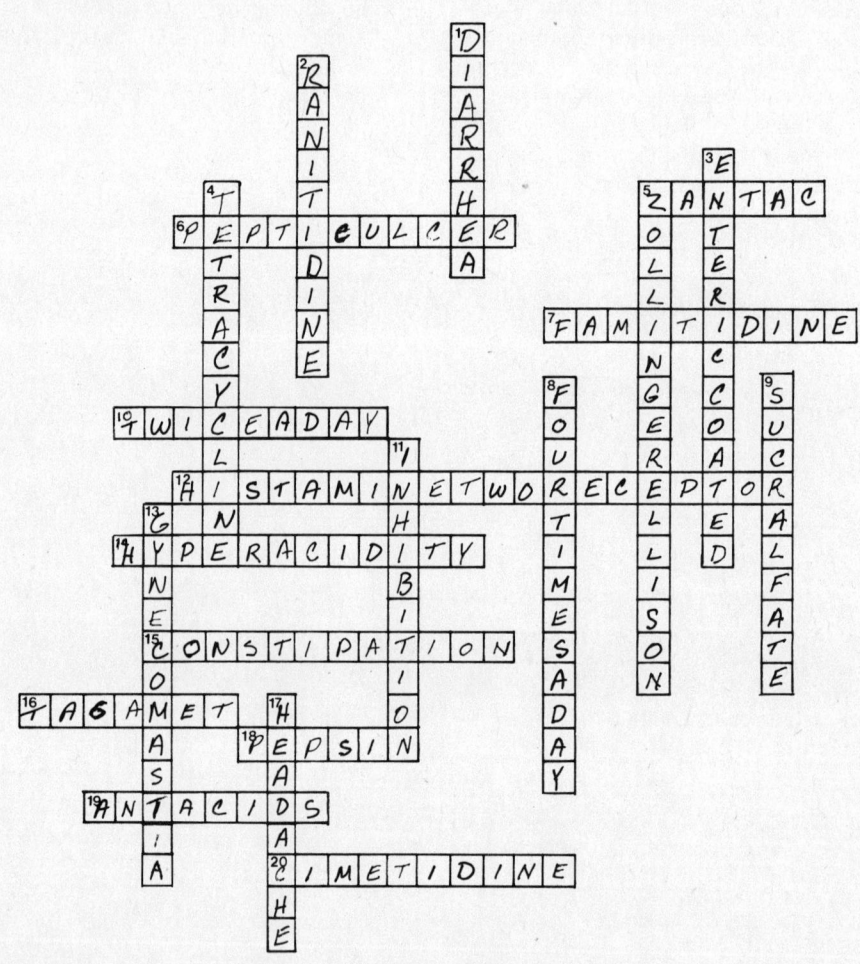

Correct the False Statement

1. T
2. F; whether they are applied topically or are ingested for systemic effect
3. F; age 6 years and older
4. F; sugars and starches
5. F; 15 minutes to 30 minutes
6. F; not exceed the dosage recommended on the label
7. F; soluble
8. T
9. T
10. F; with meals
11. T
12. T
13. F; acidic
14. F; liver
15. T
16. F; fat-soluble
17. T
18. F; histamine
19. F; act on different receptors than do the antihistamines
20. F; less than
21. T
22. F; do not readily cross
23. T
24. T
25. T
26. T
27. F; does not rule out
28. F; have not been established as safe
29. F; are not free from adverse side effects
30. T
31. T
32. F; both a comfort and therapeutic measure; adequate use of antacids may prevent or delay the development of esophageal peptic ulcers or strictures
33. F; local rather than systemic
34. F; no analgesic action
35. T
36. F; is contraindicated
37. F; will not be absorbed in appreciable amounts
38. F; the drug should be recovered by gastric lavage
39. F; the victim should always be evaluated by a physician
40. F; water should be given by mouth
41. T
42. T

Multiple Choice Questions

1. e 2. d 3. c 4. d 5. b 6. c 7. b 8. b
9. a 10. e 11. c 12. b 13. a 14. b
15. b 16. c 17. d 18. c 19. d 20. d
21. b 22. b 23. c 24. a 25. b 26. d
27. d 28. b 29. c 30. d 31. d 32. d
33. a 34. b 35. b 36. b 37. b 38. b
39. c 40. a 41. c 42. d 43. a 44. c
45. a 46. d 47. d 48. c 49. c 50. a
51. c 52. b

Selection of Options

1. a, b, d 2. a, c, d 3. b, c 4. a, c
5. a, b, c, d 6. b, d 7. c, d 8. b, c, d, e
9. a, b 10. b, c 11. b, c 12. a, b, c, d
13. a, e 14. a, b, c, d, e 15. a, b, c, e, g
16. a, d, f, h 17. a, b, d, e 18. d only
19. b, c, e 20. a, b 21. a, b, d 22. a, c, d
23. a, b 24. a, c, d 25. a, c 26. b, c
27. a, b, c, d 28. b, c 29. c, d, e
30. a, b, c, e 31. a, c 32. a, c, d, e 33. b, c
34. a, b, c, d

Short Answer Questions

1. Mix equal parts of salt and sodium bicarbonate.
2. a. Take $\frac{1}{2}$ tsp of sodium perborate and add water to make $3\frac{1}{3}$ oz of solution.
   b. Take $\frac{1}{4}$ tsp of sodium bicarbonate and add water to make $3\frac{1}{3}$ oz of solution.
   c. Take a scant $\frac{1}{4}$ tsp of sodium chloride and add water to make $3\frac{1}{3}$ oz of solution.
3. 0.9%
4. A drug preparation that contains small amounts of substances essential for breakdown of food into soluble, absorbable particles
5. Acids, bile, enzymes, choleretics
6. Dilute the solution 10–20 times; sip it through a glass straw; practice proper oral hygiene; rinse mouth with a mild alkaline solution; consume food immediately after taking HCl solution
7. Excessive hydrochloric acid production; inadequate pancreatic secretions; inadequate mucus secretion; impaired mucosal resistance to acid; inadequacy of cardiac sphincter; hypermotility of the stomach
8. An excessive number of acid-secreting parietal cells; inadequate mucus production; mucosal susceptibility to acid penetration; metabolism favoring excess production of chemicals such as histamine that stimulate acid secretion; diaphragmatic structure susceptible to development of a hiatal hernia; stress response patterns with a predominance of parasympathetic

nervous system activity; undue sensitivity to external stimuli that trigger acid secretion
9. A resurgence of acid secretion that follows elevation of gastric pH from the use of antacids
10. These are relatively new drugs, and there are likely to be adverse reactions that have not been recognized as yet
11. Smoking; ingestion of gastric irritants; high levels of stress; overeating; increased intra-abdominal pressure (e.g., from girdles)
12. Only in small amounts (less than 4 oz), because large amounts stimulate gastric emptying
13. From hourly to four times a day (after meals and at bedtime)
14. No, the daily costs of each are roughly comparable
15. Assuming institutional policy allows it, yes, provided amounts used are monitored and the client is taught how to use the medication
16. Usually not—side effects of and adverse reactions to various preparations are usually different
17. Mostly (unabsorbed) in the feces; the small amount that is absorbed systemically is eliminated by the kidneys
18. They should be chewed thoroughly or dissolved by sucking them before swallowing
19. An emetic is a substance that induces vomiting
20. An antiemetic is a substance that reduces nausea and vomiting
21. Scopolamine
22. Hallucinations, disorientation, confusion
23. Vomiting involves the forceful expulsion of stomach contents and usually results in larger volumes of emesis than does regurgitation
24. No, because many antiemetics have adverse effects on the fetus
25. Poisoning caused by strong acids, strong alkalies, bleaches, and liquid lipids such as petroleum distillates
26. If vomiting is not contraindicated, stimulation of the back of the throat with a finger may be used to induce gagging and vomiting

Personal Exercise: Self-Medication

The consumer needs to distinguish the various signs and symptoms of upper gastrointestinal problems: heartburn, pain (sharp, burning, gnawing), distention, nausea, vomiting, regurgitation. For short-term treatment, it is necessary to match these signs and symptoms with those described by the medication label as appropriate for use of the drug. Some trial and error is required to determine the best agents for an individual. The consumer needs to know that severe or persistent problems require the attention of a physician. If more than one drug is effective, the consumer should compare the prices for comparable doses and choose the most economical preparation.

31
Agents Affecting the Lower Gastrointestinal Tract

Correct the False Statement

1. T
2. F; are contraindicated for
3. F; the bulk-forming laxatives
4. T
5. T
6. F; 1 to 2 minutes
7. F; increases sympathetic nervous activity
8. F; bulk-forming laxatives
9. T
10. F; too toxic
11. F; are not effective
12. F; removing irritants and toxins from the intestines

Crossword Puzzle

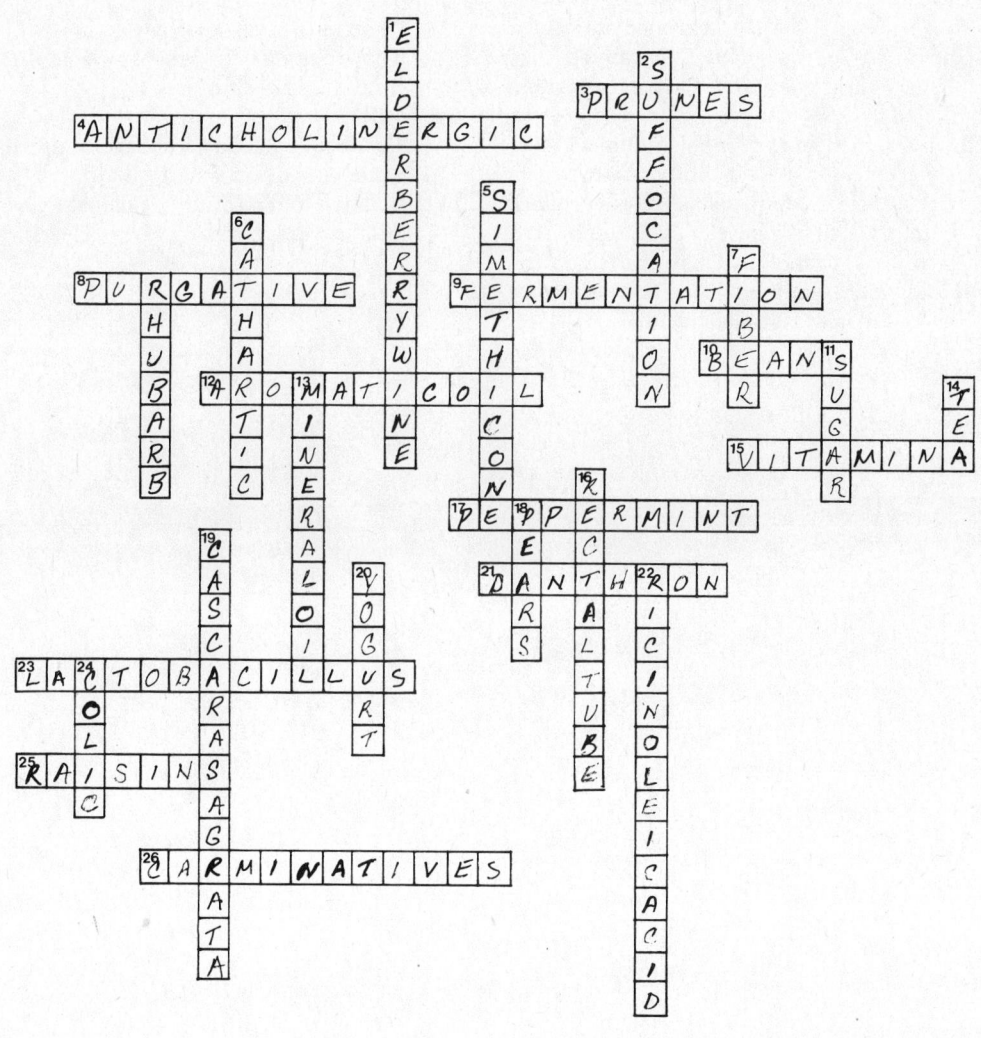

Multiple Choice Questions

1. a 2. c 3. c 4. b 5. a 6. b 7. b 8. a
9. c 10. b 11. c 12. d 13. b 14. a
15. d 16. b 17. c 18. c 19. d 20. b
21. c 22. a 23. a 24. d 25. b 26. c
27. d 28. a 29. a 30. b 31. a

Selection of Options

1. b, c, e 2. b, c 3. a, b, c 4. b, c
5. b, c, d 6. a, c, d, e, f 7. a, b, d 8. a, d
9. a, b, d 10. a, b, d 11. a, c, d 12. a, d, e, f
13. a, c, e 14. b, c 15. c, e 16. b, c
17. a, b, d, e 18. a, c, e, f 19. a, c, d
20. a, b, c, e

Short Answer Questions

1. a. The passage of frequent, semiliquid, or liquid stools
   b. The passage of infrequent, hard stools
   c. A drug that stimulates defecation
   d. A chemical able to hold other chemicals on the surface of its molecules
2. They are relative terms denoting the strength of action of the agents; purgatives are the strongest, cathartics are intermediate, while laxatives are the most gentle. (Laxative is also used as a class title to refer to all agents that induce defecation.)
3. Effectiveness in producing defecation; inability to affect the stomach; inability to produce a systemic effect if absorbed; inability to produce discomfort such as nausea or cramping
4. Figs, prunes, pears, raisins, rhubarb, coffee
5. Bile and pancreatic enzymes convert castor oil to the irritant ricinoleic acid.
6. Glycerin, lactulose, magnesium hydroxide, magnesium sulfate, sodium phosphate, sorbitol
7. Increased fiber in the diet; ample hydration; exercise; regular habits of defecation
8. Lack of exercise; lack of privacy; disruption of usual defecation patterns; fasting; fluid restriction; use of depressant drugs
9. Tea, blackberries, blueberries, elderberries
10. Charcoal, chalk, kaolin, pectin
11. They inhibit intestinal absorption of beneficial nutrients and drugs
12. Irritation
13. Gas-forming foods (cabbage, onions, beans); artificial sweeteners (saccharin or cyclamates); laxative foods (prunes, raisins, figs, rhubarb, pears, bran); coffee

32
Steroid Hormones and Their Antagonists

Matching

1. a 2. c 3. b 4. a 5. a

Correct the False Statement

1. T
2. F; do occur even though
3. T
4. F; on arising
5. T
6. F; live vaccines such as oral polio vaccine
7. F; insomnia
8. F; high concentrations of drug are not legal in over-the-counter preparations
9. T
10. F; altering enzyme function in the renal tubule
11. F; sodium reabsorption and potassium excretion
12. T
13. F; glucose tolerance test
14. T
15. F; hypertensive crisis
16. F; a 20-gauge or larger needle
17. F; fluorocortisone
18. F; more
19. F; by adrenals as well as by the gonads
20. T
21. T
22. F; anabolism
23. T
24. F; exert some masculinizing effects
25. F; increased
26. F; estrogens
27. F; less
28. T
29. F; cyproterone acetate
30. F; less markedly
31. T
32. T
33. F; chlorotrianisene
34. F; do
35. F; considerably lower than
36. T
37. T
38. F; less soap (or more oils)
39. F; fertility drug
40. T
41. T
42. F; increase

Short Answer Questions

1. General debility; hypovolemia; weak heart action; hypotension; tendency toward shock; intestinal colic; increased skin pigmentation
2. Yes, and they may produce systemic effects.
3. Hyperglycemia and increased risk of diabetes mellitus; osteoporosis and increased risk of bone fracture; hypertension; hypernatremia; hypokalemia; decreased resistance to infection; increased risk of abnormal clotting; insomnia; signs and symptoms of peptic ulcer of hyperacidity; abnormal hirsutism; menstrual disturbances; infertility; striae; delayed healing
4. Complete blood count (especially red blood count); electrocardiogram; blood pressure; blood chemistry tests (especially glucose, sodium, potassium, and cholesterol); chest and spinal x-ray; glucose tolerance test; height, weight; growth status in children; signs and symptoms of infection; intraocular pressure
5. Because response to these medications fluctuates with stress levels
6. They produce a marked increase in sodium retention and potassium excretion, a secondary increase in water retention and extracellular fluid volume, and decreases in body fluid concentrations of potassium and hydrogen ions
7. Edema, hypernatremia, hypervolemia, hypokalemia, alkalosis, increased blood pressure, cardiac enlargement, cardiac arrhythmias, headache, arthralgia, tendon contractures, congestive heart failure, cerebrovascular accident, weakness, intestinal atony or paralytic ileus
8. Tissue turgor, blood pressure, body weight, serum electrolyte concentrations, muscle strength, cardiovascular function, intestinal function, emotional status
9. Premature cessation of growth; permanent impairment of fertility; cancer of the liver
10. They are sometimes helpful, but their use should be avoided or delayed because of the risk of permanent impairment of fertility or

short stature caused by early closure of the epiphyses.
11. No, they can impair sexual response, produce permanent infertility, and increase the risk of cancer of the liver.
12. A diet abundant in fluids, high in protein, adequate for calcium and calories, high in minerals and vitamins
13. Androgens
14. Estrogens
15. Yes, unless a penile prosthesis is implanted.
16. Not until growth is complete, because estrogens can cause premature closure of the epiphyses.
17. Surgical castration prior to the age of menopause; acute symptoms of menopause such as severe hot flashes or dyspareunia; family history of dowager's hump or brittle bones
18. Cancer of the body of the uterus, hypertension, diabetes mellitus
19. Bleaching of dark hairs, electrolysis of hair roots
20. Clomiphene, tamoxifen

Multiple Choice Questions

1. d 2. b 3. b 4. d 5. a 6. c 7. d 8. b
9. c 10. b 11. b 12. a 13. a 14. d
15. b 16. b 17. b 18. d 19. c 20. a
21. c 22. c 23. c 24. d 25. b 26. d
27. d 28. a 29. c 30. b 31. b 32. b
33. d 34. d 35. d 36. c 37. b 38. d

Selection of Options

1. a, b 2. a, d, e, f, h 3. a, b, e 4. c, e
5. a, b, c, f, g 6. a, b, d, e 7. a, b, c, d
8. a, b, c, d, e, f, g, h, i, j, k, m, n 9. a only
10. b, d 11. a, c, d 12. a, b, c 13. a, c
14. a, b, c, e 15. b, d 16. a, b, d, e, f
17. b, c 18. a, c, d 19. b, c 20. a, c, d, e, f
21. a, c 22. b, c, e, g, h 23. b, c 24. b, c
25. b, d, e 26. a, b, d, e

33
Protein Hormones: Insulin and Other Drugs Affecting Blood Glucose

Correct the False Statement

1. T
2. T
3. T
4. F; never (because it is destroyed by intestinal peptidases)
5. F; do not require
6. T
7. T
8. F; more slowly than
9. F; discarded as unfit for use
10. F; generally opposite to
11. F; does not differ from
12. T

Short Answer Questions

1. Insulin, glucagon, somatotropin, thyrotropin
2. In urine by the kidneys
3. Increased blood sugar level
4. Interrupted insulin therapy; family or personal history of allergy
5. To decrease the risk of lipodystrophy
6. No, not until therapy has stabilized the diabetic condition
7. Reduced blood sugar, increased adiposity; accelerated cardiovascular degeneration; stimulation of production of insulin antibodies; (in toxic doses) hypoglycemia, sympathoadrenal discharge, headache, stroke, coma
8. Temperature of 60° to 70°F; darkness; protection from agitation; protection from freezing
9. Sugar (candy, sweetened orange juice), glucagon
10. The regular insulin
11. Every 20 minutes
12. 30 minutes
13. 1 to 2 hours

Multiple Choice Questions

1. a 2. d 3. b 4. c 5. d 6. c 7. b 8. d
9. b 10. b 11. b 12. b 13. c 14. a
15. b 16. a 17. b 18. d 19. b 20. d
21. b 22. a 23. c 24. c 25. d 26. a
27. a 28. d 29. c 30. a 31. d 32. b

Selection of Options

1. a, b, d 2. a, c, e, f 3. a, d, e
4. a, b, d, e, f 5. a, b, d 6. a, e 7. a, b, c, d
8. b, c 9. a, b, c, e, f 10. a, c 11. b, d
12. b, c 13. b, d 14. a, b, c 15. d only
16. b, c 17. b, c, d 18. a, b, d 19. a, d
20. a, b, d 21. a, b, d 22. b only 23. a, c

34
Thyroid, Parathyroid, Pituitary, and Hypothalamic Hormones

PART 1: THYROID, PARATHYROID, PITUITARY, AND HYPOTHALAMIC HORMONES

Correct the False Statement

1. F; polypeptide
2. T
3. T
4. F; Paget's disease
5. F; tetany
6. F; tyrosine
7. T
8. F; hours to days
9. T
10. F; are not appropriate for use in
11. T
12. T
13. F; with ample fluids
14. T
15. F; in tracer doses
16. F; gamma rays
17. T
18. T
19. F; increases
20. F; 1000 times
21. F; thyroid malignancies whose cells concentrate iodine
22. F; and is also effective against metastatic lesions
23. T
24. F; whenever radionuclides are employed, whether in tracer or therapeutic doses
25. T
26. F; are not effective
27. F; reacting with a receptor on the membranes of target cells
28. T
29. F; once a day for several days
30. T
31. F; warm the vial

Short Answer Questions

1. Decreased calcium ion absorption by the intestine; decreased serum calcium ion concentration; decreased bone resorption; increased calcium ion excretion by the kidneys
2. Nervousness; restlessness; insomnia; a tendency toward weight loss; hyperphagia; increased body temperature; diaphoresis; increased basal metabolic rate; an increased protein-bound iodine
3. Cretinism, myxedema, iatrogenic hypothyroidism (secondary to surgical removal of the gland or chemical ablation of thyroid tissue)
4. Generally not, although the urine will be radioactive. Following administration of the dose, it is only necessary that the client reside where a large sewage disposal system serves the residence.
5. Propylthiouracil, methimazole
6. Support of optimal hormone production; (in high doses) inhibition of hormone secretion by the thyroid and promotion of goiter formation
7. 10 days to 2 weeks
8. The Great Lakes' basin
9. Alpha particles; beta particles; gamma rays
10. Rad, curie, rem
11. Chronic progressive degenerative conditions characterized by remissions and exacerbations
12. Freezing, heat, agitation
13. Apparently not. In adults, when the pituitary gland is destroyed or removed, lack of the hormone appears innocuous even though, theoretically, hyperglyemic response to stress would be reduced.
14. Yes, for severely hypothyroid clients whose weakened hearts may fail under the stimulus of increased thyroid hormones
15. Renal tubules and smooth muscle of blood vessels

Multiple Choice Questions

1. c 2. b 3. b 4. a 5. b 6. d 7. a 8. a
9. c 10. c 11. c 12. b 13. a 14. d
15. a 16. c 17. b 18. c 19. c 20. d
21. c 22. c 23. d 24. b 25. a 26. d
27. a 28. b 29. b 30. a 31. a 32. c
33. d 34. d 35. d

Selection of Options

1. a, c, d 2. a, d 3. b, d, e, f 4. a, b, d
5. c, d 6. a, b 7. b, c 8. a, c, d
9. a, b, c, d 10. b, c 11. a, c 12. a, d
13. a, b, d 14. b, c 15. b, c 16. b, c, d
17. a, b, d 18. a, b, c, e, g 19. c only
20. a, b, d 21. c, d, e, f, g, j, l 22. f, g, h
23. b, c

PART 2: EXERCISES RELATING TO HORMONES IN GENERAL

Matching

A. 1. g 2. c or e 3. f 4. l 5. h 6. i 7. d
   8. b 9. j 10. k
B. 1. b 2. d 3. a 4. c 5. b 6. b
C. 1. c 2. a 3. d
D. 1. d 2. b 3. c 4. a 5. e 6. h 7. g

Correct the False Statement

1. F; multiple, acting on a number of sites
2. F; protein (or glycoprotein) hormones
3. F; often

Short Answer Questions

1. Steroid, glycoprotein
2.

3. Cholesterol
4. A primary deficiency of corticosteroids caused by adrenal failure
5. Drug requirements are highly variable, therapeutic goals may be variable, and hormones cause many side effects

Multiple Choice Questions

1. a 2. b 3. b

Selection of Options

1. a, e, f, g, h 2. b, d, e 3. a, b, c
4. b, c, d, f 5. b, c, e 6. b, c, e, f

Crossword Puzzle

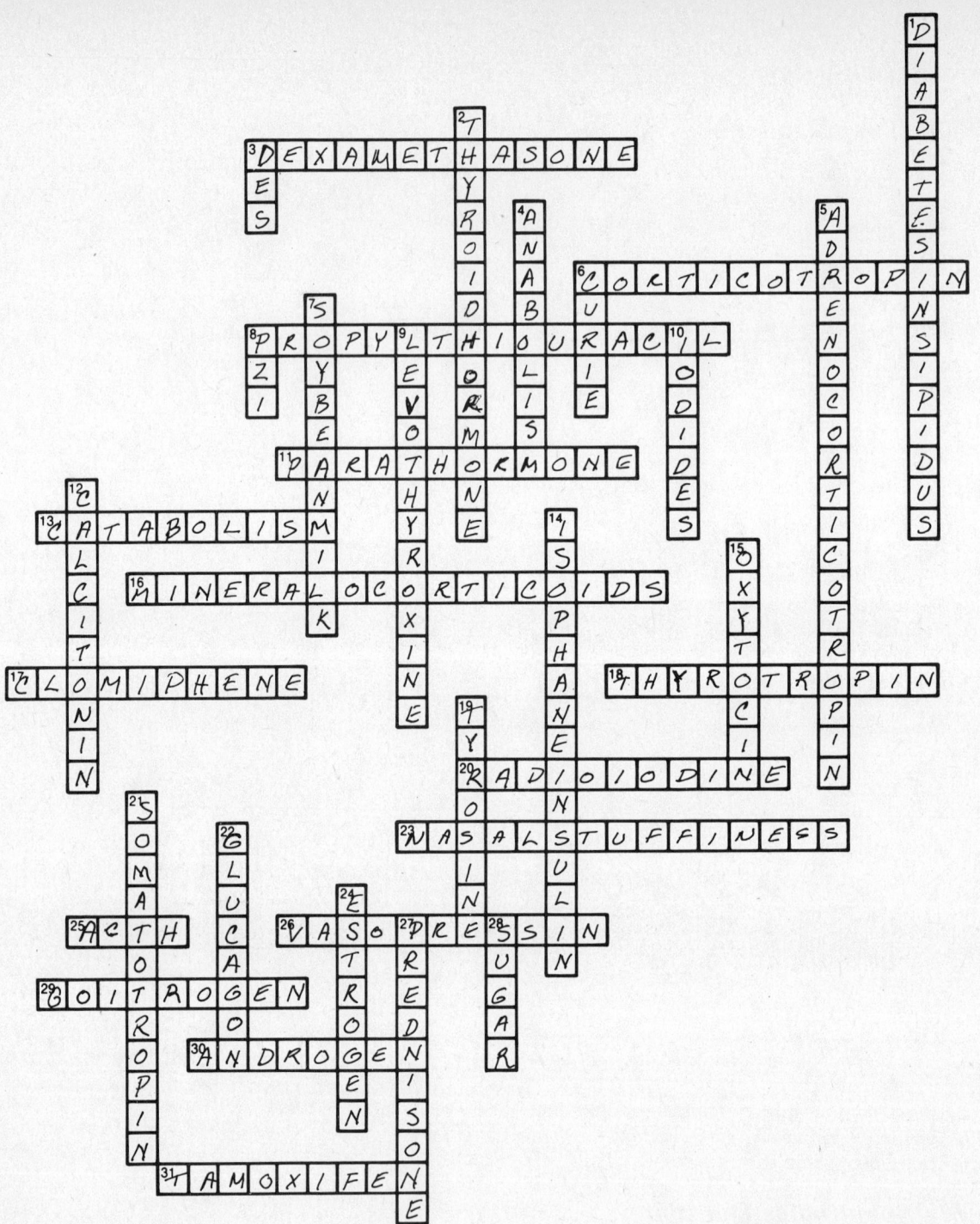

35
Drugs Affecting the Respiratory Tract

Short Answer Questions

1. a. P refers to partial pressure—tension. A gas contains molecules, and the molecules can collide with those of other gases. We breathe air that is a mixture of gases which vary as to concentration. Each gas exerts its own pressure, independently of others, on the molecules of other gases. This pressure is called "partial pressure" and is expressed as P. The amount of pressure created by any one gas is referred to as its partial pressure.
   b. PO_2 is the partial pressure of oxygen.
   c. PCO_2 refers to the partial pressure of carbon dioxide.
   d. PaO_2 refers to the partial pressure of the oxygen in the arteries.
   e. $PaCO_2$ is the partial pressure of the arterial carbon dioxide level. (Note: $PACO_2$ refers to alveolar carbon dioxide partial pressure.)
2. a. Refers to the amount of oxygen dissolved in plasma. Expressed as the partial pressure, it is the force that the oxygen molecules exert trying to escape from the solution they are in.
   b. Refers to the percent of saturation of hemoglobin with oxygen content of the blood. Blood leaving the lung usually has a pressure of 100 mm Hg.
   c. Force is required to move air along the airways because resistance is encountered to the airflow. This resistance comes from the bronchi and smaller airways. Compliance refers to the elastic properties of the lungs and wall of the chest. Compliance may change as a result of disease and this affects airway resistance. Infections, mucus, and change in surfactant can also affect airway resistance. Asthma, bronchitis, and emphysema all affect airway resistance.
   d. Refers to constriction of the bronchi
   e. Carbon dioxide narcosis is a condition where, because of disease, the person has high blood levels of carbon dioxide, which he or she is unable to remove. The $PaCo_2$ levels are high. As a result, the person may be in a coma and the driving force for breathing is no longer carbon dioxide but rather low levels of oxygen.
   f. A lipoprotein that decreases the surface tension of fluids in the alveoli and prevents alveolar collapse
   g. Decreased level of oxygen in body cells and tissue
   h. Increased ventilation; deep, rapid, or labored respiration; increased respiratory rate (normal after exercise)
   i. Decreased levels of carbon dioxide in tissue
   j. Capacity of oxygen in carbon dioxide to diffuse across pressure gradients; ability of the gases to interpenetrate
   k. Bluish coloration of the skin and mucous membranes as a result of reduced or deoxygenated hemoglobin in the blood
   l. Lack of oxygen; may be local or systemic; may be mild to total lack of oxygen (not specific in terms of amount)
   m. Cardiac disease as a result of long-standing pulmonary disease with pulmonary hypertension. Right ventricular hypertrophy results from the obstruction of airways, leading to pulmonary vasoconstriction as a result of hypoxia and acidosis.
3. It filters, warms, and moistens inspired air.
4. The air is no longer warmed and humidified and that injures the respiratory tree.
5. It carries sputum and debris up out of the alveoli and lungs whereby it can be coughed out. It also protects against infection and keeps the respiratory tract moist.
6. Smoking, emphysema, pollutants
7. Respiration is the process by which oxygen and carbon dioxide are exchanged between the atmosphere and cells of the body. Movement of air into the lung is *inspiration* and movement of air out of the lung is *expiration*. Usually this occurs passively, though we can control it to make it active, or voluntary. The body senses peripherally and in the brain the need for oxygen and alveolar ventilation adjusts to needs. The respiratory center in the brain is sensitive to changes in *acidity* and the level of carbon dioxide. Oxygen sensors in the carotid and aortic bodies monitor the oxygen level.
8. Allergic response leading to bronchospasm and constriction:

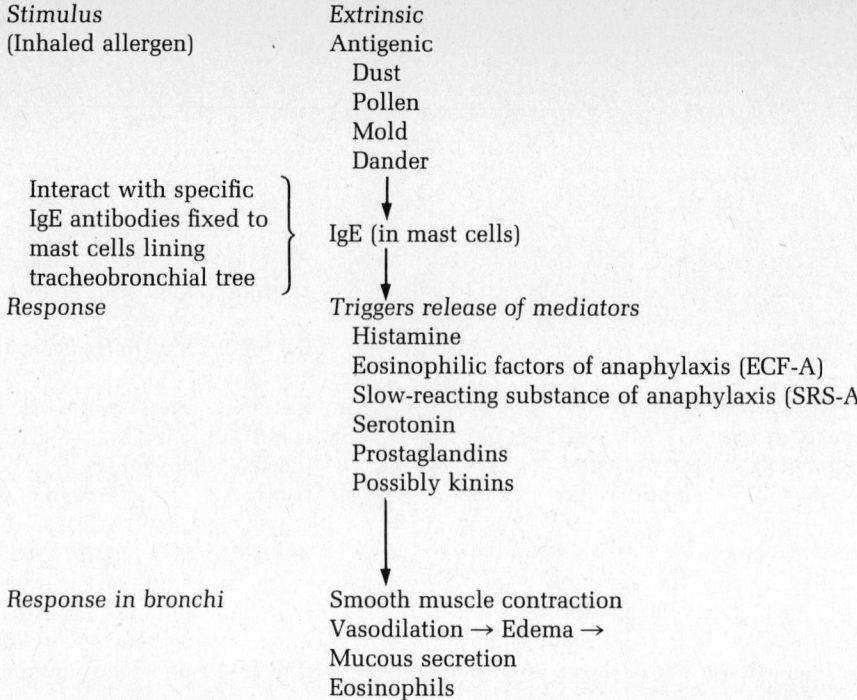

9. Theophylline inhibits phosphodiesterase. Phosphodiesterase is an enzyme that degrades cyclic 3',5' adenosine monophosphate (Cyclic Amp). If you inhibit phosphodiesterase, there is an increase of Cyclic Amp. Cyclic Amp inhibits the release of slow-reacting substance of anaphylaxis (SRS-A) and histamine and this leads to bronchodilation if it comes from bronchospasm.
10. Chronic bronchitis is associated with hyperplasia and hypertrophy of mucus-producing glands. With emphysema there is distention and destruction in the bronchioles and alveolar ducts and in portions of the lung distal to the terminal bronchiole. They become enlarged (puffed out). Airway obstruction occurs. Airways are narrowed and there is a low of elastic recoil. An increase in airway resistance occurs and expiratory flow is impeded. There is a mismatching of inspired air and blood flow. Constriction of pulmonary vessels is seen in response to alveolar hypoxia.
11. Sputum becomes very thick if a person is dehydrated. Increased hydration leads to thinning of the secretion.
12. Expectorants can increase the secretion of mucus and secretions. Expectorants can reduce the viscosity of secretions. Some liquefy secretions.
13. Anxiety will decrease the attention span and decrease learning. Fatigue will prevent learning, but most important are the changes that occur in consciousness with a decrease in oxygen and an increase in carbon dioxide.
14. Relieve anxiety; improve respiratory function (deep breathing techniques, coughing); improve hydration; preserve energy through scheduled rest; prevent infections and other complications; instruct the person to live with the disease to improve his or her level of functioning.

Sequences

4, 1, 2, 7, 5, 6, 3

Completion Exercises

1.

DRUG	RECEPTOR	ACTION	ADVERSE REACTIONS
Epinephrine	Acts on alpha and beta receptors	Relieves bronchospasm and vasoconstriction	Arrhythmias Anxiety Tension headache
Isoproterenol	Acts on beta receptors	Bronchodilation and decreased bronchospasm	Increased pulse Tremor Palpitation
Metaproterenol	More selective to stimulate beta-2 receptors	Bronchodilation	Increased pulse Headache Nervous
Terbutaline	Beta-2 stimulation	Bronchodilation	Increased pulse Tension Anxiety Nausea Vomiting

2. a. Paranasal sinuses
   b. Nasal concha
   c. Pharynx
   d. Epiglottis
   e. Larynx
   f. Glottis

3. a. Trachea
   b. Bronchus
   c. Bronchiole
   d. Alveolus

4.

DRUG	EFFECT ON THEOPHYLLINE
Cimetidine	Increases concentration and effect
Allopurinol	Increases concentration and effect
Furosemide	Increases concentration and effect
Propranolol	Increases concentration and effect
Digoxin	No effect
Phenytoin	Theophylline decreases the effect of
Lithium carbonate	Theophylline increases excretion of

Situational Exercises

1. a. Low oxygen
   b. Abnormal. Most people respond to hydrogen levels and pH of blood and increases in carbon dioxide.
   c. Change in mentation, cyanosis, apnea or coma, reddish skin color, drowsiness, headache
2. Tachycardia, anorexia, vomiting, abdominal cramps, headache, irritability, palpitations, arrhythmia. This is *above* the therapeutic level.
3. This drug is not used in emergencies. It is not used after the onset of the asthmatic attack, but rather is used to *prevent* an attack.
4. If you give oxygen, it removes the person's mechanism to breathe, which, in this case, is low oxygen and not the high carbon dioxide. The person may become apneic and go into respiratory arrest.

36
Drugs Affecting the Reproductive Systems and Sexuality

Multiple Choice Questions

1. c 2. b 3. c 4. b 5. d

Sequences

1, 7, 2, 5, 3, 4, 6

Completion Exercises

1. Estrogen; epiphyseal closure and end of transformation of cartilage into bone; results from endochondral bone formation
2. Follicle-stimulating hormone (FSH), luteinizing hormone (LH); the latter is also known as interstitial cell-stimulating hormone (ICSH)
3.

HORMONE	ACTION	TIME OF HIGHEST LEVEL
FSH	Initiates development of the graafian follicle in the ovary	Follicular phase
LH	Stimulates graafian follicle to mature and produce estrogen	Ovulation and luteal phase

Correct the False Statement

1. F; decreases sexual desire in high doses
2. T
3. F; may decrease desire, excitement, or both

Matching

1. d 2. e 3. a 4. b 5. c

Short Answer Questions

1. a. Impotence
   b. Anginal pain during intercourse
   c. Impotence
   d. Infertility
2. Nutrition, health status, age, medications, drugs, toxins, testicular temperature, body development, endocrine factors
3. Acetylsalicylic acid (aspirin): pain relief, mild inhibition of prostaglandin production; ibuprofen (Motrin), mefemic acid (Ponstel): inhibit prostaglandin production; progesterone (with or without estrogen): raises progesterone level
4. Alter diet to limit salt and carbohydrate intake; eliminate caffeine
5. High-calcium diet (1500 mg); estrogen replacement therapy
6. *Staphylococcus aureus*, sudden onset of high fever; diarrhea, vomiting, or both; rapid drop in blood pressure; sunburnlike rash and desquammation; possible sore throat, headache, aching muscles

37
Drugs Affecting the Musculoskeletal System: Skeletal Muscle Relaxants and Antispastic Agents

Matching

A. 1. d 2. g 3. f 4. h 5. e 6. a 7. b
   8. c
B. 1. g 2. h 3. c 4. a 5. b 6. d 7. e
   8. f

Completion Exercises

1. Aspirin
2. Acetaminophen
3. Aspirin
4. Aspirin; caffeine

Short Answer Questions

1. Multiple sclerosis; spinal cord tumors; cerebral palsy; "whiplash"; spinal cord injury (quadriplegia, paraplegia); herniated disc; tetanus
2. It is necessary to avoid potentially hazardous tasks, such as the operation of motor vehicles and machinery.
3. a. Allergic-type reactions because of its content of FD&C Yellow No. 5.
   b. Liver damage, hepatitis
   c. Liver damage, hepatitis
   d. Extravasation and thrombophlebitis when given IV
   e. Anticholinergic effects such as dryness of the mouth
   f. Cardiotoxic complications

38
Drugs Affecting the Kidneys: Diuretics

Correct the False Statement

1. F; hydrostatic pressure
2. F; similar in concentration to
3. T
4. T
5. T
6. F; intestinal atony and constipation
7. T
8. F; hot humid
9. F; systole
10. T
11. F; electrolyte imbalance
12. T
13. F; by the liver, especially when renal function is impaired
14. F; chronic conditions associated with edema
15. F; dilute them well

Find the Hidden Words

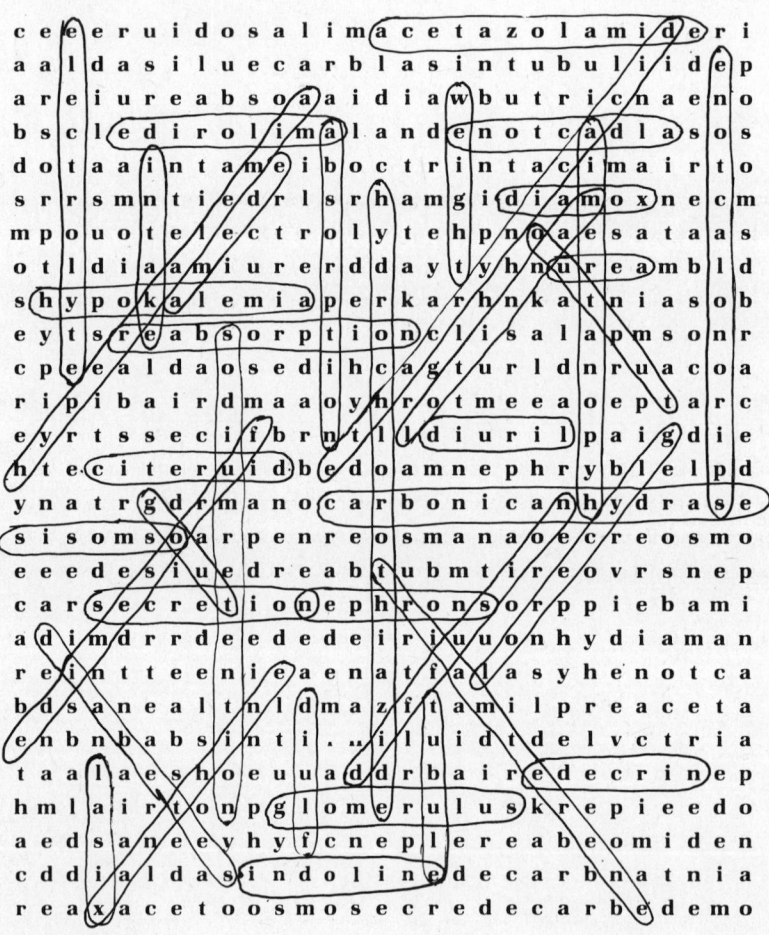

Matching

A. 1. a, b, c, d, f, g, h, i 2. a 3. m 4. e, h
   5. h, k, l 6. a, j

B. 1. a 2. d 3. b 4. c 5. b 6. b 7. c
   8. d 9. d 10. a 11. c

Multiple Choice Questions

1. d 2. c 3. d 4. d 5. a 6. d 7. a 8. b
9. a 10. d 11. a 12. a 13. b 14. d
15. a 16. b 17. c 18. c 19. a 20. b
21. b 22. c 23. d 24. b 25. c

Selection of Options

1. b, d, e 2. b, c, d 3. b, c, e 4. a, b, d, e
5. a, d 6. b, d 7. a, c, d, f 8. a, d
9. a, b, c, d 10. a, b, d 11. a, b 12. a, b
13. a, c, d, e

Short Answer Questions

1. a. A substance that increases urinary output
   b. Swelling of the tissues caused by increased interstitial fluid
2. Heart disease, nephrosis, hepatic cirrhosis
3. Glycerin (glycerol), mannitol
4. Glaucoma, seizure disorders
5. Edema associated with congestive heart failure, cirrhosis
6. Freely filtrable by the glomerulus; not readily reabsorbed by the tubule; lacking in other pharmacologic action
7. Electrolyte depletion, hypovolemia, gastrointestinal upset, impairment of hearing
8. Diabetes mellitus, gout
9. Bananas, oranges, apricots
10. Meats
11. 2.2 pounds or 1 kilogram

39
Theoretic Base for Chemotherapy, Alkylating Agents, and Antimetabolites

Essay Questions

1. The concept of synergism is being applied when combination chemotherapy is used. Drugs used in combination chemotherapy would have different sites and mechanisms of action. Using several drugs with different actions may create multiple flaws in the tumor cells, which may prevent rapid repair of the damage, delay regrowth of the tumor, and prevent or delay the development of resistant tumor cells. Differences in toxicity to normal tissues among the several drugs being used in combination may permit full therapeutic dosages of each drug to be given without unacceptable adverse reactions in the client. The rate and duration of remission obtainable with combination therapy is greater than with single drug therapy.
2. Factors that affect whether or not antineoplastic drug therapy is used include factors related to cell growth, type of malignancy, pharmacologic factors, the client's physiologic status, and history of previous antineoplastic drug therapy.

    Tumors in which a large percentage of cells are actively making deoxyribonucleic acid and dividing during a short time span are said to have a large growth fraction. These tumors are more susceptible to drug action because a large percentage of cells will be killed by the drug. Tumors in which a small percentage of cells are making deoxyribonucleic acid and dividing have a small growth fraction and will lose a smaller percentage of their cells when exposed to drugs.

    Some malignancies respond favorably to drugs in nearly all cases, and other malignancies respond only a small fraction of the time.

    The distribution of a drug within the body may influence drug therapy. Some drugs are excluded from certain areas of the body. For example, tumor cells in the brain are inaccessible to most antineoplastic drugs due to the blood–brain barrier.

    Certain drugs may not be chosen if the client has preexisting heart, liver, or kidney disease. Some drugs are toxic to these specific systems.

    If the client has previously received antineoplastic drug therapy, the choice of drugs is limited because cancer cells develop resistance to drugs by more than one mechanism.
3. Phase M: mitosis.

    Phase G_0: resting phase of interphase; normally all genetically assigned functions are performed except reproduction.

    Phase G_1: predeoxyribonucleic acid synthesis phase; cell synthesizes ribonucleic acid and protein.

    Phase S: synthesis of deoxyribonucleic acid.

    Phase G_2: continued synthesis of ribonucleic acid and protein
4. Certain tumors are treated with doses of methotrexate that are so large that such a dose would ordinarily destroy the client's bone marrow. However, the bone marrow can be protected if the client receives intravenous folinic acid. Folinic acid is a folate coenzyme that does not need reduction by dihydrofolate reductase. When folinic acid is supplied to cells, the methotrexate-induced block of tetrahydrofolate synthesis is bypassed. The folinic acid is given to "rescue" normal cells from the toxic effects of methotrexate.

Matching

1. c 2. a 3. b 4. b 5. c 6. b

Short Answer Questions

1. Triethylenethiophosphoramide, Thio-TEPA; hexamethylmelamine, HMM
2. Carmustine/BCNU, lomustine/CCNU, and streptozocin
3. a. Cisplatin (Platinol)
   b. There will be harmful effects on the ears.
   c. The symptoms would include hearing loss and possibly tinnitus.

The signs would include changes in the whisper and watch tick tests, in the Weber and Rinne tests, and in audiometric testing.

4. a. Folic acid must be reduced by dihydrofolate reductase for one-carbon transfer reactions. A folic acid analog binds with dihydrofolate reductase, which prevents the one-carbon transfer reactions essential for the purine synthesis which then interrupts deoxyribonucleic acid and ribonucleic acid syntheses.
   b. A pyrimidine analog blocks the synthesis of a substance (e.g., thymidylic acid) by inhibiting an enzyme, which leads in turn to the inhibition of deoxyribonucleic acid synthesis.
   c. A purine analog inhibits the conversion of more than one substance, which leads to altered synthesis and function of ribonucleic and deoxyribonucleic acids.
5. It is used to treat premalignant skin keratoses, superficial basal cell carcinomas, and carcinoma in situ of the vulva.
6. Avoid spicy and greasy foods; use cold meats rather than hot ones; stress a high-protein breakfast; encourage eggs and cheese; allow foods the client "craves"; use smaller servings, and even use smaller dishes; eat six meals rather than three; make sure the environment is clean, odor free, and free of unsightly items; avoid unpleasant treatments too close to mealtime; be sure the client is positioned properly; provide mouth care; encourage company during mealtime.
7. Be ever mindful of the possibility of infection, and assess for its signs and symptoms; use extremely careful handwashing technique; teach client and family the importance of handwashing; give meticulous care to invasive devices (e.g., urinary and venous catheters, respiratory therapy equipment); consider placing the client in reverse isolation; administer prophylactic antibiotics as ordered by the physician.

Completion Exercises

1. a. Anorexia, nausea, vomiting, alopecia, bone marrow suppression, hemorrhagic myocarditis and congestive heart failure, hemorrhagic colitis, stomatitis, jaundice, gonadal suppression, ovarian fibrosis, pulmonary fibrosis, hypersensitivity reactions, hemorrhagic and nonhemorrhagic cystitis, nephrotoxicity, bladder malignancies
   b. When the drug is discontinued, your hair will grow in again. Sometimes, however, your new hair may be a different texture or color. Vigorous brushing or teasing of the hair or the use of brush rollers will increase hair loss. You might like to consider using a wig because most women have found a wig satisfactory. If you choose a wig and purchase it now before your hair loss, you might be more satisfied because you could make sure that the wig is a good color match for your own hair.
2. a. Normal saline solution, hydrogen peroxide
   b. Xylocaine viscous 2%
   c. Juices high in citric acid, rough-textured foods, and hot foods
   d. Nystatin as an oral suspension
3. Malignant melanoma
4. Mercaptopurine
5. Busulfan

40
Natural Products, Hormones, and Miscellaneous Agents

Essay Questions

1. Lungs do not contain bleomycin hydrolase, an enzyme that normally hydrolyzes the bleomycin and inactivates it. The reaction in the lungs usually begins insidiously as a pneumonitis that can progress to a fatal pulmonary fibrosis. The process involves most prominently the peripheral areas of the lower lobes of the lungs. Early signs and symptoms are decreased pulmonary function, rales, shortness of breath, and cough.
2. There are two forms of cardiac toxicity: acute and delayed. The acute form occurs 1 to 3 days after administration and is not considered a contraindication to continued therapy. It is characterized by electrocardiographic abnormalities, including ST-T wave alterations and arrhythmias. The delayed form can produce a life-threatening cardiomyopathy. It is characterized by tachycardia, arrhythmias, dyspnea, hypotension, and congestive heart failure that is unresponsive to digitalis. The mortality rate is over 50%. This form appears to be dose-related and the risk is significant if total doses over 550 mg/sq m (in adults) are used.
3. Asparaginase's mechanism of action is quite different from that of other antineoplastic drugs. Most tissues need asparagine and synthesize it. The lymphoblast in acute lymphocytic leukemia does not synthesize asparaginase, but it does require it for growth purposes. The enzyme asparaginase catalyzes the hydrolysis of extracellular supplies of asparagine to aspartic acid and ammonia, thereby depleting the supply available to the lymphoblasts and leading to their death.
4. The tissues of the prostate and breast depend on the androgens and estrogens for growth and function. Carcinomas that occur in the prostate and the breast often retain the hormonal requirements of the nonmalignant tissue. It is possible to change the course of the neoplastic process to some degree by changing the hormonal environment of such tumors.

Matching

A. 1. b 2. b 3. a 4. b 5. c 6. b 7. a 8. b 9. b 10. a

B. 1. d 2. a 3. c, e 4. b, e 5. a 6. b, f 7. a

Short Answer Questions

1. Vincristine's adverse reactions involve the central and peripheral nervous systems and the autonomic nervous system. When the central and peripheral nervous systems are affected, the symptoms are paresthesias, loss of deep tendon reflexes, neuritic pain, muscle weakness, footdrop, ataxia, difficulty in walking, slapping gait, sensory loss, cranial nerve manifestations, and headache. Optic atrophy with blindness has occurred. When the autonomic nervous system is involved, severe constipation, abdominal pain, paralytic ileus, and bowel obstruction can occur.
2. Each antibiotic probably acts slightly differently, but the basic mechanism of action appears to be the formation of complexes between the antibiotic and deoxyribonucleic acid. The formation of these complexes causes alterations in the physical properties of deoxyribonucleic acid.
3. Two types of kidney damage can occur. One type is an acute renal failure that can be fatal in 3 to 4 weeks, and the other is a chronic progressive type of damage. The acute form is accompanied by microangiopathic hemolytic anemia, thrombocytopenia, and hypertension. Most of the clients experiencing the acute form had been given mitomycin in combination with fluorouracil, but some had received the mitomycin in combination with other drugs.
4. Hypercalcemia can cause renal calculi and physiologic disturbances because of an increase in the concentration of ionized calcium in the extracellular fluid. It may be so significant as to be life-threatening. Plicamycin is one agent used to lower serum calcium.
5. Clients whose tumors lack estrogen receptors do not respond to hormone administration, but clients with receptor-containing tumors benefit from hormone treatment. Antiestrogens (e.g., tamoxifen) use this concept in their functioning.

Completion Exercises

1. a. Bone marrow suppression (especially leukopenia), alopecia, mucositis, diarrhea
   b. Testicular cancer, oat cell lung cancer, Hodgkin's disease and non-Hodgkin's lymphoma
2. Chronic granulocytic leukemia
3. A rapid reduction in the levels of adrenocorticosteroids and their metabolites in blood and urine
4. Cross the blood–brain barrier, brain tumors
5. Cushing's syndrome caused by adrenal tumors
6. Mitotane
7. Lowers serum calcium

41
Drugs Used in the Treatment of Allergy

Completion Exercises

1. History; observation
2. Description of symptoms; documentation of possible factors (*e.g.*, medications, food)
3. Reaction may be severe, even fatal
4. Milk, wheat, seafood
5. Penicillin, aspirin, local anesthetics
6. Dust, pollen, industrial chemicals
7. Cheeks, antecubital fossae, popliteal fossae
8. Preventing future contact with the allergen
9. Medication (epinephrine IM or IV); life-support system (administer IV fluids, perform CPR, establish airway)
10. Adrenergic bronchodilators (including aerosols for inhalation)
11. a. Take several hours to become effective, and longer to reach maximum level of effectiveness
    b. Limited to cases that cannot be controlled by immunology or other medications
    c. Obesity; cushingoid facies; hyperglycemia; suppression of linear growth; hirsutism; thinning of skin; delayed sexual maturation; interactions with other medications
12. Taper slowly, eventually using only on alternate mornings; continue tapering to minimal dose that can be used effectively; lengthen time between doses until steroids can be discontinued totally.

13.

DRUG	POSSIBLE SIDE EFFECTS OR SECONDARY EFFECTS	POSSIBLE IDIOSYNCRASY
Pencillin	Hemolytic anemia; vasculitis; elevated fever level; malaise; vertigo; nausea, vomiting; urticaria; itching; diffuse erythema	Anaphylaxis
Anticonvulsants	Agranulocytosis; elevated fever level	
Chloramphenicol	Hematologic manifestations (thrombocytopenia, agranulocytosis, aplastic anemia); arthralgia; elevated fever level; urticaria; delayed skin allergy	Anaphylaxis
Mercurial diuretics	Elevated fever level	
Aspirin	Urticaria; rhinitis; nasal polyposis; asthma; tinnitus	Anaphylaxis

Multiple Choice Questions

1. b 2. e 3. c 4. b

42
Drugs Used for Immunity

Short Answer Questions

1. a. 2 months, 4 months, 6 months, 18 months, 4 to 6 years
   b. 14 to 16 years, every 10 years thereafter
   c. 2 months, 4 months, 6 months, 18 months, 4 to 6 years
   d. 15 months
2. Pregnancy; generalized malignancy; cell-mediated immunodeficiency disorders; current immunosuppressive therapy; sensitivity to animal species used in vaccine preparation; transfusion of immune serum globulin, plasma, or blood
3. a. Very few cases worldwide; risks outweigh benefits
   b. Measles vaccine, if given within 6 weeks before, can invalidate or cause a false-negative tuberculin test
   c. Rate of seroconversion under 1 year is variable, and therefore may not give proper ongoing protection
   d. Prevent mumps orchitis that might lead to sterility
   e. Possibility of a systemic reaction
   f. Health-care workers are at high risk because of possible contact with contaminated specimens from HBV carriers
   g. Possibility of infecting fetus
   h. Mutations may occur in some viruses, making vaccine ineffective; risk-to-benefit factors may eliminate or increase the need for a particular vaccine

Correct the False Statement

1. F; some (agammaglobulinemia results in no immunity)
2. T
3. F; through the placenta, in colostrum, by immunization with appropriate materials, or by having the disease
4. F; high

Completion Exercises

1. Interferon
2. Placenta
3. Breast-feeding
4. Lymphokines
5. Acquired immunity
6. Specific antigen
7. Siblings
8. Tuberculosis
9. 1 year of age
10. Rubella vaccine
11. An acute febrile infection or illness
12. Is not
13. Reduce the potency and effectiveness of the vaccine
14. It could cause autoinoculation

Multiple Choice Questions

1. c   2. d   3. b

43
Oral Supplements

PART 1: MINERALS AND VITAMINS

Matching

A. 1. b 2. a 3. h 4. e 5. d 6. h 7. g
   8. a
B. 1. f 2. h 3. g 4. e 5. c 6. b 7. d
   8. a

C. 1. b, e 2. a 3. d 4. a

Correct the False Statement

1. F; ultraviolet light
2. T
3. F; may be cheaper than
4. F; on an empty stomach
5. F; iron deficiency
6. F; potassium
7. F; magnesium
8. F; potassium
9. F; rickets
10. T

Short Answer Questions

1. a. An organic chemical found in food that cannot be synthesized by the human body but is essential in small quantities for health and normal growth
   b. Inorganic chemicals used by the body for essential physiologic functions
   c. The minimal intake of a nutrient that is required to prevent the development of deficiency disease in most people
   d. Levels of intake of essential nutrients considered to be adequate to meet the nutritional needs of almost all healthy persons (as defined by the Food and Nutrition Board of the National Research Council)
2. a. Therapeutic strength: vitamin preparations that contain dosages high enough to correct vitamin deficiencies
   b. Maintenance preparations: vitamin preparations designed to prevent deficiencies in people with no existing deficiencies
3. Not usually, because it is not as well absorbed when given with food—but it is given with food when necessary to reduce adverse gastrointestinal side effects

Multiple Choice Questions

1. d   2. b   3. e   4. d   5. a   6. b   7. f   8. f
9. e   10. b 11. c 12. a 13. e 14. a
15. d 16. e 17. d 18. c 19. d 20. d
21. f 22. b 23. c 24. b 25. a 26. b
27. d 28. d 29. b 30. b 31. b 32. d
33. b 34. c 35. d 36. a 37. b 38. a
39. a 40. c 41. c 42. d 43. a

Selection of Options

1. a, d, e, f   2. a, b, d   3. a only
4. a, b, c, d, g   5. d   6. b, e   7. b, c   8. a, e, f
9. b, c, d, e   10. b, c, d   11. c, d, e   12. c, d
13. b, d, e   14. a, d, e   15. d   16. b, c, d, e
17. b, c, d   18. b, d

PART 2: HEMATINICS

Short Answer Questions

1. A hematinic is an agent that improves the quality of blood either by increasing the hemoglobin level or the number of erythrocytes, or both.

2. *Ferritin* is the form iron takes when it is stored in the body. From 30% to 35% of body iron is in storage form. *Transferrin* is a plasma protein in the body that is responsible for delivering iron to specific receptors on cell membranes.
3. Women using intrauterine devices; infants experiencing rapid growth spurts (6 months to 2 years); women in the last two trimesters of pregnancy; some vegetarians; individuals with absorption problems involving the duodenum and upper small intestine; individuals experiencing unexpected acute blood loss (hemorrhage); individuals experiencing unidentified chronic blood loss greater than normal
4. Liver; kidney beans; tuna; eggs
5. Ferrous sulfate should be administered when the patient has not eaten for two hours and is not planning to eat for the next two hours.
6. If the objective is being met, the hemoglobin should increase between 0.15 g and 0.25 g/dl of whole blood per day.
7. It is difficult to evaluate an individual's response to the iron in the preparation; there is no proof to date that the combination preparations are best; iron combination preparations are inevitably much more expensive.
8. When noncompliance with oral therapy is very high; when intolerance to oral preparations is very high; in malabsorption
9. Vitamin B_{12}; parietal cells of stomach
10. Pernicious anemia
11. Inadequate dietary supply; uremia; alcoholism; hepatic disease; nontropical sprue; tropical sprue; congenital hemolytic anemias; certain drugs (some anticonvulsants, oral contraceptives, methotrexate, trimethoprim)
12. Vertigo; tinnitus; weakness; easy fatigability; faintness; drowsiness; headache; loss of libido; shortness of breath

Matching

1. d 2. b 3. c

PART 3: FEEDING FORMULAS

Correct the False Statement

1. F; should be reduced in both strength and amount to prevent indigestion
2. F; relatively common because attention is focused on the pathologic condition, and nutrition may not be monitored adequately
3. F; prepare the proper dilution of formula
4. F; no

Multiple Choice Questions

1. b 2. b 3. a 4. d

Selection of Options

1. a, b 2. c, d

Crossword Puzzle

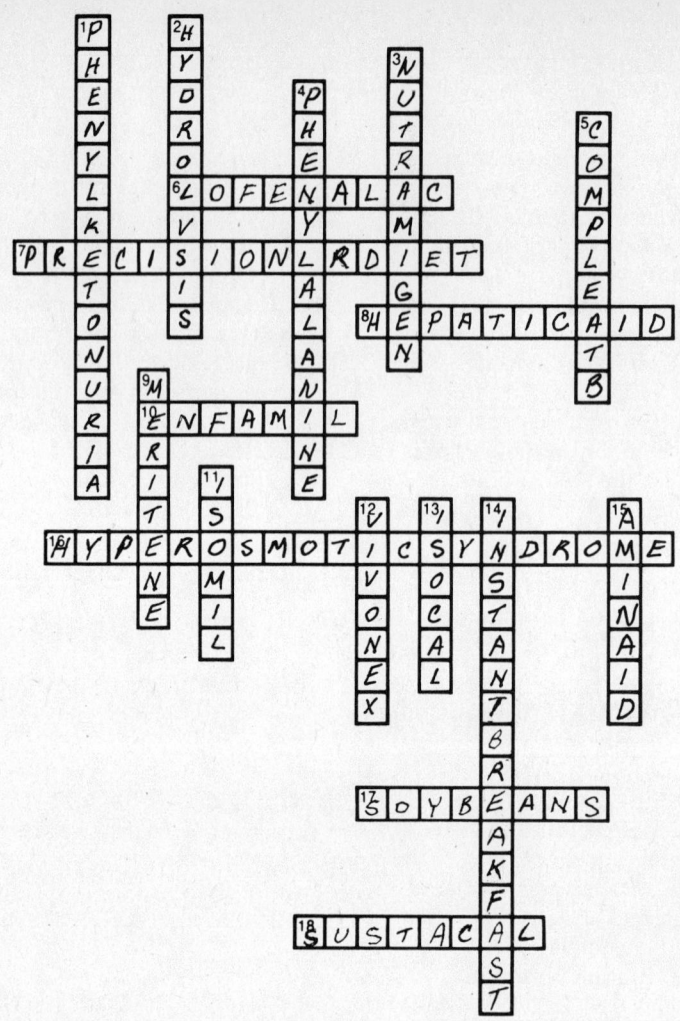

PART 4: HEALTH FOOD PRODUCTS

Correct the False Statement

1. F; are not required to adhere
2. F; seldom recommend
3. F; health food literature
4. T
5. F; sometimes
6. T
7. F; exercise caution because the preparations are not controlled by the Food and Drug Administration

Multiple Choice Questions

1. b 2. d 3. c 4. d 5. a 6. b 7. d 8. d

Selection of Options

1. a, b, d

44
Parenteral Preparations

Matching

1. b, d   2. f   3. a, c

Correct the False Statement

1. F; total parenteral hyperalimentation solutions
2. F; phthalate (or filters)
3. F; is sometimes administered in the home to clients on long-term therapy
4. F; saline solution

Short Answer Questions

1. Hyaluronidase (Wydase)
2. They tend to delay it
3. Lipids
4. One with a microscopic filter that removes aggregate particles
5. The client should be placed immediately on the left side to trap the air in the right ventricle.
6. A maximum of 3 weeks (21 days)
7. Typing and cross matching
8. In the refrigerator, away from the coils to prevent freezing
9. 18 years; 65 years

Multiple Choice Questions

1. c   2. b   3. a   4. e   5. c   6. c   7. b   8. a
9. c   10. b   11. c   12. b   13. a   14. a   15. a
16. b   17. a   18. c   19. e   20. a

Selection of Options

1. a, b, d   2. a, b, c, d   3. b, c, d   4. a, b, c, d
5. a, b   6. a, d   7. a, c   8. a, c, e, f, g
9. d only   10. b, c   11. a, b, c, d   12. a, b, d

45
Diagnostic Agents

Multiple Choice Questions

1. a 2. b 3. b 4. b 5. a 6. d 7. c 8. b
9. c 10. d 11. c 12. d 13. b 14. b
15. d 16. b 17. b 18. b 19. d 20. d
21. a 22. a 23. a 24. d 25. b 26. a
27. d 28. b 29. a 30. c 31. b

Matching

1. b, h   2. a, b, e, f, h, i   3. g   4. d   5. d
6. d   7. c

Correct the False Statement

1. F; ionize chemicals in body tissues
2. T
3. T
4. F; should fast for several hours so that the barium will remain undiluted as it passes through the tract
5. F; use of a laxative
6. F; should be screened for risk factors for adverse reactions (sensitivity tests are not recommended)
7. T
8. T
9. F; at a faster rate (because the radioactivity of the residual radionuclide also declines over time)
10. T
11. T
12. T
13. F; parenterally
14. F; very small
15. F; influence multiple body processes; multiple
16. F; allergic reaction or anaphylaxis
17. T
18. F; infrequently
19. F; minutes to days
20. F; the person has been previously exposed to the pathogen

Selection of Options

1. a, c, d   2. a, c   3. b, c   4. a, b   5. a, b
6. a, c   7. b, c, d, e   8. a, b, c, d, e
9. a, b, d, e   10. b, c   11. b, d, e
12. b, c, d, e   13. b, d   14. b, d, e   15. c, d
16. b only   17. b, c, d   18. a, b, c   19. a, b
20. a, d   21. a, b   22. b, c

Short Answer Questions

1. There is none; it is believed to be unsafe at all levels
2. Nausea, vomiting, urticaria, malaise, fever, hypotension, hypertension, bronchoconstriction, tissue necrosis (after extravasation)
3. Hypervolemia, diuresis
4. a. Containing atoms that disintegrate with the emission of electromagnetic radiation
   b. The dose of ionizing radiation absorbed per unit of mass, material, or tissue
   c. Roentgen equivalent in man (REM), or the estimated biologic effect relative to a dose of 1 roentgen of x-rays
   d. The quantity of x- or γ-radiation in air
5. Photography, scintography, use of Geiger counter
6. In lead-lined containers
7. Tissue concentration of a chemical, fluid volume (e.g., of blood, body water); cardiac output; pulmonary ventilation; peripheral vascular circulation
8. Adverse reactions to substances chemically similar to the radionuclide to be used; history of unusual or excessive exposure to ionizing radiation; pregnancy; lactation; phase of menstrual cycle in women in their childbearing years
9. Disease of the pancreas, liver, or biliary tract
10. Patch test, scratch test, intradermal injection
11. Because anaphylaxis sometimes occurs

46
Enzymes and Drugs Affecting Enzymes

Matching

1. b (asparagine) 2. a (galactose) 3. a 4. e
5. h 6. a (lactose) 7. e, g 8. d

Correct the False Statement

1. F; proteins
2. F; genetic inheritance
3. T
4. T
5. F; cells that cannot synthesize asparagine
6. F; units

Multiple Choice Questions

1. c 2. b 3. a 4. a 5. d 6. d 7. b 8. c
9. d 10. c 11. b 12. d 13. a 14. b
15. a 16. d 17. b 18. c 19. a 20. b
21. c 22. a 23. c 24. d 25. b

Selection of Options

1. a, d 2. a, e

Short Answer Questions

1. It is used to discourage impulse drinking. The ingestion of the daily dose is a ritual involving renewal of the alcoholic's pledge not to drink. When disulfiram is in the system, the alcoholic cannot drink without experiencing very distressing symptoms.
2. About 7.5 ml of absolute alcohol (15 ml of 100 proof, or 50% alcohol)
3. Add 10 drops of Lact-Aid to a quart of milk and refrigerate for 1 day before consumption.
4. Infection or inflammation in the tissues to be infused
5. They are metabolized as proteins.
6. Because they might develop antibodies that inactivate the enzymes
7. If anaphylaxis occurs, the client will need epinephrine medication. Halothane and epinephrine interact to increase the risk of cardiac arrest.
8. Anaphylaxis
9. Avoid personal exposure to the drugs because they are antigenic; protect the drugs from heat or agitation because they are protein in nature
10. Most enzyme drugs cannot penetrate cell membranes or the blood–brain barrier.

47
Complexes: Chelators and Ion-Exchange Compounds

Matching

A. 1. e 2. a, b 3. d 4. c 5. b 6. a 7. e
   8. a, b, c 9. a, b 10. c
B. 1. b 2. a, c 8. d

Correct the False Statement

1. T
2. F; are
3. F; an alkaline
4. T
5. F; trace minerals
6. T
7. F; parenterally
8. T
9. F; are not absorbed systemically; locally in the GI tract
10. F; avoid inhaling dusts or powders

Multiple Choice Question

1. d

Selection of Options

1. a, b, d, e 2. d only 3. a, b, c 4. a, c, d

48
Substance Abuse

Short Answer Questions

1. a. The self-directed use of chemical substances for nontherapeutic reasons, in conflict with generally accepted norms and cultural values
   b. The state of behavior characterized by the inability to control a craving or drive for a substance
   c. A state that exists when an increasing amount of a substance is required to produce the desired effect experienced with the original dose
   d. The altered state (physical or psychological) that results from continuous use of a psychoactive substance
2. a. Tolerance and physical dependence → metabolic changes similar to withdrawal symptoms → attempt to mediate symptoms → tolerance and physical dependence
   b. Abuse → central nervous system damage → mental capacity reduction → inability to make judgments → abuse
   c. Abuse → social disapproval → need to find like-minded companions → abuse
   d. Abuse → guilt and shame → attempt to resolve these feelings → abuse
3. a. Barbs, blue devils, downers, green dragons, goofballs, yellow jackets, nimbles, pink ladies, rainbows, red devils, reds, stumblers
   b. Scag, smack, junk, horse, H, brown sugar
   c. Snow, big C, coke, flake, gold dust, nose candy, rock, white
   d. Acapulco Gold, gold, gage, grass, hay, hemp, J, Jane, Mary Jane, Panama Red, pot, reefer, smoke, weed
   e. Hash, kif, black Russian, quarter moon, soles
   f. Acid, beast, blue heaven, brown dots, California sunshine, chocolate chips, haze, mellow yellows, orange mushrooms, orange wedges, paper acid, sugar, sunshine, white lightning, yellows
   g. Cube, hocus, first line, morf
   h. Quads, soapers, sopes
   i. Angel dust, peace pill, surfer, killer weed, hog, DOA, rocket fuel, elephant tranquilizer

Completion Exercise

SUBSTANCE OF ABUSE	PHARMACOLOGIC EFFECTS	WITHDRAWAL SYMPTOMS	TOLERANCE–PHYSICAL DEPENDENCE
Opioid analgesic (heroin, morphine)	Euphoria; drowsiness, lethargy; decreased physical activity; pinpoint pupils; constipation; decreased vision	Diaphoresis; anxiety; insomnia; lacrimation; rhinorrhea; nausea, vomiting Onset: 2°–48° Duration: 7–10 days Peak: 72°	Tolerance: + Dependence: +
Cannabis	Increased BP, dry mouth; injected conjunctivae; tachycardia; initial period of stimulation; heightened perception; euphoria; relaxation, sedation, drowsiness	None recognized	Tolerance: + Dependence: rare
Alcohol	Motor and sensory disturbance; vasodilation; in large doses—depressed respiration, diarrhea or constipation, liver toxicity	Stage 1: 8° after cessation—nausea, vomiting, headache, tremors Stage II: 8°–24°, irritability, increasing tremors, seizures, hallucinations Stage III: DTs	Tolerance: + Dependence: +

SUBSTANCE OF ABUSE	PHARMACOLOGIC EFFECTS	WITHDRAWAL SYMPTOMS	TOLERANCE–PHYSICAL DEPENDENCE
Nicotine	Stimulates release of epinephrine; also has depressant effect; increases cardiac rate and BP, respiratory excitation; vomiting; vasoconstriction; diarrhea	Variable time of onset; irritable, hostile, jittery; increased appetite; headache; fixation on smoking, craving for cigarette	Tolerance: to some degree Dependence: questionable
CNS depressants (Nembutal, Seconal)	May decrease inhibition; short-term euphoria; calming of anxiety; sedation; hypnotic; anticonvulsant in long-acting forms	Anxiety, tremors, sleep disturbance, irritability; weakness; nausea, vomiting; hypotension; seizures; myoclonic contractions; hallucinations; hyperpyrexia; delirium tremens, death Duration: up to 14 days	Tolerance: + Dependence: +
CNS stimulants (Dexedrine, cocaine)	Restlessness, euphoria, increased energy, anxiety, hyperactivity; increased BP, and pulse; cardiovascular stimulation	No gross physiologic changes, although lethargy, sleep disturbances, and depression may be seen	Tolerance: + develops rapidly Dependence: +
Psychedelics (Mescaline, LSD)	CNS overactivity; anxiety; nausea; increased BP; dilated pupils; increased heart rate; visual illusions; perceptual changes	None apparent	Tolerance: + Dependence: none known

49
Drug Therapy in Maternal Care

Short Answer Questions

1. a. Slower
   b. Faster
   c. Faster
2. a. 75 g–80 g
   b. 2.5 g–7 g
   c. 2.0 g–4.0 g
   d. Six to eight glasses
3. a. 10 mg PO tid; can increase to 25 mg qid
   b. 250 mg tid; can increase to 500 mg qid
   c. 20 mg PO bid; can increase to 80 mg PO bid
4. a. May lead to premature labor, neonatal problems (e.g., hyperbilirubinemia, respiratory depression)
   b. Oxytocic effects may precipitate labor
   c. Anticoagulation abnormalities of the fetus increases the risk of CVA and CNS abnormalities
   d. Maternal hypovolemia and reduced placental perfusion may result in low-birth-weight infants
5. Moist compresses or warm showers; manual or mechanical pumping; supporting bra
6. Exposing nipples to air; changing position of infant while nursing: lubricating nipples between feedings; releasing nipple from infant's mouth properly by breaking suction

Matching

A. 1. d 2. b 3. a 4. c 5. e 6. h 7. f
   8. g
B. 1. d 2. c 3. a 4. e 5. b
C. 1. b 2. c 3. d 4. a 5. e 6. f
D. 1. d 2. c 3. a 4. b

Essay Question

Maternal glucose goes through the placenta, while maternal insulin does not. Insulin is produced by the fetus by the 28th week. β cells hypertrophy to produce additional insulin needed to handle excess glucose. Hyperinsulinemia produces a fetus with excessive growth and storage of excess glycogen, causing fetal obesity. Hyperinsulinemia continues after birth, causing hypoglycemia.

Correct the False Statement

1. T
2. F; may cause birth defects when taken during pregnancy
3. T
4. F; gain at least 15 pounds
5. F; should not be done in the presence of fetal demise, diabetic mother, or PIH
6. T
7. T
8. T
9. F; 90 ml–100 ml/hour
10. F; some drugs cannot be used in late labor because neonatal respiratory depression may result

Situational Exercises

A. 1. a. Check fetal viability; observe frequency and intensity of uterine contractions; observe effect of contractions on fetus
      b. Check fetal age; note cervical dilation and effacement; look for fetal membranes in lower canal
      c. Complications; baseline blood studies; information on labor (e.g., ruptured membranes, bloody show)
      d. Mother in lateral recumbent position; 150 mg ritodrine in 500 ml 5% dextrose in sterile water to be used continuously up to 12 to 24 hours after contractions stop; microdrip and infusion pump for administration
   2. Check maternal pulse and BP q15min during increases of drug, and q30min during maintenance; monitor fluid intake and output; observe for side effects (dyspnea, chest pain, pulse above 120 beats/min, BP below 90 mm Hg, or decrease from baseline)
   3. Report pulse over 120 beats/min; report agitation, nervousness; report palpitations, tremors
B. 1. b 2. c 3. a, d 4. d

Completion Exercises

1. Oxytocin
2. Ergonovine maleate; methylergonovine maleate
3. Erythromycin 0.5% ophthalmic ointment; tetracycline 1% ophthalmic ointment
4.

DRUG	POSSIBLE MATERNAL SIDE EFFECTS	POSSIBLE FETAL SIDE EFFECTS
Meperidine	Nausea, vomiting; respiratory depression	Respiratory depression
Nisentil	Nausea, vomiting; respiratory depression	Respiratory depression
Hydroxyzine	Hypotension; vertigo; drowsiness	CNS depression
Valium	Hypotension; vertigo; drowsiness	Hypothermia; CNS depression; may remain active in fetus for 10 days

50
Drug Therapy in Pediatric Nursing

Matching

A. 1. a 2. c 3. b
B. 1. b or c 2. a only 3. b or c

Short Answer Questions

1. a. Calculate drug dosage using an appropriate source for a reference. Consider the toxic effects of any medication on a client with an immature body system.
   b. Assure safe administration by assessing correct patient drug, dose, route and time.
2. Knowledge of a preschooler's growth and development would include attention to child's concrete thinking, occasional resistant behavior, response to clear explanations and expectations, preference for liquid or chewable medications, response to praise and rewards, and comfort measures following painful experiences.
3. a. Play may be used to allow the child an opportunity to vent feelings and concerns about an invasive procedure.
   b. The nurse may use play to instruct a child about health care and assist the child in understanding a procedure.
4. Pharmacokinetic responses, immature body systems, cumulative toxicity, genetic endowment, age, psychologic and cognitive development, environmental factors, underlying chronic conditions
5. Fewer number of glomeruli, underdeveloped active transport system, slow rate of drug filtration, potential for toxicity

6. Clark's rule:

$$\text{Child dose} = \frac{\text{weight of child}}{150 \text{ lbs}} \times \text{average adult dose}$$

Fried's rule:

$$\text{Child dose} = \frac{\text{infant's age in months}}{150 \text{ months}} \times \text{average adult dose}$$

Young's rule:

$$\text{Child dose} = \frac{\text{child's age in years}}{\text{age of child} \div 12} \times \text{average adult dose}$$

Surface area rule:

$$\text{Child dose} = \frac{\text{surface area of child}}{1.73} \times \text{adult dose}$$

Case Example

ASSESSMENT DATA	DIAGNOSIS	GOAL
A. 1. Postoperative child. Ambulation ordered	1. Alteration in comfort related to surgical site and ambulation	1. Alleviation of pain and anxiety
B. 1. Fear of needles 2. Intravenous and intramuscular medications ordered	1. Anxiety related to needles and medical procedures	1. Alleviation and expression of anxiety

INTERVENTION	OUTCOME CRITERIA FOR EVALUATION
A. 1. Administer analgesia after teaching child about necessity of intramuscular injection. 2. Teach child alternative comfort measures such as correct positioning, relaxation techniques, breathing exercises, visual imagery. 3. Use analgesia prior to severe pain. 4. Allow child to express or play out concerns about intramuscular injections.	1. The child will tolerate intramuscular injections and be comfortable during ambulation as evidenced by normal vital signs, verbalization of decreased pain, and ability to ambulate.
B. 1. Provide an opportunity for play using hospital equipment; play may be structured or occur spontaneously so the nurse may assess feelings, concerns, and fears. 2. Information is supplied with concrete explanations; dolls or models with anatomical parts may be used. 3. Parental participation is encouraged to alleviate their anxiety and increase their knowledge. 4. Monitor intravenous infusion. 5. Monitor amount, pH, guiac of nasogastric secretions. 6. Monitor vital signs. 7. Assess mucus membranes. 8. Monitor urinary output, specific gravity, pH.	1. The child and parents will relax and be less anxious. 2. The child will play with medical equipment and exhibit his or her fears. 3. The child will be adequately hydrated as evidenced by moist mucus membranes, urinary output and specific gravity, normal electrolyte values, and vital signs.

51
Drug Therapy in Gerontologic Nursing

Short Answer Questions

1. Pharmacologic, psychologic, physiologic, economic.
2. Changing pharmacokinetic parameters; polypharmacy; chronic disease; diminishing physical, emotional, social, and economic resources
3. Physical resources, such as weakened motor function, decreased hearing, decreased vision, alterations in taste and smell, loss of natural teeth, changed nutritional requirements; mental resources such as decreased memory; material resources such as limited finances
4. Monitor drug use; suggest use of generic drugs; monitor use of over-the-counter products; interpret physicians' orders, provide counseling on drug interactions; dispense smaller portions of prescriptions as necessary; give discounts; extend credit; provide delivery service
5. a. Depressed respiratory function
   b. Angina from increased metabolic rate, enhanced effect of digoxin, palpitations
   c. Syncope from cerebral ischemia secondary to lowered BP, confusion, dizziness
6. Confusion, depression, excitation, dizziness, loss of memory, slurred speech
7. Most drugs are eliminated by the kidney. In the elderly you would expect an accumulation of drugs because of decreased kidney function. The accumulation could lead to toxicity.

Correct the False Statement

1. F; health-care professionals as well as cultural norms are too quick to prescribe medication for every ache and pain
2. T
3. F; to request regular caps from their pharmacists
4. F; of altered pharmacokinetic parameters
5. F; lack of assessment and teaching by health-care professionals
6. T

Matching

1. d 2. g 3. a 4. e 5. b 6. f 7. c 8. h

52
Drug Therapy in Community Health Nursing

Correct the False Statement

1. T 2. T 3. T 4. F; drug

Jumbled Words

KNOWLEDGE + MOTIVATION + CAPABILITY = COMPLIANCE

Short Answer Questions

1. Administration; regimen; action and effects; side effects; contraindications
2. Client's name and address; physician's name; pharmacy's name; prescription number
3. a. For client: dosage is fixed for both or all drugs and difficult to alter, may have potentiating or contraindicating effects; for nurse: difficult to assess the intended action, effects, and adverse reactions of each drug
   b. Variability of the drug's effects because of ingestion of food, physical status (e.g., stomach problems), use of alcohol or other drugs that interfere with the sustained-release drug's effects
4. Various answers may be given, including tea: tends toward constipation; yogurt: replaces intestinal flora; pears and prunes: tend to loosen stool; bananas and oranges: increase blood potassium; green leafy vegetables: increase body stores of folate
5. Various answers might be given. For example, use of an iron supplement, with or without a vitamin compound, could result in constipation, irregular bowel regimen, and possible decreased appetite and weight loss

Situational Exercises

1. c 2. d 3. c

53
Drug Therapy for Pain Relief

Matching
1. g   2. f   3. b   4. c   5. f   6. d

Correct the False Statement
1. T
2. F; may develop
3. T
4. F; sometimes helpful, but can be a very misleading indicator of subjective pain
5. T
6. F; approximately the same level
7. F; may vary greatly
8. F; more severe
9. F; are sometimes helpful when given (e.g., if a pain-producing activity is to be carried out)

Multiple Choice Questions
1. b   2. c   3. c   4. b   5. b   6. d   7. b   8. d
9. b   10. b   11. d   12. b   13. b   14. d
15. d   16. b   17. c   18. c

Selection of Options
1. a, b, c, d, e   2. a, b, c, d, e, f, g
3. a, b, c, d, e, f   4. a, d   5. a, b, c, d
6. a, b, c, d, e, f, g   7. a, c, d, e   8. b, c, d
9. a, b   10. a, c   11. a, c, d   12. a, c, d
13. a, c, d, e, f

Short Answer Questions
1. Salicylates (aspirin, salicylic acid, methyl salicylate); acetaminophen
2. a. A drug that inhibits the transmission of a pain impulse
   b. Dependence on a drug for maintenance of physical equilibrium (addiction)
   c. Progressive need for drug use for emotional well-being (habituation)
   d. The need for ever-increasing doses of a drug to produce equal therapeutic or psychotropic effects
   e. The period following abrupt discontinuation of a drug of dependence, characterized by pronounced physical or emotional disequilibrium
   f. Altered synaptic function in the neural pain pathway that facilitates passage of an impulse
3. Tolerance to the drug; withdrawal syndrome on discontinuation of the drug
4. Advantages: decrease in the client's anxiety, better control of pain, general decrease in overall quantity of drugs required for pain control, greater autonomy for the client, decreased risk of development of habit of pain, decrease in conditioned response to use drugs, decrease in the level of stress in the client; disadvantages: difficulty in maintaining security over controlled drugs; (possibly) an increased risk of tolerance and dependence in some clients
5. An opioid analgesic such as heroin, morphine, methadone, or codeine; alcohol such as wine or vodka; a nonalcoholic antiemetic such as prochlorperazine; a stimulant such as codeine or amphetamine
6. The need for expensive equipment, including infusion-control devices; increased risk of infection; inconvenience of the cumbersome equipment
7. 300 mg
8. Objective evidence of pain (e.g., vital signs, muscle rigidity, facial expression); nature of the pain (type, location, severity); physician's orders for medication; time interval since last dose of analgesic drugs; client's history of pain experience; client's usual response to pain (including coping behaviors)

Sequences

Provided that the priorities are consistent with those of the client, the order would be 4, 3, 1, 2.

Situational Exercises

1. 10 mg
2. 1.25 mg/hour
3. Greater than that dosage

Personal Exercise

Neither the nature of the biases nor their strengths are of great importance in this exercise. What matters is how well the student has analyzed and clarified these personal factors, and has prepared to counteract their influence on nursing actions.

54
Self-Medication with Over-the-Counter Drugs

Personal Exercise: Drug History

The material in this answer will be different for each student. It should reflect a wider understanding of nonprescription drugs and a greater knowledge of their risks and benefits.

Completion Exercise

TYPE OF DRUG USE	ADVANTAGES	DISADVANTAGES
Prescription	Effective for the relief of symptoms of serious as well as for self-limiting illness; definitive diagnosis of illness by health-care professional; monitoring of response to treatment by health-care professionals; choice of drugs and dosages individually tailored for the client	Relatively expensive; use of more dangerous drugs increases risk of adverse reactions; requires time and resources of professional health-care personnel that may be in short supply
Nonprescription	Effective in relieving symptoms of many self-limiting and long-term chronic illnesses; drugs are relatively safe; increased personal autonomy for the consumer; economical	Lack of definitive diagnosis by health-care professional; risk of delaying treatment of a serious illness; dosages recommended are inadequate for some people; lack of monitoring by health-care professionals

Correct the False Statement

1. T
2. T
3. F; five or six times
4. T
5. F; could not be eliminated
6. F; not all "health products"; tested for safety and efficacy
7. F; potent drugs; may

Multiple Choice Questions

1. d 2. b 3. d 4. b 5. a 6. d 7. d 8. a 9. b 10. a

Selection of Options

1. a, b   2. a, c   3. a, b, d, g   4. a only   5. a, b, c   6. a, c, d   7. a, c, d

Short Answer Questions

1. Use for self-limiting, short-term, or stable chronic conditions; consult a physician before undertaking prolonged use (more than 2 weeks); follow recommendations for dosage on the drug label; heed warnings on drug labels; seek the advice of health-care professionals about non-prescription medications
2. Laxatives should not be taken when abdominal pain is present; sedatives should warn of the safety hazard caused by drowsiness; antidiarrheal preparations should caution against taking the drug when fever is present; the label on the saccharin package must state that its use may be hazardous because it has been determined that saccharin causes cancer in laboratory animals
3. Sugar or syrup is harmful to diabetics and to those with reactive hypoglycemia; alcohol may be harmful to alcoholics, diabetics, persons on drugs causing disulfiramlike reactions, and pregnant women; sympathomimetics are detrimental to diabetics, those with reactive hypoglycemia, seizure disorders, and sensitivity to stimulants, such as people with hyperthyroidism
4. *The People's Pharmacy Two*, by Joe Graedon, New York, St. Martin's Press, 1980